BENEFITS IN MEDICAL CARE PROGRAMS

BENEFITS IN MEDICAL CARE PROGRAMS

Avedis Donabedian

HARVARD UNIVERSITY PRESS
Cambridge, Massachusetts, and London, England   1976

Library of Congress Cataloging in Publication Data

Donabedian, Avedis.
    Benefits in medical care programs.

    Bibliography: p.
    Includes index.
    1. Medical care. 2. Medical care—United States.
3. Medical economics—United States. I. Title.
[DNLM: 1. Health services. 2. Insurance, Health.
W84.1 D674b]
RA411.D66   368.3'8   75-33225
ISBN 0-674-06580-8

To Dorothy

Who has been all gifts
to one man

PREFACE

More years ago than I dare to remember, I set out to write a book that would collect and organize the key elements in medical care organization. Fortified by the assurance that came from a decade of intellectual exploration and a shelf full of lecture notes, I thought the job could be done during a sabbatical year. How wrong I was!

As I began to examine more critically what I thought I knew, it shrank under my hand, much of it turning insubstantial as dreams. What survived were the organizing principles that I had used, like the concealed armature within the clay figures of a sculptor, to give shape and meaning to my material. On this foundation, after some repairs and large extensions, I began to build again, using old materials, but also much that was new to me. It has been slow work. I had to learn as I went along; and the material I needed was sometimes difficult to find, and often refractory to being organized. Soon, I saw that the work must be done in stages and published in installments, and that it might never be completed.

The first installment appeared in 1973 as *Aspects of Medical Care Administration: Specifying Requirements for Health Care.* Now, after more than two years, there is a second volume. Each is complete in itself, but they are tied to each other by a unifying perspective, a recurrence of dominant themes and a set of organizing principles. Among the latter is the simple notion that those who plan and administer health services have certain key tasks to perform. For example, they must formulate and examine their objectives, define and measure the need for service, assess the actual and potential ability of the current stock of health resources to produce the services needed, and estimate current and future requirements for these resources. All this I discussed in the first volume.

In this second book I have fixed my attention on the question of what services should be included as benefits in a medical care program under any one of several forms of prepayment, including health insurance, whether mandatory or voluntary. This question is always with us. It is particularly pressing now, when, as a nation, we are examining how well the current system performs, and choosing among alternative proposals for national health insurance.

As was true of its predecessor, this book does not offer an answer. Instead, it develops a procedure for analysis, so that decisions can be made with greater knowledge of the reasons and consequences. To serve this purpose, I have attempted to convey the relative certainty of what is presumed to be known, to specify what is not known, and, in places, to suggest lines of further inquiry into the unknown.

There is, also, a larger purpose. Prepaid benefits are so central to health care that they cannot be understood without touching on some of the most fundamental features of the medical care process and the organization of health services. The framework for analysis becomes correspondingly embracive. Thus, a great deal that is learned in this context (such as factual knowledge, approaches to analysis, or proposals for research) has wider application. As a result, much of this book bears on the general field of medical care administration.

The organization of the material in this book reflects a particular view of what one needs to know in order to understand and act intelligently in the formulation of policy, in planning, and in administration. It can be said that knowledge begins with empirical observation. But until they are organized, empirical observations are not comprehensible, nor can they serve as guides to future action. Theory is the outgrowth of this organization, leading to generalizations that can explain the present and predict the future. But action cannot flow from either empirical observation or theory unless it is linked to them by one or more objectives. The objectives of social action are, themselves, subject to general rules that may be called values; and values occur in distinctive configurations that constitute ideologies. Empirical observations, theory, objectives, values: these are the four categories that must be fitted together to achieve purposeful action.

Prepaid benefits are introduced into the medical care system, subject to certain governing principles, in order to solve one or more perceived problems. In the first chapter I have tried to establish what these principles and problems are. Accordingly, I have examined the mandate under which social action in the health field occurs, the distribution of ill health and use of health care services in the population, and some fundamental properties of the medical care process and the health services that it purveys.

Next comes a rigorous examination of the principal effects of the provision of health benefits on the medical care system. The four affected areas studied are: use of services, substitution of services, prices, and the redistribution of income. A chapter is devoted to each effect; and each chapter takes up, in succession, theoretical expectations, empirical evidence, and implications for policy and action. This tripartite, but integrated, development, under each of the four effects, is a distinctive feature of the design, and no effort has been spared to make it work.

The progression from theory to empirical observation in each chapter, and the confrontation between the two, is, to some extent, a fiction. I knew the major empirical findings before the theoretical sections were written, and when possible, the theoretical expectations were modified accordingly. The major purpose of the theoretical section is to offer a succinct, coherent description of each effect, in an effort to help the reader understand the relatively inchoate material that follows. On several occasions, however, detailed examination of the empirical findings suggested unforeseen generalizations, which have been kept in context and advanced as hypotheses to be tested.

Whether the empirical sections have any further utility is debatable. All too frequently, the empirical studies are seriously defective, their findings inconclusive, and their collective meaning ambiguous. A case could be made for giving them short shrift. On the contrary, I have given them a place of honor in the text and lavished much critical attention on them. I have done so for several reasons. With all their defects, these studies have generated the evidence by which theory must be tested. Collectively, they embody our intellectual history, remind us of the contributions of our fellow workers, illustrate in concrete form the elusive abstractions of our theory, and demonstrate the problems of doing research in this field. But, by paying such close attention to the empirical studies, I have run the risk of losing the way in a maze of detail. To reduce this danger, I have tried always to keep in view the integrating threads of theoretical expectation and have offered frequent summaries to help us keep our bearings.

The importance attached to values and objectives is established from the very start, in considering the social mandate for health care. Later, values and objectives serve to connect the effects of prepayment with the implications of these effects for policy and action. Finally, in the concluding portion of the text, objectives come to occupy the center of the stage, as determinants of policy and as tools for assessment.

If there is something original in this treatise, it is in the design and in the fitting of the subject matter to that design. Whatever insights I may have gained in the process, I have shared with the reader. Among these, I commend to his special attention the few small steps that have been taken towards defining more precisely the risk against which insurance is sought and the tentative exploration of the epidemiology of price changes as a social phenomenon transcending economics.

These accomplishments, modest as they are, I am happy to share with all who have helped me so generously with my work.

Primarily, I am indebted to the Carnegie Corporation of New York and to the Milbank Memorial Fund for financial support. With that support has come a flexibility in procedures, an informality in relationships, and a degree of personal interest that would delight any investigator. As a result, I feel that I have had not only sponsors, but also friends: Leroy Burney and David Willis at the Milbank Memorial Fund, and Sara Engelhardt at the Carnegie Corporation. Margaret Mahoney, before she left the Carnegie Corporation, played a key role. It was she who, after my illness, when I had all but abandoned my plans for this book, continued to press forward with the arrangements for it and, finally, challenged me to action with an offer that I could not refuse.

The School of Public Health at the University of Michigan has been an equal partner in sponsoring this book by releasing large amounts of my time and making the necessary accommodations to my intermittent absences. This has required a rare degree of good-will and understanding on the part of Eugene Feingold, department chairman, Myron Wegman, former dean, and Richard Remington, current dean.

As in all my previous work, I have had to lean heavily on the Reference Collection of medical care materials at the School of Public Health. I am particularly indebted to Jack Tobias and Lillian Fagin for their expert stewardship of the collection and their constant readiness to respond to my demands, no matter how unreasonable.

I am also indebted to Barbara Black for her supervision of my finances, which have always been a mystery to me. As a result of her good management we have remained solvent to the end.

The text, as it now stands, owes a great deal to Harry Foster, editor at the Harvard University Press. In addition to performing superlatively well the more obvious editorial functions, he was able to spot with uncanny accuracy every weakness or ambiguity in my reasoning, and challenged me to set the matter right. As a result, the text has gained in clarity and rigor.

The usefulness of the book has also been enhanced by the index which was prepared by Joseph Lovett. He has drawn on his previous experience and his knowledge of the field to fashion what we hope is an effective key to whatever riches are to be found in the text.

The labor of writing a book falls heavily on the author, but the privations that it entails are shared by his wife and children, who are almost widowed and orphaned while the ordeal lasts. Therefore, my greatest indebtedness is to my family for their loving loyalty and support.

And now, at last, it is time to stop; to cut the final moorings; to let go. The book, dear reader, is now no more mine than yours; may it fare well in your hands.

Avedis Donabedian
Ann Arbor

CONTENTS

PART ONE

Some General Considerations

1

Introduction and Background

Introduction

In considering any medical care program, two questions are likely to be of greatest concern to a consumer: whether he is eligible, and what services he can get. As we shall see, the scope of benefits and the conditions governing eligibility are so intimately related that it is difficult to speak of one feature without becoming involved, to some extent, in the other. The discussion can begin, arbitrarily, with either. We have chosen to begin with benefits.

The administrator may have to deal with program benefits in three contexts; the three are related, but call for somewhat different points of view and impose somewhat different tasks. The first, and perhaps most demanding context, is the design of a new system or package of benefits, to be made available through some mechanism that governs eligibility; the mechanism may be insurance, service, or welfare. The second context is when the administrator is called upon to evaluate benefits that are already in force in one or more programs. This evaluation may be a prelude to the formulation of new policies, which may eventuate in new benefits. If so, the frame of reference is similar to that used for the design of a new package; but the task is likely to be more manageable, since piecemeal improvement rather than total reform is usually the order of the day. The administrator may also become involved in an evaluation on behalf of clients (a labor union, for example) who have a choice of participating in one program or another. More usually, perhaps, the administrator is in charge of a facility or program that provides care; and he is, therefore, vitally concerned with the impact that a system financing a set of benefits may have upon his program or facility. In the third and most frequent context, the administrator is implementing and managing, on a day-to-day basis, whatever benefits are in force. This context applies whether the administrator is in an agency that only finances care, one that only provides care—for which it is reimbursed by a third party—or one that does both. Because of a bias in the author's interests, and limitations in his experience, the emphasis in this book will be on the broader issues relevant to benefit design and evaluation. However, the implications of policy choices to the implementation and management of benefits will be pointed out wherever possible.

Background

Attempts at analysis and evaluation are often based on a view of reality and a set of expectations that are not made as explicit as they should be. In this section we shall briefly describe our own view of relevant aspects of the medical care scene, so that the reader can judge at the very outset where we stand, and where we are likely to go. We shall do this under the following headings: (1) the social mandate and objectives pursuant to which benefits are provided, (2) the distribution of the need for care and the use of service, (3) aspects of the medical care process, (4) the interrelationships among health services, and (5) the definition of a health service.

Social Mandate and Objectives

In an earlier volume, to which this is a sequel, we described the general value orientations that underlie many policy decisions in medical care (1, pp. 1–27). In particular, we emphasized the distinction between the libertarian and egalitarian orientations, and we declared a preference for the latter. Elsewhere, we have proposed a set of criteria to be used in the evaluation of medical care programs in general (2). The gist of these arguments is that medical care services should be organized so as to result in a use of service that is proportionate to need, rather than to ability to pay. This formulation recognizes certain assumptions, postulates, and empirical observations that should now be considered.

"Need," as we have pointed out, may be defined in a variety of ways (1, pp. 61–69). We will take it to mean a situation or condition that requires medical care, or the aggregate of such situations or conditions. We shall discuss, a little further on, what kinds of care may be legitimately considered to fall within the ambit of the medical care system. For now, there is a prior question: who decides what situations or conditions require care, what kinds of care are required, and how much? The traditional answer is that the decision is made by individuals who consider the value to themselves of medical care services as compared with the alternatives they might buy, and who make decisions in a manner that best expresses their own preferences. Given a specified distribution of incomes, and certain assumptions concerning the production and pricing of medical care services, it can be shown that such individual decisions lead to an optimal situation, in the sense that the preferences of any one individual cannot be better met without diminishing the extent to which another individual can satisfy his. This view assumes that need for medical care is only one of a wide set of needs, that it is not possible to satisfy all needs of all people, and that each individual is the best judge of what needs he will satisfy, in what order, and to what extent, within the limits imposed by his means.

The libertarian values implicit in this formulation are commandingly powerful and should be contravened only for the most compelling of reasons. In our earlier volume we summarized the ways in which the free market model does not apply to medical care services and, consequently, why there are precisely such compelling reasons for social intervention (1, pp. 15–23). The basic moral argument was that, since good health is necessary to success in a society that makes a central value of personal achievement, access to the means necessary to health cannot be conditional on prior achievement, without discrediting the entire system. The more pragmatic arguments made against the libertarian position were that individuals do not know enough about health and medical care to make the choices they would make if they had that knowledge; that, accordingly, many decisions are made for consumers by their physicians; and that the health of individuals is of social concern because it influences the health and welfare of other people too. Of all these reasons, economists seem to find the last to be most persuasive: namely, that there are "external benefits" to medical care received by individuals. Hence, a great deal has been made of the instances in which infection has spread from untreated persons, or where the infirmities or disabilities of some workers have exposed other workers, or customers, to undue risk. However, as Pauly points out, all that is necessary to the argument of "external benefits" is that people, individually and collectively, derive some satisfaction from the receipt of medical care by others (3, pp. 11–19). The basis for the satisfaction is immaterial. For all we care, it could arise out of the conviction that people who need medical care should receive it!

The postulation of external benefits, irrespective of whether the benefits are received in the form of health, virtue, or of some other kind of personal satisfaction, is attractive because it keeps social policy firmly rooted in individual preference, or in some collective expression of this preference. There is no need to appeal to any higher order to determine what is good for people. A more general argument, but one that achieves the same purpose, holds that all medical care decisions are composed, in part, of the choices that are made by individuals alone and, in part, of the choices that are made by individuals through legitimate social instrumentalities, including government. To the extent that any given government represents the wishes and aspirations of individuals, its choices and decisions may be regarded as extensions of individual choice. However, to the extent that government or any other social instrumentality does not represent individuals, its choices are, at best, benevolent paternalism and, at worst, tyranny. We must see to it, therefore, that individuals can and do participate effectively in decisions concerning the features of medical care programs, including benefits and eligibility.

To hold that government action represents the aggregate of individual choices is one defense against the accusation that those who feel they know better are making decisions that they consider to be good for others. Another defense goes as follows: The receipt of medical care has low priority, relative to other commodities and services, because individuals are, ordinarily, occupied with the present or the immediate future, and have neither the opportunity nor the knowledge to take a lifetime view of their health. One could argue that if they could see their health in this longer perspective they would make certain choices that the short-term view does not lead them to make. The social arrangements for the provision of health services help individuals make more prudent choices by providing the knowledge and the opportunity to institutionalize the appropriate choices. Under these arrangements, individuals may be seen to put certain resources aside, out of reach of the immediate competing pressures of other needs, in order to assure highly valued things for themselves, now and in the future.

Thus, two conditions are necessary to guard against paternalism in social programs for medical care. One is that these programs should embody the long-term preferences of individuals, and another is that they be arrived at, and maintained, in as democratic a fashion as possible. The legitimacy of medical care programs does not, under this formulation, rest on what physicians, other health experts, or political leaders consider to be good or proper. It rests on nothing other than the basis for all our social institutions: free and informed consent.

Through such a train of thought we arrive at the conclusion that the program benefits we seek are those that are most likely to satisfy the long-term preferences of individuals and that are most likely to adjust use of service more closely to need. The further assumptions that pertain to the adjustment of use to need are: (1) it is not possible to meet every last bit of need; (2) needs can be arranged in some order of priority; and (3) at present, need and use of service are not congruent in our population.

If these assumptions are correct, one has to ask how various needs may be ordered in the hierarchy of priorities. This is a difficult question to answer. However, if we have accepted the formulation that the medical care system has institutionalized the lifetime preferences of individuals, we can propose that these preferences are based on the ability of services to generate health and well-being. In other words, those services that are preferred (or would be preferred if individuals were given the opportunity for informed and deliberate choice) are those that are most effective in assuring health not only immediately but over a lifetime. It follows that the priority of needs corresponds to the amount of health that can be generated, using current technology, from the receipt of care appropriate to each need. This begs the questions of what health is, and how it can be measured so that it can serve, at least in theory, as the yardstick for priorities. We have dealt with this subject at some length in our earlier volume (1, pp.

136–150); here, it is sufficient to indicate that what is envisaged is a weighted index of person-years of functional capacity, and the object is to maximize this measure.

It is easy to see that each individual, given limited means, would elect to use those services that are most likely to assure the greatest returns to himself in terms of lifetime health, especially if some system of discounting were introduced so that immediate gains would acquire somewhat greater value than deferred gains. The rule that governs the social distribution of health is much more controversial than that which governs individual choice. Elsewhere, we have proposed that the social objective of medical care programs should be to distribute health services so as to bring about the greatest equalization in lifetime health among population subgroups (2). Implicit in this formulation is the recognition that health depends on many things other than medical care, and that medical care has only a limited capacity to preserve or restore health. Furthermore, while equalization is still our preference, we are bound in real life by the social decisions that emerge from our system of government.

There is a second objective to the provision of benefits under organized auspices. This is the protection of individuals and families against the financial ravages of unpredictable and unpostponable medical care expenditures. Each year a small proportion of families suffers the impact of relatively large medical care expenditures. Severe illness of some duration in any one member can financially cripple a family for many years, making it impossible to maintain an accustomed standard of living or to achieve aspirations. These eventualities are considered particularly cruel and unfair because illness usually occurs through no fault of the sufferer. The provision of benefits in a manner that permits the spreading of risk among consumers at any given time, and for any given consumer over a longer period of time, is a major defense against one of the more captious cruelties of the human condition.

Obviously, the two objectives, of adjusting services to need and protecting financial integrity, are interrelated. They do, however, represent two different emphases in social policy and in the corresponding program design. Those who emphasize financial protection are more willing to accept, as given, whatever distribution of health services is current, even though they may concede that this distribution may be altered by the mechanisms that bring about protection. Those who emphasize the adjustment of use of service to need are more concerned with implementing the socially most desirable distribution of services, and they would use benefit design as one device to bring about the desired distribution. Throughout this monograph we shall have to proceed in the presence of these two objectives, and our study will be subject to the tension that is created by their divergent emphases.

Need, Use of Service, and Unmet Need

The established view of the distribution of health status is that the poor, and the otherwise underprivileged, suffer from more prevalent and more intense ill health, and that ill health itself causes poverty and deprivation. A proverbial vicious circle is set up, and many people become ensnared in it. There is little doubt that this picture has been true of all societies at some time during their history, as it has been of ours in the recent past. What is now being questioned is whether the picture is still accurate today. The question arises because recent reviews of the evidence suggest that the distribution of health has changed remarkably in the more developed countries. Both Kadushin (4) and Antonovsky (5, 6) agree that the health distinctions among classes have been greatly reduced. They disagree, however, on the extent of the reduction. Kadushin holds that distinctions have been virtually eliminated, while Antonovsky emphasizes that, in spite of considerable equalization overall, a wide gap still separates a group at the top from a group at the bottom.

The precise social distribution of ill health in many societies, including the U.S.A., is remarkably difficult to plot for the following reasons: first, with rising expectations, attention has shifted from levels of mortality to the prevalence of morbidity; second, morbidity itself can be viewed either in terms of diagnostic categories or in terms of the social and physical disability that it brings about; and third, data on the prevalence of illness in large population groups are not often available and, when available, suffer from deficiencies that make the findings less than conclusive. For example, in the U.S. the household interview and the health examination components of the National Health Survey exclude persons in institutions, who are precisely those who are most likely to be ill. The household interview survey depends, of course, on the respondents' ability and willingness to report. Further, definitions of illness and disability include components that are themselves likely to be correlated with social class variables. For example, the definition of acute illness is based on a restriction of activities during at least one day, the receipt of medical attention, or both. Absence from work is an equally important feature in the definition of disability. Recognition by the respondent of items on a list of "chronic conditions," and another list of "impairments," is critical to the reporting of illness. Such recognition is most likely to be related to the educational attainment and other social circumstances of the respondent, including the receipt of prior medical care and its nature.

It is difficult, a priori, to predict the net direction of bias introduced by all these features. It has been argued, for example, that manual labor, more common among the lower classes, requires higher levels of fitness and that, as a result, the lower classes are more likely to report disability relative to the demands of their work. It has also been argued that persons with low income are often unemployed or only episodically employed and, therefore, are more likely to report that illness has caused inability to work. Both these arguments, if true, would lead to an expectation of higher levels of disability among persons of lower income compared to those of higher income, given equal levels of biologically defined "health." On the other hand, one might argue that persons in the higher income groups are more aware of the consequences of neglecting an illness, have greater discretion to attend or stay away from work, and are more likely to have income protection during illness. All these would lead to expectations of greater reported disability among the well-to-do.

As to the ability and willingness to report illness, it would seem reasonable, though hardly established, that the poor and less educated would be less able or less willing to report. One could speculate that part of this unwillingness results from the suspicion with which the poor regard their interrogators, and part is due to the lesser saliency of minor illness in a life overburdened with more pressing problems. Underreporting would also ensue if, as seems likely, the poor receive less medical care in proportion to the amount and severity of illness that they suffer, if the care they receive is of lower technical quality, and if the care is less well understood by them, either because the physician will not explain as fully, or because they are less able to understand the physician. Under these circumstances, the poor would be less likely to qualify as having had an "acute condition" and less likely to know that they have a "chronic condition." Thus, we are left with the presumption that, on balance, the findings of the household interviews conducted by the National Center for Health Statistics tend to underestimate ill health in the poor. This is, however, only a presumption; and it is curious that a question of such importance to health policy has not been conclusively settled by empirical study.

The problems of method that have been described so far have to do with the definition and reporting of illness. There are also difficulties in defining the socioeconomic variable, especially when a time series is being examined. Income, education, occupation, residence, ethnicity, age, and other variables are highly intercorrelated. It is, therefore, difficult to know which factors account for observed differences in health. Over time, the significance of a given level of income in accounting for variations of health can be expected to change, even when corrections are made for inflation. It is possible that income, per se, may become relatively less significant, and education or race relatively more significant, in distinguishing levels of health (7).

With these difficulties in method firmly in mind, we can now turn to an assessment of the situation in the U.S. in the 1960's, as reported by Lefcowitz (7), who based his study on information published by the National Center for Health Statistics. A national study of births during 1964–1966 suggests that infant mortality, after correction for education of parents, shows a consistent relationship to family income for blacks but not for whites. This is a remarkable finding since infant mortality, in the past, has been very sensitive to socioeconomic differentials. As to the distribution of professionally-defined abnormalities, the Health Examinations Survey of samples of the civilian population who are not in institutions shows that there are no clear gradients relative to family income for impairments of vision and hearing, or for conditions as varied as diabetes, anemia, coronary heart disease, osteoarthritis or rheumatoid arthritis; nor is there a regular relationship between income and hypertension or hypertensive heart disease when race and sex are accounted for.

Although these professionally-defined abnormalities are only weakly related to income, when it comes to disabilities reported by the civilian, noninstitutionalized population, the relationship to income is clear and strong; the more severe the disability, the greater the relative differential among income groups. Furthermore, the differential is present within each age group, although it is more marked in middle age than among young persons or the aged (8, 9). National data that have become available since the assessment by Lefcowitz show that these relationships have, in the main, remained unchanged. In fact, the disparity between the lowest and the highest income groups (uncorrected for changes in purchasing power or age structure) is even greater in 1971 than it was in 1965–1966 (10, pp. 13–14). In explaining such disparities, Lefcowitz suggested that equivalent illness has more severe consequences in terms of loss of work and loss of income among the poor than among the rich. While this seems plausible, it is also likely that illness is more severe, or becomes more severe, among the poor, resulting in greater disability.

In summary, until more reliable and refined data are available we shall proceed with the conclusion that disease in its more severe and disabling forms is more common among persons of lower income. Accordingly, the need for medical care should be greater for such persons. The next order of business must be to examine the extent to which services are distributed according to income and according to need.

We are interested in the relationship between income and the consumption of health services because we can draw from it inferences concerning two issues of major importance to social policy: one issue is access to care and the other is the burden of expenditures for care. Somewhat parallel to these two concerns, there are two ways of measuring consumption: in physical quantities (such as visits to a physician or days in a hospital), or in expenditures. But the purpose of analysis and the method of measurement do not always correspond. The choice between measuring by expenditures or by physical quantities is often determined mainly by the availability of data: expenditures, for example, may be used as a proxy for services. When expenditures are used, it should be remembered that the poor are more likely to receive care at reduced prices and to have payments made on their behalf by government programs or private charity. On the other hand, middle and higher income persons are more likely to have insurance, so that medical care charges are not paid out-of-pocket (11). When adjustments are made, as they should be, to account for the foregoing variables, expenditures may be a truer reflection of access because the remaining price differentials may indicate more service, higher technical quality, or improved amenities (12).

On the other hand, when expenditures are measured in order to determine their financial impact on families with different incomes, the decision may be made to include only actual outlays and debts incurred during a specified period. If so, the accounting should include insurance premiums paid by the family as well as some adjustment for the tax deductions they receive for medical care expenditures (11). Employer contributions towards insurance premiums are usually not included, although it could be argued that if these contributions were not made, an equal sum, less tax, would be available as disposable income. Nor is consideration given, in this context, to that portion of personal taxes that finances public medical care programs.

In establishing the relationships between income and the consumption of health services, there are also problems in the measurement of income. One theory of consumption postulates that persons consume services, including health care, in accordance with established patterns that correspond to their permanent income rather than to temporary reductions or increases in their more usual income (13). If one makes the additional assumption that at the low end of the range of observed incomes one is more likely to find temporary reductions in income, and at the higher end of the observed income range temporary increases, the consequence is that the effect of income on access is underestimated if observed income rather than permanent income is used to establish the relationship.

Income is further distorted because illness itself reduces income through temporarily or permanently interfering with earning power. This phenomenon will also result in an underestimate of the effect of income on access, by showing, at the low end of the income range, levels of use that are higher than one would otherwise expect. It follows that, without corrections for the effects of transitory income and for the effect of illness on income, the effect of income on access is underestimated. However, if one were interested in the financial impact of expenditures for health care on families, observed income rather than corrected income could be the more appropriate variable to use.

A further refinement in establishing the relationship between income and consumption is to correct for family size, since family size both reduces income per family member and increases the use of health services per family (12). Further corrections are necessary if one is interested in the effect of purchasing power per se, as distinct from the characteristics that are correlated with income and that, collectively, distinguish the poor from the more prosperous. Such characteristics include age, education, and race. Among other effects, older age is associated with higher levels of need and lower income; education is associated with a greater valuation of health and health services; and race is associated with institutional barriers to the receipt of service. In every instance, the corrections that are necessary depend on the inferences that are to be drawn from the analysis. If one wishes to measure the differential impact of medical care spending on different income groups, it is appropriate to relate observed income to out-of-pocket expenditures, plus medical debts, plus premium payments (with or without adding employer contributions), plus tax payments for medical care net of medical deductions. If the interest is in measuring differences in access to care, it is sufficient to relate services or the monetary value of services (corrected for price differences that do not represent quality) to observed or adjusted income. If, on the other hand, it is desired to find out what accounts for the differences between persons in different income groups, it is necessary to refine the measure of income and to separate its effects from the effects of factors that are associated with it. Thus, one must distinguish the use of income as a rough and ready marker for socioeconomic status from its use as a measure of the ability to pay out of current earnings or substitutes for such earnings.

Now that the reader has been alerted to some of the problems inherent in studies of the relationship between income and consumption of health services, let us next turn to what is known about this relationship. The established view, and the one that corresponds to theoretical expectation, is that with increasing income there is increasing consumption, whether measured in services or expenditures, although the rise in consumption is proportionally less than the rise in income. This means that the poor receive less care than the rich, but expenditures for care represent a greater share of family income for the poor. Economists use the word "elasticity" to designate the percent change in one quantity as a ratio of the percent change in another. In this instance, the income elasticity of the consumption of health services would be less than one, since a one percent increase in income is associated with a less than one percent increase in consumption. An elasticity of one would mean that income and consumption increase proportionately; an elasticity of more than one would mean that a one percent increase in income would be accompanied by a more than one percent increase in consumption; and an elasticity of zero would mean that consumption remains unchanged irrespective of differences in income.

There is ample evidence, limited by imperfections in method, that in the recent past the income elasticity of medical expenditures has been less than one (11, 14). Feldstein and Carr have critically reviewed ten studies, done between 1917–1919 and 1960, all of which have come to this conclusion (11). The elasticities that were discovered ranged from 0.496 for farm operative families in 1941 to 0.957 for urban families in 1935–1936. A more recent review by Klarman reports that studies of data for time periods within a span of almost 50 years have found the elasticity of demand for physicians' services to range from 0.21 to 0.62, when demand was measured in visits, and from 0.17 to 0.82, when demand was measured in expenditures (14, Table 1, p. 363).

Some aspects of studies on the elasticity of demand for medical care can be illustrated by reviewing briefly a small selection of these studies. Feldstein and Carr, after pointing out some of the problems in measurement, add the findings of a study of their own, in which they introduced a number of refinements in method (11). The data were obtained from the 1950 Bureau of Labor Statistics survey of consumer finances; the authors showed that for each 1,000 dollar increase in income there was a 34.3 dollar increase in medical care expenditures, corresponding to an income elasticity of 0.699. When corrections were made for family size, education of head of household, number gainfully employed in each family, and the presence of health insurance, the income elasticity was reduced to 0.501, corresponding to an increase of 24.6 dollars in expenditures for each 1,000 dollar increase in income. In other words, part of the effect of income is attributable to other variables associated with income. Even more important, income accounted for only 16 percent of the variation in spending.

Feldstein and Severson have reported an analysis of more recent data with essentially similar results (15). The data were from a survey of the civilian, noninstitutionalized population of the U.S. in 1958, conducted jointly by the Health Information Center and the National Opinion Research Center. Through the use of a multiple regression equation, the effect of income was estimated while various other factors were held constant: age and education of head of household, percent of families with one or more members sixty-five years or older, percent of families with one or more members under five years of age, percent of single-person families, percent of families living in urban areas, the proportion of the bill covered by insurance, and the amount of free care received. Findings are given concerning the relationship of income to expenditures and use of service for different components of medical care. The income elasticity of total medical care spending was 0.590 (lower estimate), corresponding to a difference of $29.00 in expenditures for each difference of $1,000 in income. The degree to which the variables used in the regression, including income, were able, all together, to account for differences in expenditures or use varied considerably by type of care, being highest for hospital admissions (75%) and lowest for drug expenditures (8%). Only 25 percent of the variation in total spending could be accounted for by the variables used. Nevertheless, inclusion of variables other than income modified considerably the effect attributed to income. For example, without including other variables in the regression equation, a 10 percent increase in income appeared to be associated with a 1 percent increase in total physician visits. When the other variables, plus price, were added to the regression, a 10 percent increase in income was associated with a 6 percent increase in total physician visits. In this instance, the variables were correlated with income so as to mask its true effect on use of service.

The distinction between observed and permanent income in measuring the income elasticity of medical spending appears to be a matter of considerable concern to economists. Transitory elements in observed income have generally been corrected by using grouped data, rather than data for individual families. The rationale is that grouping tends to equalize transitory variations in income. Accordingly, Feldstein and Carr recomputed their data for 1950 and added data for 1960, using cities as the unit of analysis (11). The elasticities computed in this manner were higher than those computed using families as the unit of analysis. For 1950, the value rose to a shade above 1. Presumably on the basis of this experience, Feldstein and Severson's analysis of the 1958 national sample grouped family data into the primary sampling units (metropolitan areas and counties) of the original area probability sample that was used for the survey. The values cited above, in our review of this work, have been corrected for the effect of transitory income.

More recently, Silver analyzed data pertaining to all employed persons in the U.S. during July through December 1962; the data were grouped into 24 cells by region, sex and age. His values for the income elasticity of medical expenditures are the highest encountered in the literature reviewed by this author, ranging from 3.19 for dental care to 1.82 for hospital care, with a value of 2.53 for total expenditures (16). Silver argues that the use of grouped data reduces the biases that arise from errors in measurement of income, from the association of health status and income, and from interrelationships among expenditures for different health services (16). However, grouping also masks variations within groups, possibly resulting in erroneous findings concerning the presence, magnitude, or even direction of relationships—a phenomenon recognized in areal analysis as the "ecological fallacy" (17).

Thus, it is not clear precisely how to account for the larger elasticities found in studies using geographic areas as units of analysis. In contrast to such studies, Andersen and Benham took the family as their unit for analysis and used "two-stage instrumental variable analysis" to obtain an estimate of permanent income and then to relate this estimate to observed and standardized expenditures for care (18). As expected, the elasticities were somewhat larger when the permanent income estimate was used, although not in all cases.

The study reported by Andersen and Benham is the most recent that we have reviewed, and for that reason the findings are of particular interest. The data pertain to the civilian, noninstitutionalized population in 1963. The income elasticity of physician charges was 0.41 for observed income, and 0.63 for permanent income. However, when corrections were made for the comprehensiveness of insurance benefits, the propensity to use specialists, the propensity to use preventive services, and for certain demographic characteristics, the income elasticities were reduced to 0.22 and 0.17, respectively. Thus, in this instance, variables other than income accentuated, through their correlation with income, the differentials in medical care spending.

An additional interesting feature of Andersen and Benham's study was their use of two measures of expenditure, one observed and the other standardized. Standardization was achieved by applying the California relative value scale for 1960 to data on use of physicians' services. Without accounting for factors other than income, the elasticity of standardized charges relative to observed income was 0.31, as compared to 0.63 when observed charges were used. The authors tend to favor the explanation that the difference is accounted for by differences in price and that, therefore, "expenditures significantly underestimate the proportion of all physician services consumed by low-income families" (18, p. 91). However, as the authors also recognize, the differences could be, at least in part, due to the better care received by higher income families.

Comparisons of income elasticities for different expenditures and for the corresponding services can also be found in the work of Feldstein and Severson (15). For 1958, after accounting for the variables already described, the income elasticity for physician expenditures was 0.558 and for total physician visits 0.622, whereas the elasticity for hospital expenditures was 0.508 and for hospital patient-days 0.471. Needless to say, the correspondence between expenditures and services in these instances is not complete, since physicians provide services other than visits, and hospitals provide inpatient services other than patient days.

The conclusion to be drawn from all these studies is that, until

1963, the income elasticity of medical care services and expenditures, in general, and for the services of physicians, in particular, was less than 1 and probably in the vicinity of 0.5. Thus, the poor had less access to care but spent a higher proportion of their more meager income for health services. Since then, Medicare has been introduced and public welfare care has been expanded under the Medicaid program. These two programs are thought to have increased the care received by the aged, many of whom are poor, and the care received by poor families with dependent children; thus, they should have brought about equalization in access to medical care by income. For these reasons, and possibly for others, one would expect a narrowing of the gap between income groups.

The data that are relevant to this expectation come from two time series: the continuing reports of the National Center for Health Statistics, and the periodic surveys that were conducted, in cooperation with the National Opinion Research Center, first by the Health Information Foundation and later by the Center for Health Administration Studies of the University of Chicago. So far, there have been four surveys, in 1953, 1958, 1964, and 1971 (19–21). Recently Bice et al. (22), and Lefcowitz (7) have examined, and commented on, the trends as revealed by the reports of the national center; Andersen et al. (21) have reviewed the findings of the four national surveys spanning the years 1953 to 1971. Only in the report by Andersen et al. (21) is there an attempt, at least occasionally, to correct for inflation by adjusting the income brackets—which they designate low, middle, and high—for each decade.

The information summarized by Andersen et al. (21) and Bice et al. (22), when combined, shows that between 1963 and 1970 there has been considerable equalization among income groups in the percent of persons who visit a physician and in the number of visits per person per year; but the equalization has been achieved in somewhat different ways. Table 1 shows the data. The percent who visit a physician has remained the same in the high income group, but has increased in the low income group. For the number of visits per person per year, the opposite has occurred. The low income group has maintained its position, but the high income group has reduced its consumption to the level of the poor. This

TABLE 1. Percent of Persons Who Visit a Physician during a Year, and Visits per Person per Year, by Income, U.S.A., Circa 1963 and 1970

Use of Service and Income	Circa 1963	Circa 1970	1970 as Percent of 1963
Percent who visit physicians			
Low income	56	65	116
High income	71	71	100
High as percent of low	127	109	—
Visits per person per year			
Low income	4.3	4.3	100
High income	5.1	4.3	84
High as percent of low	119	100	—

Source: Reference 21, Table 4 and Reference 22, Table 2.

Note: The data for percent who visit a physician come from the University of Chicago surveys of an area probability sample of the civilian, non-institutionalized population. Visits exclude inpatient hospital visits and telephone calls. Income categories for 1963 are less than $4,000 and $7,000 or more, and for 1970 they are less than $6,000 and $11,000 or more. The data for Visits per Person per Year are from the National Health Survey of the civilian, non-institutionalized population for 1963–64 and 1969. Visits exclude hospital inpatient care but include telephone calls. Income groups are less than $3,000 and $10,000 or over.

suggests that, given a relatively fixed complement of practicing physicians per unit population, increased access by the poor has been adjusted for by a reduction in the number of visits per person for all persons, rich or poor, after access has been achieved. The reduction has resulted in a net redistribution of the total volume of care in favor of the poor. However, this conclusion is tentative, since the data from the two sources are not completely comparable, as indicated in the footnote to Table 1. For that reason, we turn to data drawn exclusively from the National Health Survey, which are shown in Figure 1. The patterns portrayed conform closely to those already described, with the major exception that the visits per person in the lowest income group appear to have risen to a moderate degree. It is possible, from the data cited in Figure 1, to compute the number of visits per person for those who made at least one visit. When this additional information is obtained, one is led to conclude that recent changes in the health care system (possibly the introduction of Medicare and Medicaid) have been particularly favorable to those recognized as "poor." In

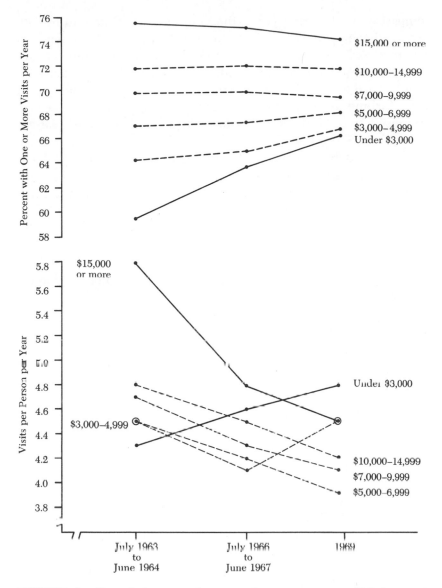

FIGURE 1. Use of physicians' services by income group, U.S.A., specified years.

Source: Reference 23, Tables A and B, pages 4–5.

comparison with earlier years, the poor are more likely to initiate care, and there is less likely to be a reduction in the amount of care received once care is initiated, so that the total volume of care received per person has increased. To some extent, these gains appear to have occurred at the expense, in health care, of persons in other income groups, who are about as likely to initiate care as they used to be, but are likely to make fewer visits once care is initiated.

When the data are classified simultaneously by income and age groups, it appears that lower income children have improved their access to care, but remain less likely to see the physician during a given year. Furthermore, lower income children make such a small number of visits when they do see the doctor that the total care received per child per year has remained considerably less than for children in the higher income group. In early adult life and middle age, the lower income group have increased their propensity to receive care to a moderate degree and have also increased the number of visits per person among those who see a physician. The consequence is that lower income persons who do receive care now receive more care, on the average, than do higher income persons of comparable age. In the age group 65 and over, there has been an increased propensity to seek care and a reduction in the number of visits per person in all income groups, so that income differentials in volume of care received have remained essentially unchanged.

Table 2 summarizes the situation in 1970, based on the data reported by Andersen et al. (21). It is clear that, for the total population, although the well-to-do are more likely to seek care, they are likely to receive less care in terms of their average number of visits to a physician. The total volume of physician services outside the hospital is now inversely related to income. However, this relationship does not hold in all age groups; children and the aged are exceptions to the general trend. Little children in the "high income" group are more likely to see the physician, make more visits if they do see a physician, and chalk up 44 percent more visits per person than do children in the "low income" group. Among those 65 and over, the differences are not as marked. Although persons in the "high" group are more likely to seek care, they make fewer visits per person who sees a physician,

TABLE 2. Specified Measures of Use of Physician Services, by Age and by Income Group, U.S.A., 1970

Age and Income Groups	Percent Who See a Physician	Visits per Person Who Sees a Physician	Visits per Person
All persons			
Low income	65	7.5	4.9
Middle income	67	5.9	3.9
High income	71	5.1	3.6
High as % of low	109	68	73
Age 0–5			
Low income	80	4.0	3.2
Middle income	86	5.1	4.4
High income	90	5.1	4.6
High as % of low	112	128	144
Age 35–54			
Low income	65	7.8	5.1
Middle income	67	6.0	4.0
High income	69	5.4	3.7
High as % of low	106	69	73
Age 65 and over			
Low income	73	8.6	6.3
Middle income	86	7.4	6.4
High income	85	7.9	6.7
High as % of low	116	92	106

Source: Reference 21, Table 8. Values in column 1 computed as follows:

$$\frac{\text{Column 3}}{\text{Column 2}} \times 100.$$

Note: See footnote Table 1 for definitions.

so that the total visits per person are only slightly greater than in the low income group. If one ignores the finer detail, the conclusion is that the poor now receive more non-hospital physician services than the well-to-do, except for the aged, among whom the well-to-do enjoy a smaller advantage, and children, among whom the well-to-do are considerably ahead.

The data for hospital care, as reported by Andersen et al. (21), also show a shift in favor of the poor. In 1953, admissions to short-term hospitals were about equal in all income groups. Increasingly, the trend has been toward more frequent admissions for the poor, with the result that, in 1970, there is a marked inverse gradient relative to income. In 1970, there were 19 admissions per year for each 100 persons with a family income of under $2,000, compared to 9 admissions per 100 per year for those with a family income of $17,500 and over. Unfortunately, Andersen et al. do not cite data on length of stay or patient days in their report. However, knowing that the poor generally stay longer in the hospital once they are admitted, the gradient in patient-days is expected to be even sharper. When the trends for admissions are examined by age groups, it appears that the reversal in gradients relative to income occurred prior to 1963 for persons aged 18–54, and between 1963 and 1970 for persons aged 0–17. Quite unexpectedly, the findings for persons 55 and over show either no change in relation to income, or an increase in admissions by persons in the higher income group, so that, in 1970, there is almost no difference in admissions by income.

The data for dental care, reported by Andersen et al. (21), are particularly interesting because they stand in such contrast to those for the services of hospitals and physicians. Here, the traditional positive relationship to income has remained virtually unchanged. Thus, one can broadly rank three services in descending order of personal and social saliency: hospital services, physician services, and dental services, respectively. One can also distinguish three age groups: persons in the working years, children, and the aged. It would seem as if the services pertaining to the more serious and urgent needs have been the first to be redistributed, and that redistribution has gone farthest for these. It would also seem that redistribution was earlier, and has been more extensive, for persons in the working years, whereas children and the aged have lagged behind. This may be a rather fanciful order imposed upon such incomplete data. It is, nevertheless, very tempting to interpret the data observed as a consequence of interactions, as yet not fully elucidated, among differential social provisions of health benefits and differential perceptions of seriousness and urgency of need.

As to the factors responsible for the patterns observed, and the changes that have occurred during the last two decades, one can only speculate. Dental care may be assumed to have maintained its traditional positive relationship to income because it has been regarded by individuals and by society as a more discretionary item, more akin to a luxury than a necessity. Hence, it has had a lower personal priority in comparison to other needs or wants; and society has made little provision for it through health insurance or public medical care programs. Hospital care has been at the other extreme in terms of perceived necessity and of the provision for coverage under voluntary health insurance, as well as under governmental programs. Thus, the reversal in its gradient relative to income has occurred early, and has been most socially pervasive. The services of physicians, exclusive of inpatient care, have occupied an intermediate position in individual and collective priorities, somewhere between dental care and inpatient hospital care.

The expansion of benefits under health insurance, and the nature of the benefits, could conceivably explain part of the remarkable change in the relative health care position, by income group, of young and middle-age adults. Bice et al. suggest that the improvement in access to physician services for poor children mainly concerns therapeutic services, and that the increment of services received by well-to-do children is largely accounted for by preventive services, including health supervision (22). Insufficient coverage of preventive services under Medicaid in the recent past may have contributed to this differential. As to the possible impact of Medicare on the aged, it appears that the higher income groups have taken at least as much advantage of its provisions as have persons of lower income, in part because for the latter the deductible features of Medicare may have posed a barrier to access. It may also be that the greater coverage of hospital services in this program has substituted inpatient for outpatient care. If so, this seems to have occurred to a greater extent in the higher income groups. The result is that one finds, in 1970, a persisting small income differential for physicians' services, and almost no differential in hospital admissions. It is also possible that this relative equality in use of service reflects a relative similarity in disability among the aged irrespective of income group, as some surveys have reported (8, 9). It may be that, among the aged who survive, socioeconomic differentials in the need for care are overshadowed by the ravages of the aging process itself.

So far, we have tried to explain recent trends and differences in use of services in terms of arrangements for the financing of health services. It may be that more pervasive social changes are also at work. For example, Lefcowitz has emphasized that, currently, education rather than income is the more important influence on use of service (7). This is somewhat difficult to substantiate, since the relationships observed are so dependent on where the education and income breaks are made in grouping the data. But let us assume that Lefcowitz's observation is correct. If one makes the further assumption that, within broad income groups, the traditional relationship between income and education is not as close as it used to be, one can explain at least part of the attenuation of the relationship between income and use of physician services. This speculation is salutary because it broadens our sights beyond the medical care system itself. More importantly, the question of whether education or income has more influence on use of services has very important implications for medical care policy in general, and for benefit design in particular.

Let us now turn to some additional features of the methods used to examine the reported trends. One such feature is the fineness of the income breaks, and another the purchasing power of specified incomes. The data cited by Andersen et al. for physician services do make an adjustment for purchasing power, but the income groupings are so broad that they may conceal differences in use of services, especially at the higher end of the income range. The breaks used for 1970 were below $6,000 for "low" and $11,000 and over for "high." The income intervals used to examine hospital admissions are much finer, but are not available in the same detail for all the survey years, nor do they adjust for purchasing power. Further, when cross tabulation of two or more variables is made (for example of age and income) the groupings have to be drastically reduced in number in order to achieve reasonably stable rates for each cell. Needless to say, the persistence of the more traditional patterns of use at the extremes of income, assuming these were found to exist, would not mean that considerable redistribution has not occurred. It would simply identify groups that need special attention in program design.

Other aspects of method that must be considered are the possibility of differential reporting by income at any given time, and the presence of trends in the propensity to report over time. We know very little about trends in reporting. As to differential reporting by income group at any given time, we have surmised that the poor are less likely to report illness as well as receipt of service. If so, the error of reporting would reduce not only the reported prevalence of need among the poor, but also the reported prevalence of services received in response to need. Whether this means that the ratio of reported service to reported needs thereby adjusts itself so as to correspond to reality, no one can say.

Finally, and most importantly, one needs to consider the implications to medical care policy of the change in the relationship between income and use of service. This does not mean that benefit design is not relevant. On the contrary, as we have speculated, much of the change we have seen is probably the result of changes in the nature of health care benefits in voluntary and governmental programs in the recent past. The question now is how to adapt benefit design to the changing situation. Here, two important inferences may be drawn. The first is that, as use of service by income is equalized, the potential inequities in medical care spending relative to income become magnified, and the alleviation of these inequities assumes even greater saliency as an objective in benefit design. Second, as ability to pay becomes less important as a barrier to access, other barriers, such as education, race, or geographic location, become more important concerns in the design and operation of medical care programs (7, 22). But these speculations, though valid, are somewhat premature since one last, and most important, piece of evidence necessary for the formulation of policy has not yet been brought in for examination.

So far, we have dealt with use of service without direct reference to need for medical care. The critical piece of information for the formulation of policy is whether use of service corresponds to need. If we accept the view that need is more prevalent among persons of lower income, the trends in use of service that we have described suggest increasing congruence between need and demand. The question is whether there is still a gap, how large it is, and in what groups of people it is localized. Unfortunately, data on this important point are quite meager. The surveys reported by Andersen et al. do give some information (21). During 1971, the poor were slightly more likely to report the occurrence of a disability that kept them in bed or made them unable to carry on their usual activities because of illness or injury. The poor were even more likely to have a disability of long duration. The difference between income groups was more marked in days of disability per person with a disability, than in the sheer likelihood of a disability. The propensity to seek care among persons who reported a disability was not very different by income. What was very different was the amount of care provided by a physician relative to the duration of disability. Contact with a physician, either in person or by phone, for each 100 days of disability showed a regular, and rather steep, progression as follows: 9 contacts for the rural poor, 11–12 for the urban poor, about 14 for the rural nonpoor and 17 for the urban nonpoor. This certainly suggests that the poor do not receive care proportionate to the severity or duration of their disability.

The data reported by Andersen et al. (21) do not give findings on disability by age group. Bice et al. (22) report findings, from the National Health Survey, which relate age to use of physicians' services (exclusive of inpatient care) by severity of disability, but not by its duration. In 1969 there were no consistent differences within each disability category, by age, except for children (0–16) and, to a lesser extent, for the aged (65 +). Table 3, which gives part of the data cited by Bice et al., shows that for these two age groups, differences in favor of the well-to-do tend to persist when controlled for disability status. One would expect the magnitude of income differentials in the use of physician services outside the

TABLE 3.   Ratio of Physician Visits per Person per Year for Low Income Persons, to Physician Visits per Person per Year for High Income Persons, by Age Group and by Disability Status, U.S.A., 1969 [a]

	Ratio by Age Group	
Disability Status	Children (0–16)	Aged (65+)
No limitation of activity	0.65	0.69
With limitation, but not in major activity	0.33	0.51
With limitation in amount or kind of major activity	0.59	0.95
Unable to carry on major activity	—	0.72

Source: National Center for Health Statistics, Health Interview Survey. Cited in Reference 22.

[a] The income groups are less than $5,000 and $10,000 and over. Physician visits include telephone calls but exclude inpatient visits.

hospital would be reduced as the severity of the disability increases, but the data do not reveal a consistent relationship of this
kind. This may be in part due to the possibility that the more
severe grades of disability are, to some extent, established and
stabilized, so that they no longer elicit demand for care. It could
also be that hospital care is relatively more frequent or more
lengthy among the more disabled, and substitutes to some extent
for care by the physician outside the hospital.

So far, we have dealt with the relationship between volume of
care and need for care. It may also be that the poor are at a disadvantage with respect to the content or quality of care. Information
concerning this matter is largely inferential, and, to that extent,
open to question. It can be summarized as follows (24): The poor
are more likely to receive care at the emergency and out-patient
clinics of hospitals. While it is not possible to generalize about the
technical quality of this care, it is likely to be less personalized
than care received from the family's physician. The physicians
who provide the bulk of care to welfare recipients tend to be a
subset of physicians who have characteristics that suggest lower
levels of technical performance. At least in the larger cities they
tend to be generalists, to have tenuous hospital affiliations, if any,
and to carry very large case loads. By and large the poor, irrespective of welfare status, are more likely to receive care from generalists than specialists, again suggesting lower levels of technical
performance, though not necessarily of personal attention. Past
studies have also shown that the poor have a greater propensity to
consult practitioners such as chiropractors or pharmacists, who
might be considered as less adequate substitutes for the physician.
There is also reason to believe that a given practitioner, or institution, may treat the rich differently from the poor, to the disadvantage of the latter. In fact, it may very well be that current differences in the "amenities" and quality of care separate income
groups more sharply than do differences in volume of care, even
when the latter is related to need. This is only an informed guess,
and it would be difficult to document. It does not mean that the
poor never have access to good, or even superior, care. It may well
be that care received at teaching hospitals or at the better neighborhood health centers is quite comparable, or even superior, to
care received by the majority of well-to-do patients. Unfortu-

nately, opinions on this are speculative and based on circumstantial evidence.

It is now time to summarize our conclusions concerning the distribution of need and unmet need for medical care. The summary represents our view of reality and, therefore, the frame of reference which will structure much of what is to follow: We believe that much progress has been made toward a more equitable distribution of health, but that health, defined as functional ability, is still more widely prevalent among the well-to-do. Similarly, although use of service is now more proportionate to need, the poor continue to receive less service relative to their functional incapacity than do the rich. In this respect, children and possibly the aged continue to need special attention. Finally, to the extent that ability to pay becomes a less important barrier to receiving care, attention shifts to (1) the financial impact of medical care spending relative to income, (2) the qualitative aspects of the care received, and (3) those characteristics, other than ability to pay, that continue to pose a barrier to care.

A final question remains to be settled. Which level of care is appropriate relative to need? Should we design benefits so that use of service among the rich is reduced or that the use of service among the poor is increased? The current presumption is that even care for the well-to-do falls below professional norms in many respects. If so, the goal would be to improve the quantity, and certainly the quality, of care for all, but with proportionately more improvement for the poor. It is conceivable, however, that if the total resources to be allocated to medical care are severely limited, a distributive rule that makes care proportionate to need will reduce care for the rich while it increases care for the poor.

We should also remember that "use of service proportionate to need" is not necessarily synonymous with "use of service proportionate to disability or dysfunction." As we have pointed out, there might very well be a weighting or ordering of "needs" that takes into account not only the magnitude of disability or dysfunction but also their amenability to prevention or amelioration, as measured by the life-time "health potential" generated in response to appropriate health care. In this section, the occurrence of disability and dysfunction was used only as a rough indicator of the more refined concept of "need," which unfortunately remains difficult to measure with any degree of precision.

Aspects of the Medical Care Process

The current distribution of need, and of services relative to need, is one of the important considerations that go into the design of eligibility and benefit features in a medical care program. Another consideration is how the medical care process works: who initiates it and terminates it; who makes the critical decisions and on what grounds; what motivates health professionals and clients; and how professionals and clients interact. A detailed discussion of this subject would require a volume in itself; but the key features, as we see them, can be simply stated.

Outreach workers, nurses, physicians, and other workers in a medical care program can stimulate the initiation of care. However, initiation is more generally the almost exclusive responsibility of the patient or his family, who may be influenced by many personal, social, and cultural factors. The initiation of care usually occurs in response to intimations, often ambiguous, that something has gone wrong and requires medical care. The determination of what exactly calls for medical care depends on individual perceptions and accepted social definitions. The initial step in seeking care is taken with some hesitation, and with little knowledge of what its consequences will be. Thereafter, the physician and other functionaries of the medical care system are responsible for defining the nature of the problem, and deciding what needs to be done. The client is, of course, not totally without voice in these matters; but more often than not he is guided by his physician in the course that he follows.

In the light of our overall objectives, several consequences seem to flow from this formulation. We begin with the assertion that use of service must be proportionate to need, and that need is defined partly by individuals for themselves, and partly by the social instrumentalities that the individuals have chosen to act on their behalf. But the nature and extent of need or of the benefits that are likely to flow from care cannot be determined unless a competent professional evaluation is made. It follows that access to such an evaluation, with a minimum of obstacles, is an important feature of benefit design. Only in this way can one be certain that care is adjusted to need. The objective, then, is to achieve the least possible friction at entry into the system, and only subsequently to introduce the measures that are needed to ration ser-

vices according to need. In fact, there may have to be inducements to entry, so that conditions not known to the client, or not
regarded by him as important, can be subjected to appropriate
evaluation and care. If this argument is accepted, benefit design
should encourage, rather than discourage, the initiation of care,
and should provide the services necessary for the detection and
evaluation of need.

A second set of consequences follows from the key role of the
physician in determining the course of care after it has been initiated. Program benefits, as we shall see, are a system of incentives,
not only to the client, but also to the physician and to the institution where he works. Hence, a great deal of attention should be
given to the manner in which benefits might subvert or distort the
decisions of physicians and other professionals so that they depart
from what medical science would dictate to be the most appropriate and effective care. Such distortions of medical judgment are
made more likely by certain interrelationships among the components of health care, and we must now give some attention to
these interrelationships.

Interrelationships among Health Services

Medical care services are not marbles in a bag, from which one
can pull out a few without altering those that remain. On the contrary, there are such intimate functional and operational interrelationships among the services constituting medical care, that interference with one can result in profound, and sometimes
unexpected, consequences to another. This can come about in a
variety of ways and for a variety of reasons. First, some services
are prerequisites to others. For example, care by a "primary practitioner," usually a physician, is a prerequisite to most other care,
including diagnostic services, drugs, and the use of hospitals. Similarly, a means of diagnosis, at least provisionally, is a necessary
first step to instituting therapeutic and rehabilitative services.
These are sequences based on functional necessities. Sometimes
they also correspond to administrative or operational features. For
example, if an administrative decision concerning eligibility for
benefits requires prior assessment of health status, it becomes self-
defeating to exclude that prior necessity from the benefits covered. This sequence is well recognized in programs that provide

diagnostic services irrespective of ability to pay, but that require a means test prior to further care. These include Crippled Children's Programs, Children and Youth Projects, and vocational rehabilitation services. Since the decision as to "medical indigency" depends, in part, on an evaluation of the need for care, it would seem absurd to withhold service until medical indigency is established.

Second, some services are dependent on other services for a share of their effectiveness and perhaps their safety. For example, maternity services cannot be considered complete or safe unless they include prenatal and postnatal care, and perhaps family planning as well. Similarly, successful surgery depends significantly on appropriate care before and after surgery.

Third, some services are more or less complete substitutes for others. For example, inpatient hospital care may be a complete substitute for ambulatory care, whereas ambulatory care is a substitute for some, though not all, of the care provided to inpatients. There is a similar relationship between inpatient care in a hospital as compared to a nursing home. Drugs and visits to a physician may also, on occasion, substitute for each other, so that when limits are placed on visits to a physician more drugs are prescribed for a longer period of time. Dental fillings and extractions can also substitute for one another; either "destructive" or reconstructive dentistry may be encouraged, depending on what benefits are offered. Two kinds of substitutions are at issue; in one, a less expensive modality of care is substituted for another that is more appropriate, so that quality suffers; in the other, the substitutes are equal in technical effectiveness, but a more costly service replaces one that is less costly, resulting in waste. Both substitutions are inefficient since they are likely to reduce the total amount of health that is generated for a given cost. Substitution is useful if it leads to better care, or to care of equal quality at less cost. It is merely wasteful if quality remains the same, but the cost of care is increased. It is positively harmful if quality is impaired, many would say irrespective of cost, although some might be willing to give up some degree of quality, for certain savings in cost.

The conclusion to be drawn from these considerations is that medical care benefits cannot be viewed as an assemblage of independent items, but should be seen as a system of subtly interacting parts. If so, one logical course to follow is to provide "comprehensive benefits." Another course is to study carefully the interrelationships among benefits and to identify those that are most important. The most important interrelationships would be those that are most frequently observed and that have the most serious consequences when disrupted. In a later section of this volume we shall discuss what is meant by "comprehensive care," why less than comprehensive benefits are frequently provided, and what the consequences of this are to clients, providers, and to the program as a whole. In an effort to tease out the tissue of medical care services so that natural interconnections can be seen, major reliance has to be placed on the opinions and experiences of expert practitioners. Curiously enough, there has been little systematic, empirical work along those lines. What work has been done has been done in the context of explaining and predicting use of service, rather than in the context of benefit design.

Wirick is among the few investigators who have explicitly recognized that the receipt of certain kinds of services is contingent upon, or associated with, the receipt of others and has incorporated this recognition into a predictive model (25). Wirick found that the most highly predictive interactions usually occurred between the dependent variables—components of utilization—rather than between a dependent variable and any of the independent variables generally assumed to explain differences in use of service. Hospital care was the best predictor of physician care; doctor visits were the best predictor of dental visits; doctor visits were by far the best predictor of expenditures for prescribed drugs; and expenses for prescribed medicines were the best predictor of hospital care.

Kalimo et al. have also studied the interrelationship among services as a factor that might explain differences in utilization (26, 27). They attempted to identify intercorrelative clusters of services and to determine whether different modes of organizing care have an effect on clustering (27). Data were used from household interview surveys in 12 study areas in 7 countries, including the U.S. Although there are many deficiencies in the data, as the authors recognize, it appears that services cluster into three groups. One cluster, considered to include physician-dependent services, comprises physician visits, hospital admissions, and prescribed medicines. Another cluster of services, considered to be more dependent on client initiative, includes physical examinations, vision examinations, preventive immunizations, and visits to the dentist. This second cluster also differs from the first in being more preventive, rather than therapeutic, in its purposes. These two clusters were also intercorrelated, especially through relationships with physician visits. Physicians' services occupied a central place by virtue of being most highly correlated with the largest number of services. A third cluster, which contained only one member, nonprescribed medicines, had very tenuous relationships with any of the other services. Of great interest was the observation that, with respect to the clusterings described, similarities between medical care systems were more striking than differences. Thus it may be possible to distinguish at least three types of services: (1) those typified by nonprescribed medicines, that are client-determined and lie outside the organized medical care system proper; (2) those that are central to the medical care system and are heavily influenced by the decisions of the physician; and (3) those that occupy an intermediate position by virtue of being preventive rather than therapeutic, being less dependent on the decisions of the physician and more dependent on client initiative and on influences in the medical care system other than those of the physician.

The Definition of a Health Service

One more feature must be added to the frame of reference that will be used in analyzing the benefits of medical care programs. This final feature is the set of considerations determining whether a given service is within the purview of a medical care program and should be included as a benefit. At the most fundamental level, the question arises because health is not a clearly defined concept and because many factors make a contribution to health, however defined. Thus, health has not only physical or physiological aspects, but also includes psychological and social well-being. Even when health is defined very narrowly, the scope of services that contribute to it can be very wide. For example, nutrition, recreation and a safe working and living environment can make a greater contribution to health, and be more urgently sought after by clients, than the traditional healing arts of the physician or nurse. The former are examples of services that make an independent contribution to health. There are other services that have no independent effect but are necessary for the effective application of more traditional health services. Transportation is a good example.

One can view health, and the services that mediate it, as a set of concentric circles. The innermost circle comprises the most traditional view of health and the services relevant to it. Each successive ring, moving outward from the center, comprises broader definitions of health and the services that correspond to these definitions. There is constant pressure to expand the area subsumed by the concept and to stretch the perimeter to include additional kinds of services relevant to it. The question is: Where does one stop? What functions are assigned to the health care system, and what to other social instrumentalities?

In my opinion, there is no conceptual solution to the problem posed by the ambiguous and extensible definition of health. Consequently, there is no absolute standard for the designation of an activity as a health service. The solution rests on pragmatic grounds. It depends on what objectives are sought, what needs to be done to achieve these objectives, and what social agencies are available to do what needs to be done. Thus, the solution may differ in different locales, populations, and time periods. In some areas, people face many problems, often intertwined, that interfere with successful, healthful living. They may face them in the absence of the social services that could help them cope with these problems. The solution, in such a situation, could be to expand the definition of health and of health services to include components that are not usually combined in one program. The justification may be: (1) that such components are necessary to the effectiveness of the more traditional health services; (2) that they make an independent contribution to the attainment of health; (3) that the inclusion of services under a single program results in considerable efficiencies; or (4) that their identification with "health" makes them more likely to be implemented for political, social or cultural reasons. Accordingly, neighborhood health centers have expanded their services to include transportation, work counseling, job placement, legal aid and advocacy, community organization, and the like. A new social agency, the "multiservice center," has emerged (28). Along somewhat similar lines, Geiger describes how professional personnel charged with developing a health program in rural Mississippi found health services to be far behind work, food and shelter in the priorities of local inhabitants. As a consequence, the health program had to expand its concerns and become a means for community organization and development (29). Unfortunately, there is little room in a national program for such adaptations to local situations, unless a considerable degree of decentralization is built in.

A subset of the more general problem is the allocation of functions and service responsibilities, either to the public health agency or to the medical care agency, assuming these are separate in whole or in part. The partition of functions and responsibilities between these two branches of the health system has usually come about as a result of historical developments, so that vested interests and tradition are the most powerful determinants of what services are included in the medical care program and what services are left out. While this separation is recognized, the question we wish to examine is whether there are some general "principles" that can rationalize the distinction. One such possible principle is the distinction between environmental health services and personal health services. The former involve manipulations of the environment; these constitute public, collective or social goods. This means that the benefits can be enjoyed by one consumer without thereby reducing the availability of the benefit to another. However, environmental services are not always public goods and, to the extent that they are not, they could constitute a personal health service. For example, public health nursing or sanitarian services that reduce household hazards for an individual family could very well be benefits in a medical care program (30). On the other hand, environmental as well as nonenvironmental services could be provided through an agency other than the medical care program, for a variety of reasons. Perhaps the most general, and most vague, principle is that of the "scope of interdependence." Alfred de Grazia writes: "According to this theory, the policy of maximum effectiveness can be obtained in an organization whose scope includes all persons or events directly connected with the plan" (31, p. 355). Thus, the jurisdictional domains of the agencies in question determine which is most suitable to assume responsibility for a given service. Another consideration could very well be scale as a determinant of cost. Local programs may not be able to assume responsibility for functions that require large size in order to be performed efficiently and well. Somewhat allied to scale is the issue of large risks which need to be spread as widely as possible. An additional consideration would be the need for consolidation to assure special emphasis. It is conceivable, for example, that multiple screening and allied case-finding procedures could be provided separately from other personal health services in order to assure that the former receive sufficient emphasis, and also because these procedures require large scale if costs are to be reduced. A final consideration in the allocation of functions is the issue of functional interdependence among benefits. For example, although preventive services might receive more emphasis if performed under separate auspices, the need to integrate preventive and therapeutic services, to the mutual strengthening of both, would probably argue for their provision within the same program.

Needless to say, the "principles" or considerations that we have enumerated above would favor one or another agency depending on the manner in which the competing agencies are organized. For example, it is quite possible to visualize a medical care program in the United States that is organized along national and regional lines and therefore would have greater potential for large scale action than the local health departments have. The reverse could also occur if personal health care is highly decentralized and assigned to a multiplicity of "health maintenance organizations." Finally, a service need not be excluded as a benefit simply because it is performed by a separate agency, if provision is made for the purchase of such service on behalf of persons who are eligible.

PART TWO

Effects of Providing Benefits

In the previous section we presented a backdrop, so to speak, for our discussion of program benefits. In this section we shall try to understand the impact of benefits on some key features of the medical care system. These key features are selected because they will help specify the objectives to be sought and the undesirable side-effects to be avoided. These features should also help determine those properties of benefit design that increase the likelihood of attaining the specified objectives while reducing the likelihood of incurring the side effects. The features selected for discussion are: (1) use of service, (2) price, (3) substitution, and (4) redistribution. Under each of these four features we shall first present a set of theoretical expectations of what the impact of benefits would be. Second, we shall review selected empirical findings that bear on these expectations. Third, we shall discuss the policy implications of the findings; and fourth, we shall describe and discuss implications for implementation and control.

Use of Service

Theoretical Considerations

Short-run Effects

It seems reasonable to postulate, as we did in the preceding section, that use of health care services is the joint consequence of three major features: (1) states of health and ill-health, (2) client decisions, and (3) provider decisions. In the short-run, states of health and ill-health can be taken to be relatively constant. Hence, whatever proximate effects the provision of benefits might have would be attributable to their influence on the behavior of clients and providers, including, in particular, physicians. As Feldstein has pointed out, benefits affect the client in two ways: through an effect on income and an effect on price (12). The provision of benefits means that the price of a service at the point of purchase is reduced. Since consumption of almost all goods and services, excepting certain prestige items, increases as price is lowered, the presumption is that medical care services will be affected in a similar way. Two consequences follow. The first is that the consumption of all medical care services is enhanced, because lowering the price of some services increases the ability of the consumer to consume all services. This is the "income effect". The second is that the consumption of the services that are provided as benefits is selectively increased in relation to other services which are not provided, or are covered to a lesser extent. This is the "price effect" (12).

The impact on the provider also shows the operation of the income and price effects, if some of the physician's decisions are presumed to be influenced by their financial implications for the client. In addition, the provider is influenced by his own financial interests. Thus, in addition to the "income" and "price" effects, one must consider the net "revenue" effects on the physician and on the institution where he works. Lower costs to the patient mean less resistance on his part to the receipt of service and fewer constraints on the physician with regard to the care he recommends. Thus, the volume of service is increased. The pattern of care may also change, because there is no single acceptable way of combining diverse medical care services to manage a given situation. This gives the physician a clinically legitimate range of choices within which he can select the course of action that will reduce the immediate out-of-pocket cost to the patient, increase his own revenue relative to his costs in money, time, or effort, or do both (12). In this context, one potent elementary consideration could be that for insured services the physician is better able to impose an acceptable price, and has greater assurance of collecting a fee, than for uninsured services. The effect of marginal revenue to the physician "net of the marginal costs to the physician of providing the service (including both opportunity costs and direct payments)" has received more extended theoretical and empirical attention by Monsma (32). He emphasizes, as we have, the dependence of the consumer on decisions made by his physician, and the range of discretion that the physician enjoys in recommending a course of action that can be both financially advantageous to himself and probably useful to the client. The concept of technological ambiguity or discretion appears to be a particularly useful analytic tool. Consequently, Monsma hypothesizes that marginal revenue to the physician will have the greatest effect on the use of procedures concerning which the client has the least capacity to make independent judgments, and which are least likely to be harmful to him. He might have added that the physician has the greatest discretion where practice is least clearly defined or standardized.

In addition to the "income," "price," and "revenue" effects, there may also be a kind of "multiplier" effect because of functional interrelationships (complementarities) in medical care. Anything that brings the client within the orbit of the care-providing system appears to predispose to the detection of new needs, and to the provision of additional services the need for which is generated by having received prior care. Thus, a visit to the physician or an admission to the hospital initiates a train of activities, often leading to largely unanticipated destinations.

Long-run Effects

So far, we have dealt with the short-run effects. Certain long-run effects might be postulated to occur through changes in the tastes of consumers, in the numbers of physicians and other facilities, and in health status. As clients accumulate experience of care, they could be expected to become better informed about need for care, and more demanding of it. In this way, a tasting of benefits may be said to generate an appetite for more. Similarly, the numbers of physicians, hospitals and other commodities that are generated in response to increased demand, themselves become instrumentalities for the generation of new demand. One can envisage an upward spiral set in motion, which seems to describe reasonably well the medical care market in recent decades. Needless to say, it is likely that beyond a certain point checks will be imposed in the form of higher prices or restrictions on benefits and on supplies. Another possible effect, in the longer run, could be a geographic redistribution of supply to accord with new purchasing power in areas where, prior to the availability of program benefits, the demand for care was low. The extent to which this redistribution occurs may depend, in part, on whether prices are allowed to rise. If they are, the relative availability of resources in the underdoctored areas may remain unaltered.

The long-run effects of changes in health status are difficult to predict. There has been a presumption, which has had a marked influence on policy, that the provision of services will improve health and will either lower the need for care or stabilize it at some level. However, the provision of care, to the extent that it contributes to longevity, also creates new needs. This is because older people suffer from illnesses that we have been unable to prevent or to cure. The development of technology has also obscured the picture, partly by enhancing our ability to deal with health problems, but also by creating new and more costly modalities of care. In the future, the need for care may stabilize at some level, which will almost certainly be higher than the current level. The most reasonable prediction is that such stabilization will not occur without the imposition of constraints upon the medical care system.

Normative Concerns

So far, we have only attempted to describe the possible effects of the provision of benefits on use of service, without attention to normative concerns, namely, what is desirable or undesirable. We shall now consider this very important aspect of the possible impact of benefits under three headings: the efficiency of production, the efficiency of allocation, and the quality of care. With respect to the efficiency of production, it is clear that social costs will increase if, in order to lower out-of-pocket expenditures by the client, or to increase revenues to the provider, more costly services are substituted for less costly ones without a corresponding increase in effectiveness. This is said to occur, for example, when inpatient hospital care, which is covered by program benefits, is substituted for ambulatory care, which is not. The efficiencies of allocation pertain to distribution of services among income groups and among levels of need. One can postulate that the income and price effects of program benefits have a greater impact on the poor than on the rich and that, therefore, the provision of benefits will reduce the gap between income groups and bring use of service more in line with the need for care. Use of service may also become adjusted to need if judgments of clients and physicians come to similar opinions concerning need. The hypothesis here is that as the propensity of the client to initiate care increases, there is a greater likelihood that a clinical assessment of need for care will be made, and that the client will concur with this assessment. Through this process, redistribution occurs to the extent that certain groups have a generally different view of need for care than other groups. It also follows that the influence of the physician on health behavior becomes proportionately greater; this is a matter of great consequence to policy and administration, because the physician assumes greater control in the distribution of care.

With respect to allocation according to levels of need, it is possible to arrange needs in a scale according to two properties: urgency and importance, in terms of consequence to health. Urgency refers to how soon care should be instituted if it is to be helpful; importance refers to the consequences to health of receiving care or not receiving it. At one end of the scale are needs that are both urgent and important, or are perceived by the client or the physician to be urgent and important. At the other end of the scale are those needs that are neither urgent nor important. The provision of benefits is more likely to influence use of service in response to the less urgent and less important services than in response to the more urgent and more important. One can postulate that as price to the client is reduced, and as revenue to the provider is increased, there will be a higher proportion of (1) less urgent and less important services, (2) unimportant but harmless services, and (3) unimportant but possibly, or definitely, harmful services. The provision of less necessary or less important care may represent misallocation. The provision of care that, in the best judgment of competent physicians, is "unnecessary" or possibly harmful represents both misallocation and poor quality.

The literature on commercial health insurance makes much of another, seemingly normative, concern, which it calls "moral hazard." Stripped of the heavily moralistic judgments which often accompany its presentation in this literature (3, p. 42), "moral hazard" appears to be nothing more than the propensity of persons who have insurance against a given loss to incur that loss as a consequence of some change in their behavior. In this sense it is pervasive, since it is a consequence of the provision of benefits. However, it is also predominantly a characteristic of certain categories of people who by virtue of sex, occupation, or personal habits and propensities, are more likely to exhibit the behavior in question. Thus "moral hazard" is a characteristic of benefits and of persons. It is a "hazard" because it increases the probability or the magnitude of loss to the insuring agency (33). It is "moral" because the behavior that produces it is generally considered to be reprehensible. The behavior is reprehensible because of certain ways in which it is seen to arise. The person who is insured may, because he feels more secure, or because of carelessness, or from a desire for monetary or other advantage, expose himself to a greater degree of peril. In the health insurance context this could mean incurring an accident, becoming ill, or, more realistically, deciding to have a baby after maternity benefits are in force. Alternatively, or additionally, the insured, having become ill, may demand more service, or more costly service, than he would have asked for in the absence of insurance. Under certain circumstances, through misrepresentation or other means, there may even be an attempt to defraud. Thus "moral hazard" is seen to arise, at best, out of human frailty and, at worst, out of reprehensible greed. According to Dickerson, some have attempted to make a distinction between "morale hazard," arising out of carelessness, and "moral hazard," arising out of dishonesty. Dickerson considers the distinction not useful, since, according to him, the difference is only a matter of degree (33, p. 541).

This stern moralism on behalf of the insurance industry ill befits its own practices. More importantly, it ignores several facets of the situation. First, it gives scant recognition to the role of the physician in determining levels and patterns of use. Second, increased utilization of a desirable commodity when its price is reduced is, according to the industry's own free enterprise gospel, nothing other than enlightened self-interest. But most important of all, it shows no comprehension of one of the basic objectives of health insurance: opening access to care and adjusting use of service to need. Thus, the phrase "moral hazard" is factually misleading and represents a concept of little analytic value. It should be dropped or be replaced by a morally neutral word such as "behavioral hazard" or "utilization hazard." Perhaps the only usefulness of the concept of "moral hazard" is in reminding us that not all utilization generated by the provision of benefits is socially desirable, or at least not desirable to the same degree.

Thus, one arrives at a general normative postulate concerning the effects of program benefits: (1) that they bring about important social benefits; (2) that there are diminishing returns; and (3) that there is an element of inefficiency and even harm. Therefore, a central concern in program design, in general, and in program benefit design, in particular, is to realize the maximum of what is good and incur the minimum of what is inefficient or harmful. What ways there are to accomplish this will be our subject in a later section. First, we must examine some empirical observations that have been made about our more theoretical speculations concerning the effect of benefits on use of service.

Empirical Observations

The empirical observations that have a bearing on health care benefits are so extensive and varied that a thorough review of the literature is prohibitive. We shall have to be highly selective, emphasizing the logical development of the evidence. Some regard will be shown for the methods used to obtain the evidence, so that the reader can have some feel for its credibility. However, the very fact that we have selected our own evidence lays us open to a charge of bias, which we hope we do not deserve, but which we are unable to refute.

Price-Elasticity of Demand

The assumption basic to our theoretical construct was that medical care was a normal good, so that a lowering in price at the point of consumption would increase use of service. Surprisingly, direct evidence bearing on this matter is rather sparse. In a 1958 study of a sample of the civilian, non-institutionalized population, Feldstein and Seversen (15) examined, among other variables, the effect of price on the use of hospital and physician services, and on expenditures for these services. They concluded that the effect of price on total physician services, including that portion provided outside the hospital, was as expected: an increase in price led to decrease in use of services. But the decrease was not proportional; a 10 percent increase in price would bring about a less than 2 percent decrease in visits. Paradoxically, as price increased, hospital admissions became slightly more frequent, although hospital days showed a negligible reaction. If it is true, as these findings suggest, that physician and hospital services are, to a large degree, obtained irrespective of price, then it could be concluded that the primary interest in the provision of benefits should be to mitigate the financial impact when the use of services is an almost inescapable necessity. However, in interpreting the findings one should remember that Feldstein and Severson, in order to correct for the transitory element in income, grouped their data into primary sampling units and aggregates of such units. The degree of heterogeneity within each of these ecological units could influence the magnitude, and even the direction, of the associations observed (17).

A study that does not have this limitation has been reported by Phelps and Newhouse (34). They measured the effect, on use of ambulatory and impatient physician services, of the introduction into a prepaid group practice plan of a 25 percent coinsurance feature, which amounts to a corresponding increase in out-of-pocket price. In this setting we have the unusual advantage of observing how a given population responds to a change in price, as distinct from observing the responses of several populations to different prices. The disadvantages are that (1) it is not clear that plan members perceive the change from zero out-of-pocket payments to a small copayment as a 25 percent increase in price; (2) it is not known what services are received outside the plan and whether a change has occurred in these; and (3) there are also incentives to the physicians to reduce services under a prepayment system. Under these circumstances, the arc elasticity of demand was found to be −0.137, which means that "a 10 percent increase in price would result in a 1.37 percent decline in visits" (34, p. 23). This is quite similar to the value computed by Feldstein and Severson (15). However, Phelps and Newhouse argue that such values are an underestimate of price elasticity since they do not include costs additional to fees, such as the costs of travel and of time. If these are included, one finds that a small additional increase in the form of fees has brought about a relatively large decrease in services consumed. Usually, benefits are only meant to reduce out-of-pocket payments for care, and only this price is relevant to our concern. However, as Phelps and Newhouse point out, the impact of a package of benefits, or a new system for delivering care, depends on how it affects a broader range of costs.

We shall return to the subject of the relationship between price and use of service in a subsequent chapter that deals with the possible effects of insurance on price and, through the intermediacy of price and other variables, on the supply and consumption of services.

Use of Service by Insured and Uninsured

Indirect evidence concerning the relationship between price and use comes from studies of health insurance. These studies can be roughly classified, according to method, into those that compare insured with uninsured populations, and those that examine the effect of introducing insurance or, rarely, of withdrawing benefits. When one compares experience before and after a change in benefits, one needs to account for the possible effects of other related or unrelated changes that have occurred concurrently. When one compares insured and uninsured populations one needs to take into account the effect of characteristics that are associated with the propensity to have insurance and also have independent effects on use of service. Prior to Medicare, persons with health insurance were less likely to be aged and more likely to be white, to be better educated, to have higher incomes and to live in urban places (35 and 20, pp. 76–84). All these associated characteristics, except lower age, are likely to encourage use of service and, therefore to reinforce the effect of insurance. Two characteristics of particular theoretical interest, and of relevance to policy, are, as we have indicated earlier, income and the severity of need that is likely to be associated with low income, low education, and being black.

The Effects of Having Insurance. Periodic surveys of the civilian non-institutionalized population have shown that families and persons with insurance, which usually covers hospital services and the services of physicians in the hospital, tend to receive more hospital and related services than those who do not have insurance (19, 20, 36, 37). From 1953 to 1963, persons with insurance were decidedly more likely to be admitted to short-term hospitals. Although insured persons stayed somewhat fewer days in the hospital, they accumulated a larger total of patient-days of hospital care. Table 4 shows that, in 1963, the insured as compared to the uninsured had 67 percent more admissions, a 20 percent shorter length of stay and a 20 percent larger total volume of short-stay hospital care. In the early 1950's this pattern (more admissions, shorter stays, more patient-days) held within each age and income group examined with a few exceptions (19, 36). By 1963, the picture had become somewhat less clear. When cross tabulated by age, sex, income and residence, admission rates were uniformly higher among the insured in 1963, as they had been in 1953. However, in 1963, the length of stay was not uniformly lower for the insured in all subgroups tested; as a result the insured sometimes spent more patient days in the hospital, and sometimes fewer, than the uninsured. Data for 1968, for persons under 65, suggest that further changes may have taken place. There was very little difference between the insured and uninsured in the percent of persons admitted to short-stay hospitals. When examined by age group, the insured were more likely to be admitted to hospitals if

TABLE 4.   Use of Specified Medical Care Services, by Health Insurance Status, U.S.A., 1953 and 1963

Use of Service and Expenditures	1953			1963		
	I [a]	U [a]	I as % of U	I	U	I as % of U
Short-term hospital use						
Admissions per 100	14	9	156	15	9	167
Length of stay	7	8.3	84	7	8.8	80
Patient-days per 100	100	70	143	101	84	120
Surgical Procedures in Hospital						
All procedures per 100	9	5	180	6	3	200
Tonsillectomies per 100 children under 17	30	9	333	24	7	343
Percent who visited dentist	40	26	154	45	24	188
Percent who saw physician outside the hospital						
All	64	55	116	—	—	—
Made 15 visits or more	7	6	117	—	—	—
Mean expenditures for all personal health services in dollars	237	154	154	429	201	213

Source: Reference 19, Tables 18, A15, A81, A86, A88, A94, and 100; and Reference 20, Tables 67, 68, 71, and 72.
[a] "I" stands for Insured and "U" for uninsured.

they were below 17 or over 44, and less likely to be admitted if they were between those ages, especially in the lower income groups. In addition to this pattern of admissions, the length of stay was apparently much shorter for the insured, irrespective of age. The number of patient-days per person was highest for the uninsured in all age groups. However, in all income groups examined, the percent of persons admitted to hospitals was higher for those who had insurance (37, pp. 9 and 35).

To summarize, there was in 1953 a clear and plausible relationship between insurance and use of hospital services. Those who had insurance could be expected to be admitted earlier in the course of illness, and to be admitted for less serious illness; this resulted in a shorter stay per illness. However, the product of the shorter stays and the more frequent admissions was that the insured had more days of hospital care. Since 1953, the relationship between insurance and use of the hospital has not only become less uniform among population subgroups, but the net result has been a reversal, so that the insured have come to receive fewer patient days of care than the uninsured. More detailed analysis is needed to understand the meaning of the changes that have occurred. Obviously, as insurance becomes more prevalent, and as the scope of benefits changes, the population that has no insurance coverage varies significantly from one time period to another. Further, one has to consider the growing impact of the provision of benefits under programs other than voluntary insurance. For example, among persons 18-44 years old who had no insurance in 1968, there may have been a large proportion of unemployed, ill and impoverished persons who were eligible for public services. Because they were eligible for these services they may have been more likely to be admitted to the hospital and to stay there longer.

The generally higher rate of admission to the hospital among the insured is, of course, in line with the hypothesized effects of insurance, provided one can rule out the influence of variables associated with insurance, such as higher income, more education, and a greater likelihood of being urban and white. In the data described above the variables were ruled out, one at a time, by cross tabulation; with certain exceptions, insurance did increase admissions. Multivariate methods of analysis have also been used to isolate the effect of insurance when several other variables are held constant at the same time. For example, Feldstein and Seversen found that a 10 percent increase in the proportion of the bill covered by insurance was associated with a 4.5 percent increase in admissions, a 2.5 percent increase in patient-days and a 4.8 percent increase in hospital expenditures, when age, income, education, and residence of the population, as well as price, were held constant simultaneously (15).

The effect of insurance on length of stay is somewhat more complicated because several factors come into play, with contradictory effects. As admissions rise, it is expected that less serious cases are admitted, so that the average length of stay would go down. This should be counteracted to some extent by the hypothetical tendency of the insured to want to stay longer; in the absence of insurance or other benefits, patients may be expected to leave the hospital sooner. However, the tendency of uninsured patients to leave sooner is counteracted by the expectation that admissions of uninsured patients are more likely to be for serious illness. Moreover, the uninsured may be more likely to use public hospitals or the teaching services of voluntary hospitals, and to have unfavorable home conditions, physical as well as social. These characteristics would also tend to lengthen, rather than shorten, hospital stays among the uninsured. Some studies have been made in an attempt to correlate length of stay with some of these factors. Rosenthal has reported findings in a sample of discharges from short-term hospitals in 5 New England states in 1962 (38). Patients were grouped by age, sex and ICDA diagnostic category. Analysis of a selected subset of these groupings suggested that price was negatively related to length of stay, but that the length of stay was more strongly related to the average daily charge than to the ratio of out-of-pocket charges to total charges. Rosenthal suggests that this is so because the patient is more aware of the former than the latter, and that behavior is regulated accordingly. For each 10% increase in average daily charges there was a 2 percent or more reduction in length of stay in 19 of the 28 groupings examined, and a 5 percent or more reduction in 6 groupings. That there is greater discretion in some situations than in others is suggested by the fact that price elasticity was considerably higher for post-operative than total surgical stay; long stay cases showed greater elasticity than short stay cases; and tonsillectomies and adenoidectomies tended to have the highest price elasticities even though their length of stay is short. For example, in female children (age 0–4) a 10 percent increase in the average daily charge was associated with an almost equal reduction (9.7 percent) in post-operative stay. Opportunity costs may also enter into the decision concerning length of stay: surgical care has a higher elasticity for children than for teenagers; and surgical care for older adults has a greater elasticity than for younger adults. While these findings are relevant to the effect of insurance on length of stay, they do not establish that the correlations observed are caused exclusively or even partly by a change in client behavior. It could very well be that the more costly hospitals are larger, more urban, under greater pressure of demand, and operate at a much higher pace than do the less costly hospitals. Length of stay may be influenced by decisions of the providers of care, and by system characteristics that constrain both provider and client.

A more comprehensive view of the interaction between characteristics of the medical condition, of the client, and of the hospital, is taken by Ro in a study of admissions to 22 hospitals in the Pittsburgh area during 1963 (39). Because data on physician characteristics were not available, the assumption had to be made that similar hospitals have similar medical staffs. The finding that concerns us here is the relationship between source of payment and length of stay. When no adjustment was made for diagnostic category, there was a significant ordering from longest to shortest stay by source of payment, as follows: "government," "unpaid or write-off," "service (free)," "Blue Cross," "commercial insurance," and "patient." Part of the relationship is accounted for by case mix, since the strength of the association is reduced, in some cases to statistical insignificance, by correcting for diagnostic category. Nevertheless, length of stay remains shortest when the patient pays the bill; it is significantly shorter than when government pays the bill, but not significantly shorter than when insurance pays. Other patient characteristics may also play a role. For example, persons who paid their own bill were less likely to be employed and more likely to live alone; but these characteristics were generally more likely to lengthen than shorten the stay, so that the shorter stay among those who paid their own bill may be said to have occurred in spite of these characteristics. The effect of hospital characteristics was also examined, but, except for occupancy, these characteristics produced no new information. Higher occupancy in a hospital strengthens the relationship between length of stay and source of payment. We are not told, however, whether this occurs because persons who pay their own bill leave earlier, or because persons who have third party payments stay longer. We have no information about the absolute values, nor about the manner in which the ratio has changed. Further, it is very difficult to interpret the occupancy rate. Under certain circumstances high occupancy represents greater demand; under other circumstances it may represent greater success in manipulation of demand so as to keep the hospital full. Assuming a relative shortage of beds, one could hypothesize that there would be greater pressure to shorten the stay, and that those who pay their own bill would be most responsive to such pressure. Contrariwise, if there is relative surplus, there is an inducement to keep people in hospitals, in which case it can be hypothesized that those who have third party payments are most likely to be responsive. In either instance, having insurance makes a contribution to length of stay, although it is only one among many factors that do so. We shall have more to say about length of stay when we discuss appropriateness of care.

So far, the evidence is in keeping with the expectation that persons who have hospital insurance are more likely to be admitted to the hospital than those who do not, even when the effect of other factors associated with insurance has been held constant. As to length of stay, if case mix is held constant, it would seem as if insurance, or any form of third party payment, is associated with longer stays.

Effects of Having More Insurance. If insurance that provides for a service enhances the use of that service, the provision of "more insurance" should encourage even more use. By more insurance, we mean either payment for a greater portion of the charges for a given service, or coverage for a greater number of services. In either case, prices at the point of consumption are lowered; more income is released, and can be used to purchase additional medical care; increased complementarities among benefits can generate an upward pressure for consumption; and there are more opportunities to change patterns of care by substituting one service for another.

Some evidence on the effects of "more insurance" comes from the records of the health insurance program for federal employees. In this program, persons and families who have selected plans that offer more protection ("high option") are more likely to be admitted to the hospital, stay more days per admission, and accumulate a larger total of patient-days of hospital care than do those who have selected the "low option" plans (40; also 41, Table 5, p. 8). However, in this instance, the conclusion that more insurance results in more utilization is open to question, because one could argue that those who purchase more insurance expect to have a greater need for care or to use more service.

Additional information concerning the effects of "more insurance" comes from studies of persons or families who have more than one insurance policy or plan. This matter has attracted a great deal of attention because the insurance industry sees in this situation powerful inducements to "moral hazard," especially if the combined benefits of the several insurance policies exceed the total obligations incurred as a result of illness. Unfortunately, study of the effects of multiple insurance policies is bedeviled at the very outset by problems of definition and difficulties in measurement (42–46). These problems result from two distinct, though obviously related, aspects of multiple policies. The first aspect is the need to distinguish different categories of insurance coverage. The categories to be distinguished are: (1) whether a person is a potential beneficiary of one or more insurance policies, (2) whether these policies have benefit provisions that supplement each other without overlap or duplication, and (3) whether any, among two or more policies, significantly overlap so that payment from more than one insurance policy might reasonably be expected for identical health services. Luck has suggested that the term "multiple coverage" be used to designate the second of the categories listed above, and "duplicate coverage" be used to designate the third category (42). However, this distinction is seldom made, so that "multiple," "duplicate," or "duplicatory" coverage is used to designate either the third of our categories or a mix of the second and third that is impossible to disentangle.

The second problematic aspect of coverage by more than one insurance policy is the extent to which the policies actually pay for losses incurred. There are three increasingly stringent tests that measure how well a client is protected, using three different measures of the percent paid by insurance of the costs of an illness: (1) the percent of charges for benefits covered by any of the policies; (2) the percent of charges for medical care services received, irrespective of the scope of benefits included in the policies, and (3) the percent of the total cost of the illness, including indirect costs in addition to the direct charges for care. For example, if a person had one or more policies that covered hospital room and board, one could ask what proportion insurance covered of: (a) hospital room and board charges, (b) charges for all hospital services, (c) charges associated with hospitalization, including the services of physicians in the hospital, (d) all charges for medical care irrespective of whether services were received in or outside the hospital, (e) loss of income due to the illness as well as charges for medical care, and so on. One could also lengthen the analytic or evaluative perspective to include charges and other losses incurred due to several episodes of illness over the entire year (42), or even over a longer period of time. All this is important because it relates to the notion of "overinsurance" and its associated "moral hazard." The insurance industry is fearful that as the degree of protection approaches the full monetary value of the loss, the disincentive to incur the loss is progressively reduced until it is replaced by the actually positive incentive of "profit" from illness, when payments exceed the loss; and to make a "profit" from illness is not only hazardous to the insurer but also morally depraved. Excluding moral judgments, we also are interested in the extent to which the degree of protection alters the volume of care and the distribution of care relative to need. Thus, it becomes important to know how much insurance pays towards what losses. In defining this relationship, Luck has proposed that the term "overinsurance" be used to signify "receipt of benefits exceeding 100 percent of the total charges for the covered service" (42, pp. 21–22). In the scale we have indicated above, this would be a very lenient definition of "overinsurance." Full payment only for covered services could leave the major costs of care, not to say of illness, to be borne by the patient.

Overinsurance is difficult to define and measure, partly because of a lack of agreement on precisely how much protection health insurance should provide. In addition, there are problems in rendering the definitions operational. For example, what extent of overlap in the benefit provisions of two policies renders them "duplicatory"? (42) There are the problems of obtaining accurate and representative information. In compiling its data, the insurance industry relies on information from company representatives who install and service group policies, and on information provided by persons who seek individual policies. Inaccuracy and bias are likely to be present in both sources (43, cited by 42). When information comes from household interview surveys, or even from hospital patients, it can be safely assumed that the persons interviewed have incomplete knowledge of the insurance they carry, so that verification of the policies becomes important (45, pp. 17–18 and 46, pp. 33–35). Finally, there is confusion because some of the published statistics give the percent of persons who have duplicate coverage (37), and other statistics give the percentage by which enrollments or "coverages" exceed persons covered (47). In computing the second percentage, a "coverage" or "enrollment" is counted each time a person is listed as a potential beneficiary of an additional policy irrespective of how many such insurance policies there are. Hence, the second percentage is influenced not only by the number of persons who have duplicate policies (as is the first percentage) but also by the number of policies each such person has.* Thus, the two measures present related but somewhat different aspects of the prevalence of duplicate coverage. For example, in 1968 the National Health Survey reported that "of all persons under 65 years who had hospital insurance coverage, 11.4 percent had two plans or more" (37, p. 10). The Office of Research and Statistics estimates that in 1971 the excess of enrollments over persons with hospital care insurance was 37 percent, whereas the Health Insurance Association of America estimated the same statistic to be 20 percent (47). These percentages have increased markedly over time, and more rapidly than total coverage, so that the effects, if any, of duplicate coverage should have become increasingly prominent. In addition, the likelihood of duplicate coverage varies by type of benefit and by characteristics of persons, so that the effects would be expected to vary. Duplicate insurance is much more frequent for hospital services and inpatient surgical services than for other services. The relative excess of enrollments over persons enrolled, for all persons, including the aged, was 36 percent for hospital care, 29 percent for inpatient surgical services, 10 percent for inpatient physician visits, 5 percent for office and home visits of physicians, 5 percent for prescribed drugs, and 2 percent for nursing home care (47, Table 2, p. 5). If persons 65 and over are excluded, the percent of persons who have duplicate coverage increases regularly with age. This percentage also increases with income, except that

---

* Assume that there are 100 insured persons of whom 20 have 2 policies each. The number of enrollments is $80 + 2(20 = 120$. The percent of persons with multiple policies is 20 and the excess of enrollments over persons is also 20%. Now assume that each of the 20 persons who has multiple policies has 3 policies. The number of enrollment is $80 + 3(20) = 140$. The percent of persons with multiple policies is still 20, but the excess of enrollments over persons is 40%.

it appears to be lower in the middle income group ($5,000–$6,999) than at either lower or higher incomes (37, p. 10, and Table 16, p. 36). However, with respect to most characteristics, those who have single or multiple coverage are much more similar to each other than they are to persons with no insurance (46, pp. 12–20).

We are interested in the effects, or correlates, of duplicatory coverage mainly because it serves as a proxy for more insurance. In other words we are interested in establishing the extent to which the effects of insurance are a graded phenomenon in the sense that a greater degree of coverage has a correspondingly larger effect on use of service. For this purpose, it makes little difference whether "more insurance" is achieved through a single policy that provides more protection, or by a patchwork of two or more policies that are supplementary or duplicative. Duplicatory insurance may, however, give some insight into the effect of "overinsurance" that is rather narrowly restricted to some benefits. In addition, it could be that perceptions of protection, and of the financial risk involved in seeking care, would be different depending on whether "more insurance" is achieved through one policy or several.

The most definitive information on the effects of duplicate insurance has been reported by Andersen and Riedel. It concerns a sample of the civilian, noninstitutionalized population of the U.S. in 1963. "Multiple coverage was defined as coverage by two or more policies providing the same *type* of benefits, separated here into hospital, medical-surgical, and major medical" (46, p. 6). Table 5 shows the main findings. It is clear that having insurance enhances use of service, and having more insurance adds another, though relatively smaller, increment of use. As expected, these effects are partly due to characteristics, such as age group and income, that are associated with multiple coverage, although the findings usually hold, to varying degrees, even within such groups. For example, differences in hospital admissions were confined to the age group 18–64 and were most marked in the lowest of the several income groups in the sample. By contrast, the effect. of insurance on dental care, which is seldom covered by insurance, was most marked in age groups below 18 and above 64. A contemporaneous study of patients discharged from one Pittsburgh hospital during 1963 adds a few sidelights to the picture

TABLE 5. Use of Service and Expenditures, by Insurance Coverage, U.S.A., 1963 [a]

Extent of Insurance Coverage	Percent Admitted to Hospital [b]			Percent Visited Physician	Percent Visited Dentist	Percent Incurred Hospital Charges [c]	Percent Incurred Hospital Charges of $200 or more	Percent of those Incurring Charges who had Total Bill Paid by Insurance
	All	Family Income Less than $4,000	Age 18-64					
Uninsured	6	6	5	57	28	13	16	—
One policy	9	14	10	70	45	19	29	39
Two or more policies [d]	14	20	18	79	50	25	44	53

Source: Reference 46; Tables 9, 10, and 11, and text.
[a] Civilian noninstitutional population.
[b] Excludes obstetrical care.
[c] Includes hospital inpatient as well as outpatient care.
[d] Two or more policies providing the same *type* of benefit.

presented above (45). In this study "multiple insurance" was defined to include both supplementing and duplicatory insurance (45, p. 2). The main finding was that persons with multiple insurance were more likely to be admitted to private accommodation, and less likely to be admitted to ward accommodation, than persons with single insurance. However, even among persons having more than one policy, only 17 percent had private accommodation, while 21 percent were in the ward. In addition, a number of differences that did not achieve statistical significance suggest that persons with multiple insurance tend to be admitted more frequently, to receive more services, and to stay longer when admitted for maternity care.

As to the effects of "overinsurance," in the sense that a "profit" is made from illness, one has anecdotal evidence, such as the story of the medical student who financed his education by expertly feigning illness during summer vacations, and of the family that bought a new washing machine with surplus insurance payments for tonsillectomies on their three children (48, cited by 44). Such creative entrepreneurs aside, the evidence for "profit" from illness is not impressive. A study by the Health Insurance Council of 8 hospitals in 6 cities, during 1956–58, showed that 9.5 percent of the persons admitted had "multiple hospitalization coverage"; 78 percent of these had payments equal to, or larger than, the total hospital bill, and 70 percent were overpaid by 10 percent or more of the hospital bill. The aggregate of payments was 41 percent more than the actual bills. While the scale of overpayment is large, one should remember that this relates only to covered benefits, and that the findings are for a nonrepresentative sample. The sample was further biased by over 50 percent attrition in the process of obtaining verifiable data (42). A second study, under the same auspices and along the same lines, conducted in 1964, showed that "11 percent of the insured patients had multiple coverage and that these patients received approximately 23 percent more in benefit payments than the amount of their hospital bills" (44, p. 48). One suspects that the protective efficacy of multiple coverage may have undergone considerable erosion in the interval between the two studies. The study by Andersen and Riedel showed that duplicate coverage does, in fact, provide added protection. Only 39 percent of those who had one policy had their total hospital bill paid by insurance, as compared to 53 percent of those who had two or more policies (see Table 5); the differences were even more marked, 25 and 54 percent respectively, for those who had charges of $200 or more. One should note, however, that even with duplicate coverage, about half the patients did not have complete protection against hospital charges. In fewer than 5 percent of cases were insurance payments in excess of hospital charges. As a group, these 5 percent made no "profit" from illness, since average total expenditures for health services were in excess of average insurance payments. We are not told, however, if there were individual instances in which payments exceeded total charges. If so, they must have been very rare. As the authors conclude, "Even if we fail to consider other 'costs' of illness such as income loss and family disruption, these data do not seem to indicate that our health insurance benefit structure makes illness 'desirable' or 'profitable' for any significant segment of the insured population" (46, p. 28). Some duplicate coverage is fortuitous, and arises usually when several members of a family, especially spouses, obtain insurance through their employers. Most other instances occur when persons who have coverage under one plan seek further protection, probably because of doubts (generally justified) about the efficacy of the insurance they already have. Thus, fraudulent use of multiple or duplicatory insurance is likely to be a rare phenomenon, at best. However, there is little doubt that persons who have, or think they have, a greater degree of protection against the costs of medical care are more apt to use it. Insurance has a graded effect, so that the distribution of protection by its degree is an important concern of social policy.

Specific and Nonspecific Effects. It is not easy to tell to what extent the consequences of insurance are due to the "income," "price," "revenue," or "complementarity" effects. To a considerable degree the effects of insurance are specific to the service insured. For example, as we have seen, hospital insurance is associated with increases in hospital care; and the almost uniform inclusion of surgical benefits in hospital insurance is associated, as shown in Table 4, with more inpatient surgery. The inclusion of ambulatory care benefits in a health insurance plan tends to increase the use of these services to a modest degree (49–52). Insurance for prescribed drugs is associated with the much more frequent dispensing of prescriptions and a small increase in the average charge per prescription (53); and insurance for ambulance services is accompanied by remarkable increases in their use (54). On the one hand, this specificity reinforces our belief that what we observe is truly the effect of insurance itself and, on the other hand, it suggests that the price effect is important. However, one also observes that the effect of insurance is not confined to the services covered. For example, Tables 4 and 5 show that insured persons, compared to those who have no insurance, are more likely to visit a physician outside the hospital and to see a dentist, even though insurance that includes these benefits was not frequent in 1963 and was decidedly rare in 1953. The difference in propensity to visit the dentist persists even when income and age are controlled simultaneously (20, Table 71, p. 135). Since dental services and hospital care are rarely related functionally—that is, dental services are seldom performed in a hospital and are rarely a supplement or complement to hospital care—the explanation for their association must reside in the income effect or in some characteristic of the client, including the valuation he places on health. The relationship between hospital care and the services of physicians in and out of the hospital is much more complicated, affording an opportunity for the play and interplay of all the effects we have mentioned, including the effects of income, revenue, price, and complementarity. Because health insurance tends to cover mainly the services of physicians in the hospital, one would think that the services of physicians outside the hospital would be reduced because the substitution of hospital care for outpatient care would tend to reduce out-of-pocket outlays by the patient and increase revenue to the physician. On the other hand, the income and complementarity effects would encourage the use of services outside, as well as inside, the hospital. The values observed in Tables 4 and 5 can be presumed to be the net resultant of the effects of these diverse forces. The study by Feldstein and Seversen, which we have cited so often, suggests the dominance of the substitution effect, by showing a negative relation between insurance and physician visits in the home when other factors are held constant (15). We shall return to this important point when we examine studies that deal with incentives to the physician. In the meantime, we shall describe briefly a study by Weisbrod and Fiesler that shows how benefit design may set in motion intricate exchanges within the bundle of hospital services themselves (55).

Weisbrod and Fiesler describe a quasi-experimental situation which made it possible to examine two insured populations before and after one of them became eligible for more benefits. The populations were employees (including dependents) of two firms which, by virtue of being in the same area (St. Louis) and being closely competitive, were presumed to be similar in their attributes, and exposed to similar influences. Seventy percent of employees in one of the two firms chose a "preferred" plan that offered them almost unlimited laboratory, diagnostic, and other ancillary services available upon admission to the hospital. In addition, there was a daily $2 increment to the standard $10 daily benefit towards the costs of a private room, which at the time averaged about $18 per day. In other respects, coverage was comparable for the two populations, both before and after the institution of the "preferred" plan in one of the two. Data were available on use of hospital services and charges both for the year during which the plan was instituted and for the year that preceded it. As expected, there was a marked increase in expenditures specific to the services covered by the "preferred plan," except that the addition to the private room benefit was apparently not sufficient to have an appreciable effect. However, the "preferred plan" also had more general effects. Hospital admissions were less frequent in the second year than the first in both populations, for unspecified reasons; but the reduction was significantly less in the group that included those with the more liberal benefits. Further, the relative advantage in utilization enjoyed by this group was mostly confined to women above 55, and to those having diseases of the respiratory, digestive, and genitourinary systems, or needing treatment for accidents, poisonings, and violent injury. Weisbrod and Fiesler suggest that such diffuse effects occur because persons who have more liberal benefits enter the hospital so as to avail themselves of these benefits. We are not told if ambulatory services are, in consequence, reduced. Older women are more likely to take advantage of liberal benefits because for them, it is presumed, the opportunity costs of hospitalization are smaller than for employed males or younger mothers. The localization of excess admissions in certain diagnostic categories remains unexplained, but one would need to look into how diagnosis is correlated with being an older female or requiring the services offered by the "preferred plan." The large relative excess in the category of "accidents, poisonings, and violence" registered by those in the "preferred plan" is particularly interesting, since the incidence of these events is not usually considered responsive to insurance, and yet they remind us so disturbingly of the traditional strictures of "moral hazard"!

To summarize, there is evidence to support the expectation that the provision of benefits increases in a specific manner the use of those services covered by the benefits. There is also evidence that the effect goes beyond these specific services and involves other related services. Weisbrod and Fiesler remind us that the effects may not be forthcoming if the reduction in price to the consumer at the point of consumption does not exceed a certain threshold. This price threshold may explain why the use of private nursing was not increased in their study. They also emphasize that the effects of benefit coverage may vary by type of disease and by category of persons, for reasons that are as yet unclear. This variance suggests that predictions of the impact of price reductions must take account of other costs, including opportunity costs, that the potential patient might incur if he were to seek and accept care.

Role of the Physician. In our description of the effects of insurance we have had to remind ourselves frequently that these effects cannot come about merely through alterations in client behavior, since they require at least the passive acquiescence of the physician. More realistically, we have postulated that the physician plays a key role in determining levels and patterns of use, and the effect of benefits depends largely on the response of physicians, and whether physicians are constrained or encouraged by the health care system as a whole. The client, the physician, and their mutual environment are an interactive system; the forces that play upon them are complex. We have hypothesized that the physician is interested in (1) serving the best interests of the patient by providing all needed services; (2) increasing his own revenue relative to the financial and other costs he incurs; and (3) winning the patients' approval, and thus reaping both immediate psychic

rewards as well as assurance of future revenue. It can be hypothesized that the provision of benefits under insurance or other programs creates a larger range of choices in the pursuit of these objectives. Under the best of all possible conditions, the physician
can at the same time provide necessary care, win the clients' approval, and add to his own net income. It would be less socially
desirable to provide insured persons with services that yield relatively little benefit, while the medical needs of some people, or
other wants of all people, receive less attention. It would be least
socially desirable to provide services in order to reward the physician emotionally or financially, while exposing the patient to actual or possible harm.

The empirical evidence bearing on these several eventualities
is meager indeed; much of it is indirect, deriving from studies of
utilization in situations where benefits are comparable, but incentives to the physician are not. The major studies of this kind compare insurance plans that pay for care by private practitioners on a
fee-for-service basis with plans that operate through group practice arrangements in which the incentives are different. The findings have been reviewed by Klarman (56), by Donabedian (57,
58), by Monsma (32), and by Roemer and Shonick (59). As we
pointed out in our section on theoretical considerations, Monsma
set out to seek support for his hypotheses that: (1) positive
marginal revenue to the physician encourages demand for his services; (2) this effect is more pronounced when the patient has less
discretion; and (3) this effect is more pronounced when the physician has more discretion. He found that differences between prepaid group practice and other modes of providing care are less
pronounced for home and office care, in which patients have a
greater degree of discretion, than in surgery, where the patient has
less discretion and the physician enjoys more revenue. He concluded also that the effect is more pronounced for certain types of
surgery, such as tonsillectomies and appendectomies, "which involve the removal of 'useless' parts of the body," thus affording
the physician a greater discretion to act. Monsma does, however,
recognize that the findings do not always fall so neatly into place.
This he attributes to the presence of additional factors that modify
the influence of the "marginal revenue" effect on medical decisions.

Our own review of many of the same studies, and of material that has become available since, confirms the observation that one almost always finds a lower rate of hospital admissions under pre-paid group practice, than under insurance plans that operate through fee-for-service private practice (49, 51, 60–66). Presum-ably because a lowering in admission rates also changes the case mix, comparisons of length of stay do not show differences that are as large or as consistent, but the resultant volume of patient-days of care is almost always lower under prepaid group practice. The rate of hospitalized surgical procedures is also generally lower in this setting. In the few studies that permit it, comparison by diag-nostic category or type of procedure suggests that prepaid group practice reduces utilization more for procedures and admissions in which there is a larger element of discretion (60, 62, 65). Among medical conditions, diseases of the respiratory system, including influenza, bronchitis and pneumonia, have uniformly accounted for relatively fewer admissions under prepaid group practice than under a fee-for-service plan. Among surgical procedures, the same reduction has been noted for tonsillectomies and adenoidec-tomies, appendectomies, and operations for varicose veins and hemorrhoids. Of all these, the tonsillectomy rate shows the most uniform and the largest difference; the rate is often several times lower under prepaid group practice than fee-for-service.

While these differences are reasonably clear, the causes are not. To determine the causes it is necessary to compare populations that are generally alike. The several studies we have cited achieve reasonable, but variable success in assuring us of the fairness of the comparisons. Under "dual choice," those who enroll in the prepaid group practice plan are more likely to demand or require care, so that the observation that certain services are less frequent for this plan tends to confirm rather than weaken our conclusions. Another factor is the comparability of benefits. Since prepaid group practice always includes ambulatory care benefits, but alter-native plans sometimes do not, the reduction in hospital care in the former could be attributed to the substitutions of ambulatory for inpatient services. But this is not the entire explanation, as can be concluded from studies in which the benefits, including ambu-latory care, are comparable for prepaid and fee-for-service plans. The provision of ambulatory care benefits under a fee-for-service arrangement does not appear to reduce hospital and surgical services to the level observed under prepaid group practice (49). There is a great temptation to attribute at least part of this difference between prepaid and fee-for-service plans to the private practitioner's incentive to increase his own revenue. If the physician performs more surgery and hospitalizes more patients, he presumably not only adds to his revenue, but also shifts some of his costs to the hospital, and he may be able to see more patients in a shorter period of time (67). On the contrary, if the group practice is paid per capita, and if the individual physician within the group is paid a salary, more work will increase costs without increasing revenue to the individual physician or the group. In fact, there may be a positive financial incentive to reduce hospital use, if money saved in this way is eventually paid to the physician or retained by the group (68). An intermediate position is also possible, where the physician is paid a salary but the group is reimbursed, fee-for-service, by the insurance carrier, with or without additional payments by the patient; needless to say, the larger the group of physicians, the less likely it is that the rewards to individual physicians will be proportionate to their contributions to revenue (69), although in some groups considerable attention is given to achieving just that (70).

In searching for the revenue effect it is necessary to obtain a very precise picture of the flow and distribution both of revenue and of the incidence of costs. For instance, when separate insurance policies cover ambulatory and hospital care, under prepaid group practice, the group physician could have a direct or indirect incentive to shift to the hospital plan some of the costs that the group might otherwise incur, for example, the cost of diagnostic services (71). In general, whatever efficiencies there might be to grouping patients in the hospital would operate for group physicians as well, especially when the hospital plan is financed separately from the ambulatory care plan. The groups that participated in the Health Insurance Plan of Greater New York (HIP) were separated in this way. Nevertheless, the groups in this plan were able to achieve a lower level of hospital use (60, 62), which suggests that the balance of financial incentives and disincentives is not easy to identify. It also reminds us that it would be a serious mistake to consider only financial incentives in examining the behavior of physicians and medical care institutions. One must also reckon with nonfinancial and professional incentives, which include properties and effects of the system in general. For example, the discovery of more disease through more aggressive case-finding would lead to greater hospitalization in a group practice plan. Factors that might work in the opposite direction, to reduce hospitalization, include the likelihood that the physician in group practice will be more subject and responsive to formal and informal colleague control and less responsive to the wishes of the client (72). In some situations, the group physician may have difficulty in obtaining hospital privileges, so that hospital use is perforce restricted to the necessities. Densen and Shapiro have reported that while this may have been a factor in reducing hospital use in several HIP studies, it does not explain many of the differences observed (73).

The problem of hospital affiliation does not arise where the group owns its own hospital, but in that case hospital occupancy and the method by which the hospital is financed become very important. There is an impression that the Kaiser-Permanente groups exercise some control over hospital use keeping hospital supply low relative to the number enrolled (68). The qualifications and training of the staff and the quality of care that is offered may also have the net effect of reducing hospital use in prepaid group practice. Because such plans tend to have a larger proportion of specialists, they would presumably be professionally more precise and discriminating, but it cannot be said for certain whether this would mean less hospital care and surgery, or more. This probably depends on who provides care in competing plans. It has also been claimed that because of preventive activities and a higher level of care, prepaid group practice improves the health of its enrollees and reduces the need for hospital care; but this assertion has been difficult to prove.

A recent study supplies an admirable object lesson of how inextricably intertwined the various factors that motivate physicians can become; some of the observations almost defy interpretation. Perkoff et al. compared a university-based prepaid group practice plan to a control group generated under nearly experimental conditions (74). As expected, members of the prepaid group practice plan used many more ambulatory services than the control group, which was covered by a more traditional hospital and major medical plan with copayment and deductible features. Also as expected, the university plan experienced lower use of the hospital for surgical conditions in children and for nonsurgical conditions in all age groups. But, contrary to observed experience in other studies, and to the hypotheses advanced by Monsma, surgical rates for adults were higher for those enrolled in the university-sponsored plan, in a manner that could not be explained by the distinction between discretionary and nondiscretionary surgery. But, in this study, surgical rates in the community as a whole were lower than usually observed; the control group was constrained by deductibles and copayments; the experimental group was exposed to a much greater degree to formal and informal case-finding activities; and the surgeons, though salaried, were consultants from the university hospital whose services generated fee-for-service income for their departments, as well as surgical training for their students. With their subjects embedded in this field of contrary forces, it is no wonder that the investigators were hard put to reconcile their findings with those reported by others.

To summarize, while the "revenue effect" is a plausible explanation for some of the differences observed between prepaid group practice and fee-for-service plans, it is not likely to be the only cause; nor can it be said for certain that it is the major cause. Thus, we need to look for more direct evidence of the importance of the "revenue effect." One of the few studies that has a bearing on this question reports surgical rates for members of the United Steelworkers Union in 7 regions of the U.S. (75). These workers were covered by a contract providing uniform benefits in all regions. There was free choice of physician, and physicians were paid fee-for-service according to a schedule. Physicians, however, tended to charge patients fees additional to the scheduled fee paid by the insurance plan. The frequency with which such additional fees were charged was inversely related to the frequency with which surgery was performed. In regions where extra charges were infrequent, surgical operations were much more frequent; where extra charges were frequent, surgical operations were much less frequent. Figure 2 shows the findings. What one sees is the traditional relationship between price and demand. In this instance it can be assumed, though there is no direct evidence to

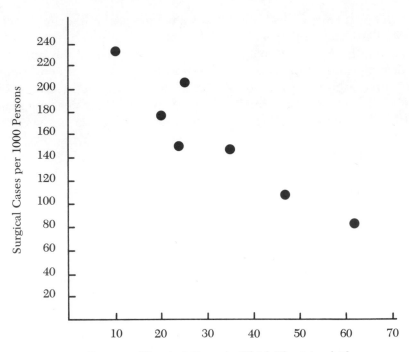

FIGURE 2. Geographic areas [a] by rates for nonobstetrical surgery and frequency of additional charges [b] (U.S.A., July 1, 1957–June 30, 1958).

Source: Reference 75, p. 75. Reproduced by permission from *Medical Care Chart Book*, School of Public Health, The University of Michigan.
  [a] The Seven geographic areas represented are (reading from left to right): Minnesota (various areas); Michigan (various areas); Detroit, Michigan; Pennsylvania (Bethlehem and Allentown); Western Pennsylvania; Ohio (Cleveland, Youngstown, etc.); and Illinois (Chicago and nearby).
  [b] For United Steelworkers covered by Blue Shield contracts.

support this, that members of the union in all regions were reasonably similar and that their health status was generally comparable. If so, the differences observed do not reflect differences in need but the impact of different pricing practices. It is difficult to say whether these represent differences in costs to the physician, in the content or quality of care, or in the expectations of physicians for income. One plausible explanation is that physicians have considerable control over their prices and may elect to achieve a satisfactory income either through performing more procedures at lower price, or fewer procedures at higher price.

A later study by Alexander suggests that this explanation is not only plausible, but likely (76). For some years prior to 1963, welfare patients in Baltimore received care by physicians who were paid on a per capita basis, irrespective of the number of services provided. On January 1, 1963, the method of payment was changed by discontinuing capitation payments and substituting a modest fee for each visit. The response was an approximately 17 percent increase in visits. Since the payments involved, whether per service or per capita, were very small, they could hardly be considered as major incentives, except to physicians who derived a large share of their income from welfare practice. Accordingly, 10 physicians, who had more than 1,000 welfare clients each, were studied separately. These physicians had also increased the number of visits, but only enough to maintain average revenue from this source virtually constant. The 10 individual physicians differed from each other in the average number of visits they had given each welfare patient under the per capita system and, therefore, in the degree to which they were threatened by a change to fee-for-service. When the potential reduction in revenue, assuming no change in physician behavior, was related to physician response, it was clear that the physicians who showed the greatest increase in number of visits were those who had previously provided the fewest visits. Thus one finds a sensitive responsiveness in physician behavior to changes in the payment system. However, if it is true that physicians tend to maintain a certain expectation of income, an increase in price, relative to cost, could lead to a reduction in service. When a broad range of benefits is provided, physicians may find it easier to earn the income they expect not by increasing the volume of service as a whole but by substituting services with greater marginal revenue for those with less. However, in offering these speculations we may have stretched our meager data beyond their limits.

Effects by Income and Social Class. So far, we have restricted our attention almost exclusively to the effects of insurance on the volume of care received. As we have said earlier, another matter of theoretical interest, and of even greater concern to policy, is the ability of insurance or any other provision of benefits to alter the distribution of use in relation to need. Two aspects of this allocative effect have been singled out: its relationship to income and to seriousness of illness.

With respect to income, we have already described recent trends which show a change in the traditional relationship between income and use of services, and have suggested that the provision of benefits under voluntary insurance and public programs may have been the major factor in bringing about the change. We have also shown that income has an effect independent of insurance, and insurance an effect independent of income. In this section we shall deal more directly with the *differential* effect of insurance on different income groups. In theory, any lowering of the price of care at the point of consumption should have a greater effect at lower incomes than at higher. It has been argued that this differential effect is further reinforced by the larger indirect or opportunity costs of receiving care at higher incomes. More specifically, one could hypothesize that the critical consideration is the ratio of the direct costs of care to the sum of direct plus opportunity costs. This ratio is presumed to be more greatly reduced by insurance at low than at high incomes. But this may not always be the case. Persons with higher income may be covered more thoroughly by insurance for income loss due to illness, may enjoy greater job security, and may be more sensitive to the threat of reduced income in the long run as a result of unprevented or neglected illness. It is not clear that consideration of opportunity costs will always depress use of service at higher incomes. The more affluent are also more likely to know what benefits are available under any set of arrangements and are better able to make any system work for themselves. In this way the enhancing effect of insurance on use of service at low incomes may be matched by an equally large, or even larger, enhancing effect at higher incomes, so that the differences among income groups are maintained or widened, rather than reduced. Alternatively, there may be no differences in the initiation of care, but the rich may opt for more intensive and effective care of shorter duration.

We have been assuming that program benefits are comparable for rich and poor. If, however, as seems likely, the rich have more insurance for a wider range of services, there is even greater reason why income differentials are maintained. Additional factors acting to preserve such differences are deductible and copayment features of benefits, a rise in prices for covered and non-covered services, and the presence of structural barriers of a socio-organizational or geographic nature that impede receipt of care by the poor. The resultant of these several tendencies must vary from one situation to another, and is a matter for empirical determination.

Even when the facts are known, it may be difficult to interpret the findings because absolute differences in use of service between the insured and the uninsured, by income class, may be larger or smaller than the relative differences. This is a special instance of a situation that is often observed in comparative studies. There is no general rule by which one may decide whether the absolute or the relative differences are more meaningful to the analysis. Hence, as we present our data we will show both aspects of the comparison.

Much of our information comes from the periodic national surveys we have referred to earlier (19, 20, 21). Table 6 gives some data for 1963 and 1953. The data for hospital admissions in 1953 show most clearly that insurance enhances use of service in all income groups, but particularly in low income groups. Income has almost no effect on use of service by the uninsured, whereas among the insured there are fewer admissions as income goes up. Thus, insurance appears to have brought about a gradient more in line with what is believed to be the distribution of need by income. In 1963 (1) admissions were reduced as income rose, for the uninsured as well as the insured; (2) as in 1953, admissions were more frequent among the insured in all income groups; and (3) the differential effect of insurance by income group was not consistently evident when one considers the relative differences in rates of admission (insured as percent of uninsured), but the effect was consistently present when one examines the absolute differences (insured minus uninsured). When the data for 1963 were tabulated by number of insurance policies carried, it was found that the service-enhancing effect of multiple insurance was present at all income levels, but was greatest for persons with family incomes of less than $4,000. "At this income level 6 percent of uninsured were hospitalized compared to 14 percent of the singles and 20

TABLE 6. Use of Specified Services, Expenditures, and Outlays, by Insurance Status and Family Income, U.S.A. (Civilian, Noninstitutionalized Population), 1953 and 1963

Services, Expenditures or Outlays	Family Income in Dollars						
	Under 2,000	2,000– 3,499	3,500– 4,999	5,000– 7,499	7,500– 9,999	10,000– 12,499	12,500 and over
Hospital admissions [a] per 100 per year, 1953							
Insured (I)	21	16	13	13		12	
Uninsured (U)	9	9	9	8		10	
I as percent of U	233	178	144	162		120	
I minus U	12	7	4	5		2	
Hospital admissions [a] per 100 per year, 1963							
Insured (I)	25	15		15		11	
Uninsured (U)	12	9		10		6	
I as percent of U	208	167		150		183	
I minus U	13	6		5		5	
In-hospital surgical procedures per 100 per year, 1963							
Insured (I)	7	7	5	6	8	5	5
Uninsured (U)	2	2	2	4	4	2	3
I as percent of U	350	350	250	150	200	250	167
I minus U	5	5	3	2	2	3	2
Mean family expenditures for health, 1963 [b]							
Insured (I)	$292	$337	$322	$438	$501		
Uninsured (U)	162	144	212	253	317		
I as percent of U	180	234	152	173	158		
I minus U	130	193	110	185	184		
Outlay for health services as % of family income, 1963 [c]							
Insured (I)	23.7	11.5	7.7	6.1	3.9		
Uninsured (U)	10.0	5.1	4.6	3.1	2.5		
I as percent of U	237	225	167	197	156		
I minus U	13.7	6.4	3.1	3.0	1.4		

Sources: Reference 19, Table 15, p. 59, and Reference 20, Tables 67, 70, and 72, pp. 129, 133, and 137.

[a] Short-term hospitals.

[b] Charges for personal health services, including health insurance benefits but excluding health insurance premiums.

[c] Outlays are essentially actual out-of-pocket payments for health services and premiums.

TABLE 7. Percent of Persons Admitted to Hospital,[a] by Insurance Status and Family Income, U.S.A. (Civilian, Noninstitutionalized Population under 65), 1968

Percent Admitted to Hospital	Family Income in Dollars					
	Under 3,000	3,000– 4,999	5,000– 6,999	7,000– 9,999	10,000– 14,999	15,000 and Over
With hospital insurance (I)	11.3	10.5	9.8	9.2	8.2	7.5
Without hospital insurance (U)	10.0	9.2	7.9	8.6	7.3	6.9
I as percent of U	113	114	124	107	112	109
I minus U	1.3	1.3	1.9	0.6	0.9	0.6

Source: Reference 37, Table 15, p. 35.
[a] Short-stay hospitals.

percent of the multiples" (46, p. 22). The National Health Survey has reported data for 1968 that give the percent of persons who were admitted to short-term hospitals rather than the number of admissions per person-year. Moreover, the report includes only persons under 65. The findings, given in Table 7, show that the insured remained more likely to be admitted to hospitals irrespective of income. Relative differences by income group show no clear trend, but absolute differences appear to be somewhat larger below an income of $7,000 than above. One suspects, however, that both the differences between insured and uninsured, and the differential effect of insurance by income group have become further attenuated, when one compares data for 1968 with the data for 1963 and 1953.

Needless to say, admissions data must be supplemented by information concerning length of stay. The data for length of stay are very equivocal, partly because of the difficulty in controlling for case-mix. Thus, there is no proof of the expectation that, when severity of illness is held constant, insured persons who have higher income will receive more intensive care and will stay in the hospital for shorter periods of time, than insured persons with lower income.

Table 6 also gives data showing the impact of insurance on the use of in-hospital surgical procedures, and on family "expenditures" and "outlays" by different income groups. For in-hospital surgical procedures, insurance appears to make a greater absolute and relative difference at lower than at higher incomes, as expected. Family expenditures for personal health services, which are charges incurred irrespective of whether they are paid by insurance or not, are always higher for insured families; and those expenditures are higher at the upper end of the income range than at the lower end, irrespective of insurance. However, insurance does not have a differential effect on family expenditures by different income groups. But there may be a differential effect that is obscured, because total expenditures as defined in this study, include both insured and uninsured services, and reflect income differentials in price and quality of care. Thus, the relatively higher charges for insured services received by the poor could be counteracted by the relatively higher charges for uninsured services, and higher prices for all services, received by the more affluent. The data for 1963 were analyzed by Andersen and Benham using relative value scales, rather than expenditures, to measure volume of care received (18). When corrections were made for insurance coverage, there was a reduction in the income-elasticity of standardized amounts of care received, suggesting that insurance enhanced, rather than reduced, the differences among income groups. This was attributed to the fact that persons in the higher income groups had more effective insurance as evidenced by higher premiums and a greater likelihood of group rather than individual enrollment.

The data on outlays as percent of family income, which are also given in Table 6, show a different facet of the picture. Outlays are essentially out-of-pocket payments for charges and premiums; they represent the cost of buying insurance plus obligations that insurance has not covered. These outlays constitute a much higher percentage of family income among the insured than the uninsured, and they are higher among low income groups than high income groups, irrespective of insurance. There are also clearly differential effects of insurance by income. At low incomes, insurance increases the proportion of income spent on health outlays much more than at high incomes.

These observations support the general conclusion that, insurance affects the use of covered health care services more at low incomes than at high incomes. However, this differential effect may not be as clearly demonstrable now as it has been in the recent past. When the volume of total services is considered, the greater enhancement in the use of covered services by the poor is counteracted by the purchase of more complete coverage by the more affluent. This does not, however, negate the expectation that with equal insurance the poor will experience a greater improvement in care than the rich. But this relatively larger improvement in care appears to also increase out-of-pocket expenditures relative to income to a much greater extent at low than at high incomes. Thus, the relatively greater access to care accorded to the poor through the purchase of insurance, carries with it the burden of larger out-of-pocket expenditures relative to income. Insurance that covers a relatively small part of expenditures appears to take away with one hand what it gives with the other. But even if all expenditures were covered, the poor would still spend a larger share of their income on health care as long as they paid a premium reasonably proportionate to the cost of the health care they need. As we shall see in a subsequent chapter, this situation can only be remedied through some form of redistribution of income or its substitutes.

The general conclusions we have drawn are subject to limitations in the data. When income groups were compared, no correction was made for the effect of associated characteristics (such as age, education, occupation, or race) or for differential reporting to the household interviewer. When comparisons were made over time, there was no correction for price inflation, so that comparability of income groups was not assured. Even more important, the increasing availability of benefits under programs other than voluntary insurance tends to obscure differences between the insured and uninsured that were previously evident. The data from the National Health survey (Table 7) differed from the other data (Table 6) with respect to the age of the population and the measure of hospital use. Finally, in none of the data do we have information on really high incomes. Accordingly, the conclusions we have drawn must remain tentative, even though they accord reasonably well with expectation.

Some studies of prepaid group practice provide evidence that social class differences tend to persist, though narrowed, even when benefits are rather extensive, and that special effort is necessary to close the social gap. This may be partly because even the best of insurance plans does not cover all costs, or even the majority of costs, to the patient. Partly, it is evidence that factors other than cost play an important role in use of service. In their study of prematurity and perinatal mortality, Shapiro et al. obtained information on the percent of women who received prenatal care during the first trimester, for three populations: (1) a sample of New York City residents, (2) persons in the New York City sample who received private care, and (3) a sample of subscribers to the Health Insurance Plan of Greater New York (77). The comparisons were between whites, nonwhites and Puerto Ricans. The findings are summarized in Figure 3. The effect of social factors can be inferred from the observation that in all samples whites were most likely to receive early prenatal care, nonwhites very much less likely, and Puerto Ricans least likely to do so. The effect of successively better insurance coverage can be inferred from the observation that the greatest ethnic differences were found in the general population sample, a considerable equalization was noted in the sample that received private care, and there was still further equalization in the sample of group practice enrollees. However, even in this last sample, all of whom had reasonably broad coverage, including office care, the pattern of ethnic differences remained, even though the degree was lessened. A more recent study by Roemer et al. compares experience under selected insurance plans representing prepaid group practice, provider-sponsored plans, and commercial health insurance (52). Although the prepaid group practice plans offer the broadest range of benefits and the fewest barriers to care, use of service among lower class members, as compared to upper class members, tended to be more favorable in the provider-sponsored plans than in the group practice plans. Under prepaid group practice, persons in the "upper" and "lower" classes were equally likely to consult a physician, but "upper class" persons made more visits and received more preventive services. The presence of self-selection and other limitations in study design make an interpretation of these findings rather hazardous, but the authors suggest that "lower class" enrollees may find it difficult to "work the system" when dealing with the more complicated and formalized group practice arrangements. This interpretation is supported by the observation that ed-

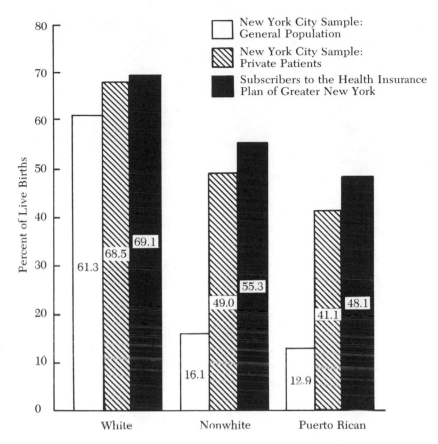

FIGURE 3. Percent of live births with prenatal care begun in the first trimester of pregnancy, by color and specified population group (New York, 1955).

Source: Reference 77, p. 175. Reproduced by permission from *Medical Care Chart Book,* School of Public Health, The University of Michigan.

ucation and occupation, rather than income, are responsible for differences in the use of physicians (52, pp. 31–32). Two reports from the Kaiser-Permanente group in Oregon suggest that the group practice system can be made accessible to disadvantaged populations, but that distinctive patterns of use will persist (78, 79). Utilization rates and patterns of the general membership of this group were compared with those of a small subset enrolled under arrangements with the Office of Economic Opportunity

(OEO). The OEO members were found to be comparable to the general membership in the propensity to initiate care and the likelihood of doing so as soon as symptoms occurred. The number of visits per person was greater for OEO members, the excess being largely made up of self-initiated walk-in visits, which demonstrated effective access in response to felt need. On the other hand, the system appears to have lost some measure of control over client behavior, as shown by the greater propensity of OEO members to make unscheduled visits, to break appointments, to seek care after hours as well as on Sundays or holidays, and to be seen by a physician other than the regular attending physician. The data on equalization of opportunity to receive care should also be accepted with some reservations because the OEO membership was selected by giving priority to families who were known to need a great deal of care. This may mean that use of service by such families should have been even greater than that observed.

A comparison of mental health services received by the same two populations in the Portland plan also leads to the conclusion that the provision of benefits can go a long way towards equalizing access to care (80). In this instance, the "poverty population" made a larger number of visits for diagnostic categories for mental disorders considered to have no defined organic cause; relatively more persons who received such care were referred to the mental health clinic of the plan; and a greater proportion of services was received in the mental health clinic. The greater propensity to refer persons in the "poverty population" to the mental health clinic may have resulted from the provision of this benefit without copayment, whereas other plan members had to pay 20 to 50 percent of the cost of such care. But, as the investigators suggest, there may have been other reasons, such as the possibly greater severity of the illness among the poor, or a difference in the physician-patient relationship in the two groups. Finally, it is not known to what extent unmet needs for such care have been equalized in the two populations, even when use of service for mental illness is greater among the poor.

From these studies one may tentatively conclude that the provision of a broad range of benefits under prepaid group practice plans will usually go a long way towards reducing social class differences in volume of care received, but that the socially disadvantaged may continue to receive less care relative to their needs, and have difficulty in conforming to acceptable behavior in an organized program. In some situations, the plan, while it reduces the financial barrier, may raise new barriers of bureaucratic complexity so that the socially disadvantaged remain relatively handicapped in access to care.

Effects by Severity of Illness. If insurance has a larger effect at lower incomes than at higher, the presumed consequence is more efficient adjustment of use to need. However, insurance may lead to a less efficient allocation of use according to disease severity. This would happen, according to our hypothesis, if insurance has a more marked influence on the use of service for less severe illnesses and if it increases the proportion of care that is of doubtful utility, unnecessary, or even harmful. To some extent, these inefficiencies may be counteracted by the encouragement of preventive services and the initiation of care earlier in the course of illness.

The data bearing on these speculations are meager. Andersen and Anderson report, without citing details, that "the relationship of surgical insurance to surgical rates is strongest where 'elective' procedures are involved" (20, p. 130). Our review of the revenue effects of insurance tends to support this contention. More detailed, though not completely convincing, evidence is cited by Richardson in a study of receipt of service for illness episodes reported by residents in three urban, low-income areas (81). Respondents rated each episode as "very serious," "fairly serious," or "not serious at all." Based on the clients' description of the episode, a physician subsequently rated each episode as "serious," if in his opinion it required that a physician be seen, and "not serious," if there was no need to see a physician. Respondents were rated as "poor" or "not poor," apparently using eligibility for care under the standards of the poverty program. According to the author, the availability of third party payment, usually through Medicare or Medicaid, enhanced service more for the poor, and for illnesses rated by the physician to be "not serious." While this accords with our expectations, the data do not regularly support the authors' interpretation, and the conclusion must remain tenta-

82 | Benefits in Medical Care Programs

tive. It should be noted, however, that in this study of predominantly disadvantaged populations, the range of incomes must have been unusually narrow.

Appropriateness of Care. More direct evidence on the adjustment of use of service to need comes from professional assessments of the appropriateness of care under different payment systems. A key study was made in Michigan in 1958 concerning the appropriateness of length of stay in a sample of hospital admissions for 17 selected diagnoses (82). Appropriateness was judged, initially, by evidence in the hospital records of compliance with criteria formulated for each diagnosis by a competent panel of physicians. When deviations were found, further information was obtained from the attending physician, and the judgment concerning appropriateness confirmed or amended accordingly. The key findings are shown in Figure 4. When the patient paid the entire bill, 16.7 percent of admissions were judged to involve understay and 6.3 percent involved overstay. When there were other sources of payment, with or without participation by the patient, only 5.6 percent of stays were judged to have been too short, whereas 11.8 percent were judged to have been too long. These findings can be taken as representative of a large proportion of hospital admissions in an urban state with considerable insurance coverage. A more limited study, using the same methods, was subsequently conducted in Nassau County, New York (83). Because of peculiarities in the research design and analysis, the findings do not represent any defined universe. Nevertheless, as shown in Table 8, one finds

TABLE 8. Percent of Hospital Admissions Who Stayed in Hospital for Longer [a] or Shorter Periods than Considered Necessary, by Source of Payment of Hospital Expenses, Nassau County, N.Y., 1962 [b]

Source of Payment	Percent with Overstay	Percent with Understay
Patient paid entire bill	14.3	14.3
Health insurance paid more than 75% but less than 100% of bill	26.3	7.8
Health insurance paid entire bill	22.2	6.2

Source: Reference 83, Tables 4a and 4c, Appendix B.
[a] Overstay includes inappropriate admission.
[b] Patients with one of 5 selected diagnoses in 5 selected short-term general hospitals.

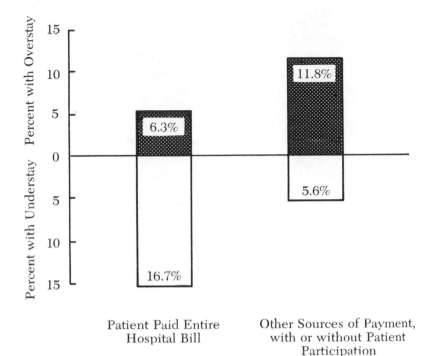

FIGURE 4. Percent of hospital patients who stayed in hospital for longer and shorter times than considered necessary, by sources of payment of hospital expenses (Patients with 17 selected diagnoses, Michigan hospitals, 1958).

Source: Reference 82, Table 221, p. 490. Reproduced by permission from *Medical Care Chart Book*, School of Public Health, The University of Michigan.

once again that when the patient pays the entire bill there is greater likelihood of understay and less likelihood of overstay than when health insurance pays the entire bill. The slightly higher proportion of overstays when the patient pays a relatively small part of the bill, as compared to when he pays no part, is probably not significant. It does, however, raise intriguing speculation about the effect on behavior of small charges that are insufficient to suppress demand but are sufficient to motivate the patient to expect more care.

So far, we have dealt with a rather tangential aspect of the quality of care, length of stay. This aspect does, of course have important consequences for the cost of care. But it is also possible that the availability of payment on behalf of the patient, or of revenue to the physician, can bring about changes more central to what is understood to signify quality. A study of primary appendectomies in Baltimore City, during 1957 and 1958, certainly suggests this (84). In this study, a comparison was made between university and community hospitals for each of four categories of payment. Whether the appendectomy was necessary or not can be judged, in part, by whether the tissue removed was normal or not. Since, even under the best of circumstances, there is an acceptable margin of "error," one could use performance in the university hospitals as a realistic standard. The findings are shown in Table 9. In the university hospitals, about a third of appendices removed when the diagnosis was appendicitis did not show clearly abnormal tissue on pathological examination, irrespective of who paid for the operation. In the community hospitals this proportion was higher, and it seemed to be sensitive to the source of payment. The proportion of normal appendices removed was highest when Blue Cross paid the bill. These observations support previous findings suggesting that under insurance, when there is a revenue incentive, there is an increase in discretionary surgical procedures affecting "useless" organs. But in the university hospitals, irrespective of source of payment, as well as on the ward services of community hospitals, certain influences and safeguards are in force that are capable of counteracting this effect. However, all these conclusions must remain conjectural, since neither the comparability of the samples nor the comparability of the pathological examinations has been established. Another deficiency is that we

TABLE 9. Percent of Primary Appendectomies Classified Pathologically as "Unnecessary" or "Doubtful" in Two University and Three Community Hospitals, by Type of Hospital and Patient's Payment Status, Baltimore, Md., 1957 and 1958

| | Type of Hospital | |
Patient's Payment Status	University Hospitals	Community Hospitals
Welfare (N = 96)	33	40
Private Payment (N = 186)	35	42
Insurance other than Blue Cross (N = 165)	35	50
Blue Cross (N = 555)	34	55

Source: Reference 84, estimated from Figure 2.

are not told about the errors of omission; namely, what happened to those who might have needed surgery but did not receive it. An error in surgery is unlike an error in the length of hospital stay, where we can measure error in both directions and decide, assuming we cannot precisely adjust use to need, whether overstay or understay is socially more desirable. In calculating the appropriate length of stay one must include not only the immediate costs of care, but also consequences to health and the costs attached to these. Further, it is necessary to examine the incidence of costs: whether these are borne by the patient, his family, the providers, the financing program, the local community, or some larger unit of society. For example, it is conceivable that understays may mean delayed recovery and larger post-hospital expenditures for the patient; and lower occupancy coupled with reduced efficiency for the hospital. On the other hand, while the higher cost of overstays could represent a burden to a national or regional financing program, it could produce revenue for the local hospital and could, under certain methods of financing, represent a net benefit to the local community. We shall have to deal with such redistributive phenomena in a subsequent chapter of this book.

Effects of Introducing Insurance

Almost all the studies that we have described so far have involved comparisons between insured and uninsured populations; from these comparisons conclusions have been drawn about the effects of providing benefits under insurance or other arrangements. It might be useful now to review some reports of the short-term impact caused by the introduction of large-scale health programs. This will allow us to see whether our expectations are supported by events, or whether our hypotheses require alteration or refinement. Unfortunately, the introduction of such programs is rarely accompanied by careful assessments; only in a few cases can we draw even tentative conclusions about their impact.

British National Health Service. It was only through a happy coincidence that the introduction of the National Health Service in Britain corresponded with a national health survey. From this survey one can glean some information concerning the impact of the Health Service scheme. Stewart and Enterline have summarized the main findings (85). It appears that there was an increase in use of the services of physicians during the first two years following the introduction of the National Health Service in those segments of the population that were not previously covered by national insurance for working people: females, the aged of both sexes, and persons of lower income. Among persons in the highest income group there was a reduction in the number of visits made to physicians. Figure 5 shows the findings by sex and by income. At first sight, these findings suggest not only a differential effect on the previously uninsured and the poor, but also a redistribution that is probably in accord with need, since the poor are more likely to have illnesses that are more disabling. It should be noted, however, that the data are for "visits per 1,000 ill or injured," so that the incidence of need, though not its severity, has been taken into account. This leads one to wonder whether, given a limit on the capacity of physicians in the short run, rationing according to ability to pay has been substituted by rationing according to ability to incur other costs, including the opportunity costs of seeking care.

Finnish National Health Insurance Scheme. In contrast to the relatively small attention given to documenting the impact of the Health Service in Britain, specific plans were made to assess the effects of introducing a national health insurance scheme in Finland in 1964 (86, 87). Since hospital care was already provided under a publicly-supported system, the new scheme confined itself to covering a portion of the costs of ambulatory care and of necessary travel. In addition, it included a daily cash allowance for those who were sick for more than seven weekdays. Household surveys provided data on use of service and expenditures during May–June 1964, before the introduction of the insurance scheme, and during May–June 1968, about 3.5 years after the scheme was implemented. The findings so far published refer to use of service by persons 15 years or older. They show, once again, a differential effect on categories of persons who were heretofore disadvantaged, resulting in a redistribution of service which is probably in accord with need, but which stops short of erasing inequalities in this respect. First, it is important to note that the overall increase in physician visits outside the hospital was very

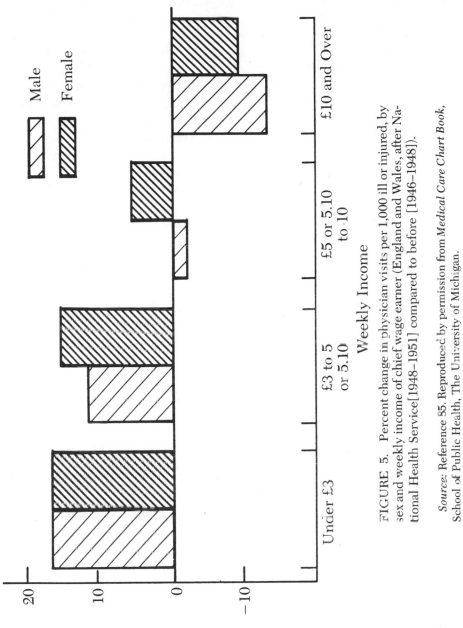

FIGURE 5. Percent change in physician visits per 1,000 ill or injured, by sex and weekly income of chief wage earner (England and Wales, after National Health Service[1948–1951] compared to before [1946–1948]).

Source: Reference 35. Reproduced by permission from *Medical Care Chart Book*, School of Public Health, The University of Michigan.

small: about 8 percent. This may reflect, in part, the limits imposed by the capacity of physicians to provide service and, in part, the less than complete removal of barriers to care. Unfortunately, we are not told what happened to inpatient care. In Finland, as elsewhere, use of service has been lower in rural than in urban regions, and lower for men than for women. Arranged from low utilization to high, the order has been: rural men, urban men, rural women, urban women. In general, the introduction of the ambulatory care scheme may be said to have reduced these differentials without altering the ordering of the categories. However, more detailed examination shows fascinating differences of response which have a bearing on our hypothetical formulations. The findings are shown in Table 10. The much greater absolute, as well as relative, improvement in rural areas may be explained by the greater effect of new purchasing power on relatively impoverished persons, the greater impact of payment for travel costs where distances to physicians are longer, and, possibly, the presence of a larger reserve capacity to provide service in rural areas. The redistribution of services in urban areas that resulted in a large increase for men, and an actual small reduction for women, can be explained by the presence of new demand on physicians working at

TABLE 10. Visits to a Physician per 100 Adults [a] per 100 days, and Absolute and Relative Changes in Frequency of Visits, by Residence and Sex, Finland, 1964 and 1968 [b]

Category of Persons	1964	1968	1968 minus 1964	1968 as percent of 1964
Rural men	44	48	+4	109
Urban men	48	53	+5	110
Rural women	52	60	+8	115
Urban women	72	69	−3	96
All men	46	50	+4	109
All women	60	64	+4	107
All rural	48	54	+6	112
All urban	61	62	+1	102

Source: Reference 87, Table 1.
[a] Persons 15 and older.
[b] Civilian, noninstitutionalized population, May–June 1964 and May–June 1968.

capacity, and a reduction not only of direct costs, but also of the opportunity costs of sickness for employed men. The large increase in use by rural women, relative to men, is difficult to explain. Nyman and Kalimo suggest that it is accounted for by a greater propensity of women to take advantage of opportunities for care. However, one would also want to examine other characteristics of the rural population, including age and type of occupation.

Prior to the introduction of the health scheme in Finland, the distribution of visits by income appeared to favor the poor when no correction was made for the number of days of sickness experienced by persons in each income group, but not after this correction was made. This is not unlike the current situation in the United States, as we have described in an earlier chapter. The introduction of the insurance scheme in Finland increased use of service in all income groups, but more so for lower incomes, so that utilization became more congruent with "need," but not fully so. The data are shown in Table 11. Further analysis of magnitudes of change, by income, within each category of severity of illness, as measured by number of days of sickness, suggests that the equalizing effects of insurance may have been more marked for illness of long duration. When diseases were characterized as

TABLE 11. Visits to a Physician per 100 Adults [a] per 100 days, by Income, With and Without Adjustment for Days of Sickness in Each Income Group, Finland, 1964 and 1968 [b]

Family Income in Finnish Marks	Not Adjusted		Adjusted	
	1964	1968	1964	1968
All incomes	53	57	53	55
0–2,500	57	63	48	54
2,501–5,000	51	58	49	54
5,001–7,500	50	56	54	54
7,501–10,000	53	56	56	55
10,001 and over	53	55	61	59
Highest income group as percent of lowest income group	93%	87%	127%	109%

Source: Reference 87, Table 2.

[a] Persons 15 and older.

[b] Civilian, noninstitutionalized population, May–June 1964 and May–June 1968.

acute or chronic, it became apparent that increases in use of service for acute illness had occurred at the expense of reductions in use of service for chronic illness, with reductions mostly in the higher income groups. Nyman and Kalimo conclude that "The chronically ill seem to be the group by which our system of health care regulated the conflict between price and supply" (87, p. 548). These relationships between severity of illness and differential responsiveness to insurance are not in keeping with our hypothesis that as financial barriers are lowered, care is sought for increasingly less severe categories of need and that, therefore, the impact of insurance is relatively larger for the less severe categories of illness. One can only speculate on why this is so. It may be that the supply of ambulatory service-capacity in Finland is too small, and the use of physician services is at such a low rate, that there is a large reservoir of unmet need for reasonably severe illness that must be met first. Further, the physician may be able to exercise a greater control on demand so that redistribution is more in accord with what he considers to require more immediate attention. The nature of the benefits may have contributed to the results by paying not only for part of the cost of care but also for part of loss of income incurred by the more prolonged illnesses. Using length of illness as a measure of severity may have also introduced a certain circularity in the conclusions; this would occur if staying away from work, for example, is upon recommendation of a physician. Perhaps the most plausible of these explanations is the crucial relationship between supply and unmet need. One can propose that it is only when the supply can be expanded that provision of benefits encourages the use of services for successively less serious or less urgent illness.

It may be concluded from the above that the Finnish insurance plan has made a great deal of progress towards the objective of redistributing service according to the short-run severity of illness (86, 87). Less progress has been made towards achieving higher levels of use, assuming this were a goal, which it apparently was not. Among the reasons for the smallness of the overall increase might be limits on the number of physicians, controls on price, and increases in complementary or supplementary services, such as care in hospitals and chronic disease institutions, nursing care, drugs, and the like. One awaits with interest further information on these subjects.

Another objective of the ambulatory services scheme in Finland was to reduce the financial burden of illness and of care; what Nyman and Kalimo refer to as the "aim of compensation" (87). Excluding compensation for loss of income, the insurance plan made only a modest contribution by covering less than a third of total expenditures in each income group. Because, as income rose, total expenditures also increased, insurance disbursements were considerably higher for the rich than for the poor. The difference between the distribution of expenses and monetary benefits on the one hand, and service benefits on the other, occurs because the rich use more expensive services. We are not told whether this is merely because of differentials in price, or whether the quality of services received is also substantially different. In this respect the system is much less egalitarian than might be inferred from the service data alone.

Medicare and Medicaid in the U.S. In the United States, the implementation of health insurance for the aged under the Medicare program has offered an opportunity to observe changes in the patterns of use of service by persons who are 65 or older. A complete assessment of the impact of Medicare would require a volume in itself, taking us far afield into many aspects of the medical care system (88). Here we shall limit ourselves to only a few observations that are directly relevant to our speculations concerning the differential effects of Medicare on use of service. The key information, which is summarized in Table 12, comes from household interview surveys of two national samples of persons 65 and over who were also recipients of social security benefits (89). Information was obtained concerning use of service and expenditures during the year preceding and the year following the implementation of Medicare, so that we are dealing with almost immediate consequences. During this interval there was virtually no change in the proportion of persons who visited a physician, excluding inpatient care, and there was a small reduction, rather than an increase, in the yearly number of visits per person. There was, however, a change in the place of the visit, with relatively fewer visits being made in clinics, emergency rooms or health centers, and relatively more in the doctor's office. In absolute as well as relative terms, this shift away from clinics was greater for blacks than whites, and more frequent in rural than in urban

TABLE 12. Use of Specified Services Before and After Implementation of Medicare, U.S.A., 1965 and 1967

Services	1965	1967	1967 Minus 1965	1967 as % of 1965
VISITS TO PHYSICIANS				
(excludes inpatient)				
Percent who made any visits	73.2	74.3	+ 1.1	102
Visits per person per year	6.6	6.1	− 0.5	92
Percent with visits in clinic				
All aged	14.2	8.6	− 5.6	61
White	13.4	8.2	− 5.2	61
Black	25.2	14.4	− 10.8	57
Black as % of white	188	176	—	—
Large metropolitan	17.6	14.4	− 3.2	82
Rural	13.9	4.8	− 9.1	35
SHORT-TERM HOSPITAL USE				
Admissions per 100	22.2	24.7	+ 2.5	111
Days per stay	14.2	15.9	+ 1.7	112
Patient-days per 100				
All	314	392	+ 78	125
Age 65–74	314	306	− 8	97
Age 75 and over	315	540	+225	171
75 and over as % of 65–74	100	176	—	—
White	320	396	+ 76	124
Black	237	351	+114	148
Black as % of white	74	89	—	—
South	242	389	+147	161
Other	345	394	+ 49	114
Large metropolitan	312	363	+ 51	116
Small metropolitan	311	372	+ 61	120
Other urban	251	431	+180	172
Rural	353	417	+ 69	118
NURSING HOME AND EXTENDED CARE SERVICES:				
Patient-days per 100				
All	701	613	− 88	87
Extended care facilities	235	289	+ 54	123
Nursing homes	465	324	−141	70

Services	1965	1967	1967 Minus 1965	1967 as % of 1965
SURGERY				
Hospital stays per 100				
All	5.9	7.9	+ 2.0	134
Age 65–74	6.1	7.5	+ 1.4	123
Age 75 and over	5.5	8.4	+ 3.1	153
Cataract	0.34	0.89	0.55	262
Cholecystectomy	0.18	0.52	0.34	289

Source: Reference 89, Tables 1, 2, 5 and 9, pages 6, 7, 9 and 14, and text on page 9.

areas. Note, however, that the relative positions of blacks and whites were not much changed.

In contrast to the relative constancy in the use of physicians for non-inpatient services, there was a slightly more than 10 percent increase in admissions to short term hospitals, and an over 10 percent increase in length of stay during the survey year, these increases together resulting in overall increase in patient-days of about 25 percent. The extent of change in hospital use varied by demographic, social and geographic characteristics of respondents. The increase in hospital use was larger for the more aged among the aged, for blacks as compared to whites, in the South as compared to other regions, and in non-metropolitan urban areas as compared to other areas. Unlike the findings in England and Finland, income did not make much difference. And there was no clear relationship between hospital use and education. The gap in use of service between blacks and whites was reduced slightly but not eliminated. In addition to changes in the volume of hospital use, there was a disproportionate rise in admissions for surgery, which were increased by over 30 percent, as compared to the 11 percent increase for all admissions. As was true for all admissions, the increase for surgical admissions was greater among those of advanced age as compared to the less aged. There were also differences by type of surgery, with some procedures showing very large increases. Admissions for cataract surgery more than doubled, whereas those for cholecystectomy almost tripled. In the first year of Medicare, one out of every 100 aged persons had a cataract operation, and one out of every 200 persons had a gall bladder removed!

Since post-hospital institutional care was a particularly innovative feature of Medicare, it is interesting to note that there was little change in admissions or length of stay for this purpose. There was, however, a shift from use of presumably less skilled to more skilled facilities. It is not clear to what extent this change is a matter of definition, since the category of "extended care facility" was one created by Medicare.

Needless to say, the interpretation of these findings must remain conjectural. If seeking out a physician at least once during a year represents patient initiative, such initiative was apparently unchanged, at least during the first year of Medicare. Among the factors that may have been responsible for this, one might consider (1) that there was no perceived need for additional care prior to the institution of Medicare; (2) that clients wanted more care, but did not know that this was available under Part B of the Medicare program; (3) that potential clients desired care and knew of the benefits, but were effectively dissuaded by the deductible and coinsurance features of the program; and (4) that there were enough physicians to accomodate the small shift towards office practice, but no more. The increase in short-term hospital admissions, length of stay, and patient-days of care suggests some substitution of inpatient services for ambulatory care; the shortage of physicians, and possibly a revenue effect, may have contributed to this increase. Thus, while one can suggest that patients did not greatly alter their behavior in seeking care, one also suspects that physicians did alter the manner in which they provided services. This suspicion is strengthened when one observes some details of practice in those Michigan hospitals that subscribe to the Professional Activities Study of the Commission on Professional and Hospital Activities (90). During the first year following the implementation of Medicare there was an increase of about 15 percent in surgical operations in these hospitals. X-rays and laboratory tests increased, most of the latter beyond 20 percent. Blood transfusions increased by 180 percent. The new affluence was eloquently expressed by the virtual disappearance of miniature chest x-rays and their replacement by large plates. Unfortunately, there is no direct evidence concerning the appropriateness of these changes in patterns of care, to which decisions by physicians must have made a major contribution. The general tendency to excessive surgery, overinvestigation, and unnecessary use of transfusions makes at least some portion of the increment reasonably suspect. Moreover, one must view with a jaundiced eye the phenomenal increase in cholecystectomies under Medicare; although it is hard to believe that the large increment in cataract operations represents anything other than a considerable reservoir of unmet need, or of demand that was deferred pending the availability of Medicare benefits.

The data for hospital use in the national study, as well as for Michigan, show that Medicare did succeed in making care differentially more accessible to persons presumed to have been especially handicapped prior to the availability of its benefits: the very aged, the black population, and residents of the South. However, the gap between blacks and whites, though somewhat narrowed, was not eliminated during the first year. We have suggested that the short supply of physicians may have contributed to the lack of increase in physician visits and to a substitution of inpatient hospital care for care in a physician's office. Similarly, the prior level of demand on hospital capacity may have been a factor in the subsequent response to Medicare. For example, the larger increase in the use of hospital services in the South and in nonmetropolitan urban places could have been due, in part, to a relatively large supply of hospital beds in those areas. In Michigan, smaller hospitals, which tend to have lower occupancy rates, reported a larger increase in the proportion of days used by persons 65 and over (90). Finally, a redistribution of hospital services has probably occurred in favor of the aged at the expense of younger persons. In the large selection of Michigan hospitals there was a 12 percent increase in admissions and a 9 percent increase in length of stay for persons 65 or older, whereas for younger persons there was almost no change in length of stay and a small reduction in admissions. In a national sample of hospitals an 18 percent increase in patient-days of care for persons 65 and over was accompanied by a 3 percent decrease in patient-days of care for the much larger number of persons under 65 (91). The general conclusions are (1) that redistribution has occurred in favor of groups with greater unmet need; (2) that this shift has most likely fallen far short of achieving equalization; (3) that the presence of surplus capacity, or the ability to expand capacity, is a major influence on the degree and direction of redistribution; and (4) that physician decisions, rather than client initiative, are mostly responsible for changes in patterns of care and that, therefore, the nature of the incentives to the physician is a major feature of benefit design.

Health Insurance in Quebec, Canada. In the recent experience of Quebec one can see perhaps the clearest empirical confirmation of theoretical expectations concerning the effects of health insurance. Compulsory insurance for hospital services has been in force in Quebec since 1961. A similarly compulsory and universal scheme, covering the services of physicians wherever given, became effective on November 1, 1970. In anticipation of this event, a group of U.S. and Candian investigators, with support from the U.S. government, conducted studies that established a base line for use of service and physician work load in the Montreal Metropolitan Area. By gathering comparable data a year after the implementation of the health insurance scheme it was possible to obtain a clear and accurate picture of the immediate response in both the demand for, and the supply of, physicians' services (92, 93). The data on use of service were collected by household interviews; those on work load were solicited by telephone. In both kinds of surveys it was possible, by expending the necessary effort, to obtain a response rate that exceeded 90 percent. A large portion of the data assembled by these means is presented in Tables 13 and 14.

An examination of the first few entries in Table 14 reveals that the supply of physician services was somewhat decreased, rather than increased, during the first year of the new plan. Although the number of physicians in active practice remained virtually the same, the number of these actually at work on any given weekday was somewhat reduced, and the hours devoted to professional work each day were diminished by almost 15 percent. The situation, then, is that the ability of the consumer to buy medical care has been enhanced without a corresponding expansion in the supply of care available. The result, as shown in Tables 13 and 14, is that the volume of services consumed remains constant but that significant redistributions occur. The first of these is a clear reduc-

TABLE 13. Utilization, by Type of Service and Income, before and after
Institution of Compulsory, Universal Insurance for Services of Physicians,
Montreal Metropolitan Area, 1969–1972

Utilization Data	Before: 1969–1970	After: 1971–1972	Percent Change
Visits per person per year, by type			
All visits	5.04	5.04	0.0
Telephone consultations	0.81	0.70	− 13.6
Face-to-face contacts	4.23	4.34	+ 2.6
Office	2.34	2.73	+ 16.7
Hospital clinic	1.17	1.17	0.0
Home	0.44	0.18	− 59.1
Other locations [a]	0.28	0.26	− 7.1
Visits per person per year, by income			
All incomes	5.0	5.0	0.0
Less than $3,000	6.6	7.8	+ 18.2
$ 3,000– 4,999	5.5	6.0	+ 9.1
$ 5,000– 8,999	4.7	4.7	0.0
$ 9,000–14,999	5.1	4.9	− 3.9
$15,000 and over	5.3	4.8	− 9.4
Days waited for appointment to see the physician, by income			
All incomes	6.0	11.0	+ 83.3
Less than $3,000	6.1	8.5	+ 39.3
$ 3,000– 4,999	6.3	9.3	+ 47.6
$ 5,000– 8,999	5.3	10.7	+101.9
$ 9,000–14,999	6.3	11.1	+ 76.2
$15,000 and over	6.6	12.3	+ 86.4

Source: Reference 92, Tables 1, 2 and 4, pages 1175 and 1176.
[a] Includes visits at school and at work.

tion in the number of telephone consultations and a comparable
increase in office visits, presumably because the latter are considered to be more satisfactory by the client. On the other hand,
home visits, which clients would no doubt welcome, are also reduced, presumably because the physician has less time to provide
this service. More important is the shift away from hospital inpatient visits as shown in Table 14. It would seem that the availability of office care has, to some extent, reduced the need for inpatient hospital care. It is not clear what factors are responsible for
this shift. Presumably the reduction in inpatient hospital contacts
and in the time devoted to this service by physicians is not due to

TABLE 14. Work Load of Physicians in Active Practice, by Type of Service, before and after Institution of Compulsory, Universal Insurance for Services of Physicians, Montreal Metropolitan Area, 1969–1972

Work Load Data	Before: 1969–1970	After: 1971–1972	Percent Change
Number of physicians in active practice	2424	2441	+ 0.7
Number of physicians actually at work on an average weekday	2403	2327	− 3.2
Hours worked Monday through Friday per physician in active practice [a]			
All activities	51.5	44.0	−14.6
Telephone consultations	4.4	2.8	−36.4
Face-to-face contacts	35.9	32.3	−10.0
Office	15.9	17.6	+10.7
Hospital clinic	3.6	3.7	+ 2.8
Home	3.0	1.2	−60.0
Hospital inpatient	13.4	9.8	−26.9
Other professional work	11.2	8.9	−20.5
Patient contacts per physician per weekday			
All contacts	33.9	30.5	−10.0
Telephone consultations	10.6	6.2	−41.5
Face-to-face contacts	23.4	24.3	+ 3.8
Office	9.8	12.9	+31.6
Hospital clinic	4.2	4.2	0.0
Home	1.2	0.4	−66.7
Hospital inpatient	8.1	6.7	−17.3
Minutes with each patient per: [b]			
Telephone consultation	5	5	0.0
Office visit	19	16	−15.8
Hospital clinic visit	10	11	+10.0
Home visit	30	33	+10.0
Hospital inpatient visit	20	17	−15.0

Source: Reference 93, Tables 1, 2 and 3, pages 1153 and 1154.

[a] Computed by dividing total contacts per day by number of physicians in active practice, including those not actually at work.

[b] Computed by dividing time spent in each activity by number of patient contacts.

the neglect of patients who are in the hospital. If so, one must conclude that the relative increase in ambulatory services occurs because the direct and indirect costs of those services are lower than the costs of hospital services to the client, to the physician, or to both.

Equally striking, and socially significant, is the redistribution of consumption by income class. As shown in Table 13, there was an increase in physician visits by persons of lower income and a reduction in visits by persons of higher income. That this represents a genuine social redistribution is confirmed by similar shifts in consumption from those with higher education to those with less; from English-speaking persons to the "ethnic minorities"; and from proprietors, executives, and professionals to unskilled workers. Within broad income groups, there was also a reduction in services received by those under 17 and an increase for all others, especially those 65 or older. The most plausible explanation is that rationing by waiting time has replaced rationing by price. In fact, as shown in Table 13, the average number of days waited for an appointment to see the physician in his office increased from 6 days to 11: an increment of 83 percent. Even prior to the implementation of the health plan, persons in the highest income group had to wait slightly longer for an appointment to see the physician. This may have been because the physicians patronized by the rich were more likely to be specialists who were less available. After the introduction of the health plan, those in the higher income groups experienced an even longer delay in seeing the physician than did those in the lower income groups. It is not known whether this happened because the poor had relatively easier access to the physicians usually patronized by the rich and increased their work load, or whether there was a greater relative decrease in the supply of services by such physicians. It is known, for example, that there was a disproportionate reduction in the hours worked by pediatricians, and it is surmised that this may have been responsible, in part, for the shift of consumption away from young to older persons, especially to those 65 or older.

The social utility of the observed redistributions in use of service is, of course, a matter of great significance to health policy. A major criterion of social utility is the relationship between need, or unmet need, and use of service. In an effort to explore this issue, the investigators obtained information on the occurrence of a list of "important" symptoms and conditions and on whether care had been received for such symptoms. The occurrence of symptoms was unchanged by the health plan, suggesting that there was no appreciable overall improvement in health during so short a period. However, if the percent of symptoms for which care was not received may be taken to represent unmet need, there was an overall reduction in unmet need as well as rectification of an originally discriminatory social distribution. Prior to the health plan 38 percent of the persons who reported symptoms did not receive care, and there was a progressive decrease in this percentage with increasing income. After the plan, the percent of untreated symptoms was reduced to 27 percent and the gradient by income was no longer present. One can conclude that prior to the institution of the insurance plan the poor had greater unmet need than did the rich, even though the former used more physicians' services than the latter. After the institution of the insurance plan, the disparity in use of service was widened by increments for the poor and decrements for the rich. As a result, unmet need (measured as untreated symptoms) was unchanged for the rich, but was markedly reduced for the poor. The consequence can reasonably be considered to have been a net benefit to all with no loss to anyone, except that everyone, and in particular the more well-to-do, had to wait longer for an appointment; doctors were more busy, though they worked shorter hours; and the time given each patient was somewhat reduced.

As we have already pointed out, a key determinant of this configuration of consequences is the relatively fixed, or even reduced, supply in the face of rising demand. As shown in Table 14, physicians generally responded by working shorter hours; but they actually saw, face-to-face, about the same number of patients, by virtue of spending less time with each patient. The one major exception is that office hours and office contacts increased absolutely, as well as relative to care at other locations. It is notable that the physicians' working hours were reduced even though the fee-for-service incentive was retained, although it was retained in somewhat restricted fashion because of a uniform fee schedule. The investigators speculate that "with the advent of 'free' medical care, the attitude of the physicians toward work may have changed, and they may now question the necessity for working 50 or 60 hours a week. Also, it is possible that physicians found they could earn as much or more . . . by working a shorter week." (93, p. 1155). It is unfortunate that we have no direct information concerning these matters. We are told, however, that the percentage of physicians with a secretary increased from 69.1 to 79.1, and the percentage with a registered nurse increased from 12.7 to 16.3. It may be assumed that the greater use of such help contributed to the ability of the physicians to maintain service in spite of reduced hours.

An additional interesting feature of the studies reported by Enterline et al. is the information on client and physician opinions concerning the insurance plan. Physicians were asked whether the plan had good or bad effects, and what these effects had been. Twenty-eight percent of physicians said that the plan had had no good effect on care, 60 percent said there had been some good effect, and 54 percent said there had been some bad effect. The investigators conclude that the physicians had "mixed feelings" about the plan because they recognized, on the one hand, the advantages of removing financial barriers and, on the other hand, the disadvantages of the increased pressure on themselves for service. Nevertheless, a majority of physicians said medical treatment had remained the same, 17 percent said that it had improved, and 18 percent that it had become worse. Unrestrained by any vested interest in maintaining appearances, clients were even more likely to perceive and report deterioration in quality. "Only 8.0 percent of the population believed that the quality of care had improved . . . and 29.7 percent thought it was worse" (91, p. 1177). However, it is difficult to interpret this finding, since, both before and after the plan, a little over 90 percent of respondents said the care they had received at their last visit had been the best possible. That adverse opinion reflects difficulty in making an appointment when wanted is supported by the observation that persons in the higher income groups were somewhat less likely to say that care had improved and more likely to say that it had become worse, when compared to those of lower income.

Seasoning. All these changes, and the ones that we described earlier, show immediate or short-term consequences of the introduction of health care benefits. By their very nature, long-term consequences are much more difficult to study and to identify, since they require longer periods of observation. With the passage of time, so many other events intervene that it is not possible to say, with any confidence, which causes have contributed to what effects.

There are a number of factors that could be presumed to play a role in what has been called "seasoning" of an insured population—a maturation in outlook and stability in behavior which develops after some time in a plan. A new program must deal with a backlog of unmet needs, which may include care that has been postponed while waiting for the program to become operational, so that service can be obtained under more favorable terms. These phenomena, which might be called the prior deprivation and deferment effects, lead to an expectation of higher levels of use early in the program with a tapering off in time. This consequence may be reinforced by the "testing effect": a tendency, on the part of some persons, to make immediate demands on the system largely to assure themselves that it will respond when they really need it. The medical care program itself may contribute to this initial surge in utilization by instituting procedures that are primarily meant to detect unrecognized illness or to prevent future morbidity, and by a more thorough investigation of all patients. Although the amount of illness detected and the use of care generated by this means depends on prior deprivation and deferment, the recognition of a discovery effect may help account for the separate contribution of the care-providing apparatus.

Contrary in action to all these factors is the effect of initial ignorance and unfamiliarity, which inhibits early use of service, and subsequent improvement in information and familiarity, which would tend to gradually increase utilization during the first few years of the program. The trend towards greater utilization with the passage of time is, no doubt, reinforced by the aging effect. This is likely to be particularly marked in a new program that embraces a population that is very large in proportion to the number who will enroll in each of future years. In this situation, one can expect yearly increments in the demand for services as the average age of the enrollees increases, until a point of equilibrium is attained, as a result of new enrollments on the one hand,

and terminations through death or loss of eligibility on the other. The demand-enhancing effect of aging may be counteracted, at least in theory, by the "health improvement or maintenance effect" that presumably attends more ready access to good care. One particular aspect of this, which has not attracted sufficient attention, is the possible presence of a risk attrition effect, at least with respect to certain conditions that require care (94). For example, removal of tonsils, appendices, and other organs is a once-in-a-lifetime event, so that once these operations have been performed they are seldom if ever repeated. Child-bearing is another event for which the likelihood may decrease after an initial period of high risk during which those pregnancies that are wanted and planned for have occurred.

The effects of seasoning are counteracted or stabilized to the extent that there is a relatively large flow of reasonably representative or typical enrollees in and out of the program. Because of its stabilizing effect, such a flow is considered to be an important safeguard in underwriting group insurance. One should also remember that all the presumed changes in the enrolled population interact with more generalized trends in the medical care system as a whole, and prepayment contributes to those trends in varying degrees. For example, as we have described in an earlier section, a spiral may be created in which demand creates supply, and supply, in turn, creates its own demand, unless demand is externally constrained by higher prices, limits on supply, or more direct controls on use of service. The long term effects of improved health are likely to be counteracted, as we have suggested, by the additional demands of an older population, by technological advances, and by rising levels of expectation. Finally, it must be obvious to the reader that these several immediate, intermediate, and long term effects often act at cross purposes, so that it is difficult to say what their resultant would be in any given situation. However, if one were forced to predict the effects on utilization of a large, new medical care program, one would postulate a small initial peak, mainly due to unsatisfied or deferred demand, followed, after a small dip, by a slowly but steadily rising level of use.

As we have intimated, empirical evidence bearing on seasoning is difficult to obtain. In one relevant study, Avnet has reported levels of use in a voluntary program, with enrollees classified by number of years enrolled (95). The findings are shown in Figure 6. The several ambulatory and inpatient services that were examined show no consistent trend other than a general tendency for a slow increase in use; the single exception was non-maternity hospital days, which have tended to decline. The hypothetical pattern we have described (initial peak-dip-slow increase) is approximated by only a few services: hospital surgical procedures, office specialist consultations, and, possibly, office preventive services. The percent of members who make one or more claims during a given year, when shown by duration of enrollment, conforms very well to expectation (95, Table 35, p. 99). Unfortunately, Avnet's data cover only one year, with enrollees classified by length of enrollment, and do not include a follow-up of a cohort of enrollees as they season with time. Consequently, the yearly cohorts may differ not only in duration of enrollment but in other characteristics as well. Not only are we given no assurance of comparability, but are told that "a correlation not attributable to length of time in [the program] was also found between duration of enrollment and age—a finding which there was no reason to suspect in advance but which, once unveiled, eliminated duration of coverage from consideration as an independent utilization variable" (95, p. 49). It is a pity that we are not told the nature of the relationship in question so we could take account of it in the interpretation of the findings.

Cohorts of new enrollees have occasionally been observed over short periods of time, and the findings that have been reported are often difficult to interpret. Two such studies will be described in greater detail in a subsequent chapter. In a study of a program of "family-focused" pediatric care for low-income families, Alpert et al. reported an unusually large number of outpatient visits for preventive purposes, and a relatively high rate of hospital admissions during the first 6 months following enrollment (96). This suggests the influence of a "discovery effect." In another study, reported by Bellin et al., there was no evidence of an initial peaking in hospital use after the establishment of a health center in a low-income public housing development. There was, however, a steady decline in hospital use. This decline is difficult to explain, but it could have been due, at least in part, to risk attrition in a

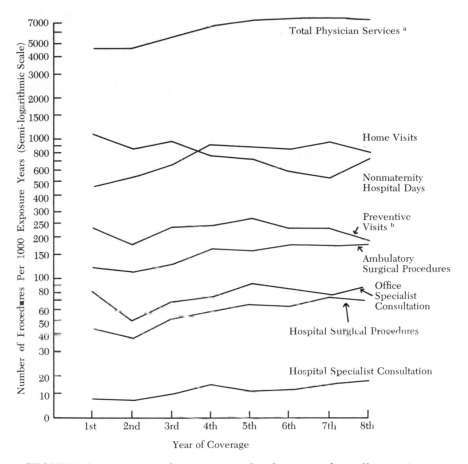

FIGURE 6. Service utilization rates, by duration of enrollment, Group Health Insurance Program (New York and New Jersey, 1954–1967).

Source: Reference 95, Tables 66, 74, 78, 84, 108 and 145, on pp. 139, 155, 162, 169, 207, 397. Reproduced by permission from *Medical Care Chart Book*, School of Public Health, The University of Michigan.

[a] Physician services include office calls and home calls, one physician service for each day of hospitalization, diagnostic x-rays, and certain laboratory tests.

[b] Preventive visits include office services not associated with the diagnosis and treatment of specific illness.

reasonably stable panel of enrollees (97). More recently, the Office of Economic Opportunity has reported on the experience in several of their programs in neighborhood health centers and prepaid group practice plans (98, 99). Almost uniformly, enrollees use ambulatory care services at a higher rate during the first six months than they do later. Unfortunately, there is no information concerning use of service prior to enrollment, and the period of observation, from a year to 18 months, is too short to indicate whether this early stabilization will be sustained. The populations in several of the prepaid group practice programs were selected in favor of "larger, high risk families with current illness or recent pregnancy" (99, p. 68). In some of the neighborhood health centers it was difficult to say who was an "active registrant," so that special procedures had to be developed to estimate the denominator of the utilization rates (98). In some programs, "outreach" activities were in effect to encourage use of service. For these, and other reasons, it is not known to what extent the findings of these studies can be generalized.

In all the studies so far reviewed, with the possible exception of the last (99), the intent is to reveal how the behavior of individuals changes as they stay longer in the program, rather than to document the aggregate experience of the program as a whole as time passes. The two experiences are, of of course, related; but the degree of correspondence depends on the rapidity of turnover in membership, and on the characteristics of the newly enrolled as compared to those who have died or have left for other reasons. Aggregate program effects beyond the first year have been assessed by Pettengill in a compilation of data on the possible effects of Medicare (91). Information was obtained from 6 different sources, including data from the Household Interview and the Hospital Discharge surveys of the National Center for Health Statistics; data reported to the American Hospital Association and published in their Journal; and data assembled by the Social Security Administration from service records and from the Current Medicare Survey. Though these sources are not fully comparable, because of peculiarities which the author describes, it is believed that the trends revealed by the different sources can be usefully examined together. One finds a substantial increase in hospital use during roughly the first year after the implementation of Medicare. During this period there was a 10 to 11 percent increase in admissions, a 6 to 12 percent increase in length of stay, and a resultant 19 to 25 percent increase in total patient-days of care for persons 65 and over. During the next two years, 1968 and 1969, admissions to the hospital continued to increase but at a declining rate; since 1969, the increase in admissions has leveled off at about 1 percent per year. However, length of stay began to decline in 1969, so that absolute values for days of care have decreased a little between 1969 and 1971. The author discusses several factors that may explain these trends, including initial access to care for the approximately 50 percent of the aged who did not have voluntary health insurance when Medicaid came into force; postponement of elective surgery until after the institution of Medicare; increasing knowledge of the benefits available under the program; and the depletion of unmet need and the establishment of a new equilibrium. Needless to say, many of these explanations are little more than conjectures. Besides, we do not know how much of the deceleration and relative stabilization in hospital use can be attributed to increases in deductibles, stricter administrative review of utilization, and a continuing increase in prices. Another peculiarity of a program for the aged, that may not apply in other cases, is the relatively rapid turnover due to mortality, and the constrained margin for further aging because of current limits on life span. However, even for Medicare, stability in the size and composition of the enrolled population cannot be assumed. It is known, for example, that between 1966 and 1971, although enrollments have exceeded deaths, the population of female enrollees in the Hospital insurance program has risen from 57.4 to 58.4 percent, and the proportion of persons 75 and over has increased from 37.2 to 39.9 percent. Both these changes would be expected to increase use of service (100, pp. xvii–xxi).

Policy Implications

It is a truism that the policy implications of the hypothesized and observed relationships between benefits and use of service— as modified by population characteristics, price, and supply— depend on the program objectives and the broader social goals that are to be pursued. So far we have considered, in one context or another, six objectives. One is the reduction of uncertainty (referred to by some as "risk") without any change in the probability of occurrence or the magnitude of loss. A second objective is the allocation of more resources to medical care. A third is the reduction of the burden of medical care expenditures, by which is meant a reduction of their effect on the standard of living. A fourth is more equal distribution of health services among classes, geographic areas, and other social divisions. A fifth objective is allocative efficiency, which may be taken to mean a principle of proportionality rather than of equality—or of equality recast as proportionality. We suggested that alternative objectives in allocation might be (a) adjustment to personal preferences, (b) adjustment to some balance of personal and social preferences, and (c) adjustment to the likelihood of generating "health potential" through health care. We also proposed that under certain assumptions these several rules for allocation might lead to very similar solutions. The sixth, and final, objective is the efficiency of production, which is the use of the least costly method of care to generate any given amount of health potential.

If the objective is merely the reduction of uncertainty, any change in behavior attributed to the provision of benefits is moral hazard, and means must be found to control it. What means there are, and how they might work, will be discussed below. The second objective—the allocation of more resources to medical care without any change in its distribution—would mean raising the lowest level of use to a more adequate level without putting limits on the higher levels. We have seen that there is some tendency for this to happen when benefits are made available, because segments of the population that already have high levels of utilization tend to make more effective use of the new benefits. This tendency is reinforced if, in addition to a basic public program, individuals may buy voluntary health insurance or pay for services out-of-pocket. The tendency is counteracted if there are constraints on buying voluntary insurance or services, or if supply is limited. Under these constraints one is more likely to attain the objective of redistribution. However, as we have seen, full equalization does not usually occur; very often, there are structural barriers to access, such as lack of information, social or cultural handicaps, and geographic barriers due to maldistribution of resources. One must also pay attention to costs other than the costs of medical care itself, including travel and the costs of staying away from work. In general, the objective of equalization, in order to be fully realized, requires much more than the simple provision of benefits. In some ways, the problem becomes even more difficult if the intent is both to increase the aggregate resources allocated to medical care, and to attain equalization, or, alternatively, allocation in proportion to need or health payoff. It is politically more feasible to adopt a policy that offers an increase of medical care for all; but if this course is adopted, one loses the use of instruments, such as limits on supply, that bring about redistribution. Greater access to all, with adjustment of use to need or to payoff, seems to require for implementation a large element of professional judgment and control over the medical care system. For this reason, and also to achieve efficiency in production, pains should be taken to assure that professional judgment is not distorted by financial incentives or by limits on the range of benefits. We shall return to this latter subject under the heading of substitution.

The objective of reducing the "financial burden" of medical care, especially for the poor, can be interpreted in more than one way. It could mean simply the reduction of uncertainty, so that expenses are predictable and budgetable, with the standard of living established accordingly. A corollary to this is that premiums should cover all or a large share of charges, so that out-of-pocket expenditures are absent or small. To the extent that this is not true, uncertainty remains, and people are subject to sharp temporary or long-term reductions in their customary standard of living because of the costs of receiving care for acute or chronic illness. Reducing the financial burden of medical care may also mean reducing the proportion of income allocated to medical care, even assuming that uncertainty has been eliminated. The object of this protection is to permit lower-income people to maintain a higher customary standard of living than would be possible if they had to pay the cost of all of the medical care they used under a program with extended benefits. In this way health benefits are used as a means to achieve income redistribution, a subject which we shall develop in a later chapter.

The empirical evidence we have described suggests that, under certain circumstances, health insurance will increase outlays for medical care (including premium payments) so that insured families in all income groups spend a greater proportion of their income on medical care. As shown in Table 6, this takes a particularly large bite out of the income of poor families who are insured. If the purpose is to reduce uncertainty without increasing the percentage of income devoted to medical care, it may be necessary to introduce deterrents to large increases in use of service because of insurance. But this raises new technical and policy questions. The technical question is what kinds of deterrents are available that do not involve out-of-pocket payments, which would only reintroduce uncertainty. The policy question is whether it is socially desirable to limit use of service by the poor.

Needless to say, we have not described all possible combinations of policy objectives and how their attainment would be influenced by the known effects of the provision of benefits in different settings. However, we hope enough has been said to indicate the types of issues that arise, and to prepare the reader for further exploration as the occasion demands. It seems to the author that social policy should aim to achieve the following several objectives *concurrently:* (1) to increase the allocation of resources to medical care; (2) to bring about a greater degree of equalization, at least to the extent of adjusting use of service to payoff in health potential; (3) to safeguard efficiency in production; (4) to reduce uncertainty; and (5) to achieve greater equalization in the proportion of income used for health care. The question of how to achieve these objectives brings us to a consideration of certain instrumentalities that are available to contain and direct the effects of insurance on use of service.

Implications for Action and Implementation

Certain devices have been traditionally used to contain and control those consequences of the provision of benefits that have been seen as a threat to the program or to its objectives. Since the emphasis in most programs has been on cost containment, the devices used have been intended to restrain the increased use of service that could be brought about by the provision of benefits. Some of these controls have been directed at the client, others at the provider, and still others are designed to have a pervasive effect on the system. Among those pervasive forces are constraints on supply, such as limits on the number of physicians trained or the number of hospitals built. Among the more direct controls on client behavior, the most prevalent is the inclusion in benefit design of financial barriers in the form of deductibles and copayments. In the past, the controls on providers have generally been in the form of price controls, particularly fee schedules or other limits on fees. Recently, attention has focused on changing the method of payment to make the physician, or group of physicians, responsible for providing to a specified population a specified range of services. These services would include not only the physician's own services, but other services as well. (101). This form of essentially contractual practice has often been advocated, but it has been implemented only in a limited way, under the misleadingly euphemistic appellation of "health maintenance organization" (102). In its most highly developed form, the health maintenance organization would correspond to certain prepaid group practices that restructure both the monetary, and the professional incentives to the physician. We have already reviewed briefly what effect such an arrangement is likely to have on use of service.

A modicum of professional supervision can also be exercised through the institution of mechanisms for utilization and quality review within the group practice, the ambulatory care clinic, or the hospital. Alternatively, or additionally, this supervision may be imposed externally by a professional association, an insurance carrier, or a public program (103). Until recently, the exercise of such control over private practice in general, and over private office practice in particular, has been very difficult to implement effectively. Under recent legislation, Professional Standards Review Organizations (PSROs) will be set up on a local area basis, with related councils at the state and federal levels (104). Certain prototypes are already in operation (105–107). The mandate of these agencies is only to review care under specified public programs, including Medicare and Medicaid, and to first review inpatient care; however, their effect could be more pervasive.

In analyzing benefits and benefit design, the possible effects of deductibles and copayments must be discussed in some detail. An attempt to deal with other controls on use of service would constitute a major undertaking in itself. It should be emphasized, however, that all controls should be judged in terms of how their expected or actual effects jibe with the objectives being pursued. As we have seen, limits on supply can aid redistribution of service while they put the lid on increases in aggregate use. Fee-for-service payments to physicians encourage over-use, while per capita payments encourage under-use. I am convinced that financial incentives and disincentives to providers, clients, or both, while effective in encouraging certain tendencies, are not sufficiently discriminating to bring about the adjustment of use to need. This fine tuning can only be brought about by introducing undistorted professional judgment as a major determinant of use of service, provided that free access has been assured in the first place. An attempt to influence professional judgment by imposing professional review over a balky and essentially hostile system is not likely to be successful. What is needed is a reorganization of the delivery of care so that the behavior of clients and providers is continuously subjected to influences that are congenial to program objectives. Formal professional review activities can then function as one element in a larger system of influences. The function of formal review is to adjust use more closely to need, and to provide continuing information on deviations from adjustment, so that action can be taken, first to find out why the deviation has taken place, and then to correct its causes.

Deductibles and Copayments

Deductibles are obligations that a consumer must assume for the initial services that he has received, before any further services will be covered by benefits under insurance, or any other programs that provide health services. Deductible obligations may be stated as a specified sum of money, a percent of charges, or a quantity of service. For example, in 1974, Medicare beneficiaries were required to pay the first $84 of hospital charges under Part A of the program and the first $60 of physicians' services and other services under Part B. Under Part A, access to extended care facilities or home health services was limited to those who had stayed in the hospital for 3 days and who had thereby, in effect, paid the deductible for that service.

Copayment, or coinsurance, refers to payment by the consumer of a portion of the charges made for care. Such payments are usually stated as a specified percentage of charges, but they may also be stated as a flat dollar sum per specified quantity of services received. For example, under Medicare in 1974, beneficiaries were required to pay $21 for each day of hospital care from the 61st through the 90th day; a daily $10.50 from the 21st through the

100th day of care in an extended care facility; and 20 percent (beyond the first $60) of the reasonable charge for the services of a physician under Part B of the program.

Expected Effects.   The insurance industry has long held that it would be an open invitation to "moral hazard" and abuse to cover all or the major share of the cost of medical care in any episode of illness. Deductibles and copayments have been the major tool in implementing this belief. While deductibles and copayments serve the same general function, their modes of action are somewhat dissimilar. Deductibles are intended to deter the initiation of care. It is expected that they will not influence receipt of care subsequent to initiation, unless the deductible is so large that it appreciably reduces the ability to pay. While copayments, may influence the initiation of care, they are intended to act after initiation to restrain the client from demanding or accepting more care or more expensive care than is considered customary or "necessary." Copayments are expected to have an increasingly inhibiting effect as charges for care mount up, because the absolute amount of the copayment increases if the copayment is a fixed percentage of the charges. In theory, deductibles and copayments should exert their influence at many points in the client-physician interaction. They are expected to restrain the client from making demands, or from complying with proposals made by the physician, if the client would not have demanded or complied in the absence of insurance. Deductibles and copayments are also expected to restrain the physician, who presumably takes costs to the patient into account, from proposing less necessary or more expensive types of care. In addition, these participatory payments may preserve a residue of consumer resistance to increased prices in the medical marketplace. Ideally insurance would cause no change at all in client or physician behavior. Since this is patently unrealistic to expect, it is hoped that deductibles and copayments would moderate increases in the use of service that are due to the presence of insurance, and that this moderating effect would differentially inhibit care that has lower priority in the estimate of the patient, the physician, or both. In this way, these participatory payments are expected to restrain expenditures for medical care, and reduce departures from efficiency. When expenditures for care are contained by restraints on the use of service and on prices, costs to the insurer are reduced, which contributes to financial solvency, higher profits, or the sale of insurance at lower prices. This strengthens the financial position of the insurer in absolute terms, as well as relative to competitors in the market. To some degree, participatory payments reduce costs to the insurer and prices to the consumer, even when they have no effect on client or provider behavior. This cost reduction comes about in two ways. First, because part of the charges are paid by the client, the insurer has less to pay. This is simply a transfer of obligations from the insurer to the client. Second, the presence of a deductible disqualifies a certain number of claims from consideration, thus reducing the administrative costs of the insurer. Since these costs are relatively fixed, irrespective of the size of the claim, the insurance agency, or the program providing benefits, reduces its administrative costs relative to the benefits it provides. To these very "practical" considerations of corporate self-interest a value ingredient might be added, to the effect that it is important to maintain in our society a modicum of personal responsibility and self-reliance in meeting the hazards of life. Finally, to return to more pragmatic considerations, one must ponder what other alternatives are open in a "free market" to the insurer who needs to control client and provider behavior. Since direct controls have not been feasible, or are ideologically repugnant, indirect controls through participatory payments become necessary and attractive.

To summarize, those advocating deductibles and coinsurance would see advantages to the insurer, the client, and society at large, as follows: (1) from the viewpoint of the insurer these devices are feasible and effective in reducing costs through (a) restraining utilization, (b) restraining increases in the price of services, (c) transferring some costs to the client, and (d) contributing to more efficient processing of claims; (2) from the viewpoint of the client they lower the price of buying insurance, certainly in absolute terms and possibly relative to benefits obtained; (3) from the viewpoint of society the advantages include (a) restraints on expenditures for care, (b) restraints on price inflation, (c) restraints on misallocation, (d) maintenance of certain social values, and (e) avoidance of more direct and more centralized controls.

Those who oppose the use of deductibles and copayments point out that they hinder access to care in proportion to need and do not help redress the disproportionate financial burden borne by the poor and the sick. First, it is pointed out that the expectation that no change should occur in client or provider behavior is based on a false premise; it is an important objective to bring about such change. Of course, the appropriateness of the change in behavior is recognized as a relevant issue, but it is contended that participatory payments do not restrain misallocation, but have the opposite net effect. This occurs when deductibles and copayments inhibit the initiation of care, making it impossible for the physician to investigate the situation and arrive at a true estimate of need. Second, copayments become larger in absolute quantity as the disease lasts longer and becomes more severe; this may represent improper allocation since, as Pauly has suggested, it is precisely in such situations that society should wish to encourage use of service (3, pp. 38–59). A third important reason why participatory payments result in misallocation is that they more thoroughly inhibit the poor, who have more need for care, than the rich, who have less. Needless to say, this effect also runs counter to the objective of social equalization in access to care. The intent to reduce uncertainty and to reduce the impact of health expenditures on the standard of living is also compromised by participatory payments. There is still uncertainty to the extent that all charges are not covered, and participatory payments are expressed as a proportion of the covered charges, which are themselves unpredictable. Participatory payments transfer obligations to the ill, at a time when they are least able to meet these obligations. Furthermore, relative to income, the payments fall most heavily on the poor, who are also more likely to be ill.

Thus, deductibles and copayments make it more difficult to achieve net transfers of purchasing power in favor of the ill and the poor. In the worst of all possible worlds, participatory payments would fail to make an appreciable impact on price or use of service but would continue to have their adverse effects on uncertainty and on transfers of purchasing power Those who rely on participatory payments by the client may have greatly overestimated the control the client can exercise on the recommendations of the provider, especially if the latter is attracted by the revenue generating prospects of insurance. Even the contention that deductibles produce relative reductions in administrative costs has been challenged, on the grounds that administering a system of deductibles and copayments has its own costs. These costs fall partly on the insurer and partly on the client and the provider, both of whom must maintain the necessary records, and who sometimes, through oversight or error, lose benefits to which they are entitled. Finally, the administrative advantages occur only if it is assumed that payments are made on a fee-for-service basis, and are made separately for each episode; fewer claims would have to be processed, since charges below the deductible would not be covered. When there is no deductible, processing can be simplified if claims are aggregated, and can be further reduced, or eliminated, if payment is not on a fee-for-service basis.

The conclusion is that deductibles and copayments are inimical to almost all the social good that is supposed to be accomplished through the provision of benefits, and that whatever needs to be done to control price or to limit less than necessary use of services will have to be accomplished in some other way. There is another conclusion that some have reached: namely, that deductibles and coinsurance are useful if their misallocative effects are corrected (3, 108, 109). This correction is made by varying participatory payments so that while they increase with income, they decrease as a proportion of charges as the total of charges increases. We shall return to these schemes in a subsequent chapter which deals with income redistribution. In anticipation of that discussion, three questions might be raised. First, can such schemes achieve the desired fine adjustment between use of service and need, or will they require the additional imposition of more direct administrative or professional controls? Second, how cumbersome and costly is implementation and administration of such programs? Finally, what steps can be taken to prevent the private purchase of additional insurance from subverting the elegantly graduated system of financial disincentives and subsidies incorporated in a public program? For example, it is ironical to see the finely constructed system of benefits and deterrents in the Medicare program become largely inoperative because of the purchase by beneficiaries of private insurance designed to neutralize precisely those features of the program that were meant to inhibit less necessary or less efficient use.

Empirical Observations. So far we have engaged in speculation concerning the possible effects of participatory payments, ar-
guing for or against them in the light of expected rather than substantiated effects. We need to turn now to empirical studies that
document these effects. But before we look at the evidence, it
might be useful to remind ourselves what it is we want to know.
First, it is important to remember that our concern goes beyond
the advantages to the insurer, to include the impact on the client,
and the consequences to the attainment of social objectives. Second, we ought to distinguish two general kinds of consequences.
One category consists of transfers of obligations from one party to
another, usually from the insurer to the client simply because the
plan specifies what the insurers will reimburse and what they will
not. These transfers are purely matters of accounting and may be
spoken of as "arithmetic consequences." This is not to say that
they are unimportant, but simply that they are thoroughly determined by the way the situation is defined. The other category of
transfers depends on how the behavior of clients or providers is
actually altered by the presence of participatory payments; it is
this category that will occupy a greater share of our attention.

A third point that needs to be made is that deductibles and
copayments should be kept distinct, since although they are often
lumped together in usage and in evaluation, they could prove to
have partly different behavioral effects. Among the possible effects, we intend to look for several that are of particular interest.
For example, we would want to distinguish effects on the initiation of care from effects on the continuation of care, and to further
subdivide these effects by type of service. These distinctions are
important because the degree to which clients or physicians play a
deciding role differs by these categories. Moreover, it is important
to know whether reduction in initiation of care is compensated for
by lengthening of care, either because illness has progressed, or
because clients are motivated to compensate for the deductible. It
is equally important to know if there are other compensatory reactions such as a substitution of services that are not constrained by
deterrents for those that are, or a rise in prices so that the provider
can recoup what he has lost through a reduction in use. Of particular importance is the need to see if participatory payments have a
graded effect. Too often one hears of participatory payments either

having or not having an effect, as if the response to this stumulus were all-or-nothing. If, on the contrary, we expect a graded response to a graded stimulus, it would be reasonable to ask if there is a true threshold below which there is no effect and above which a progressively larger effect becomes discernible. At the same time, it would be important to know what determines the magnitude of the stimulus: the absolute quantity of the participatory payment, its relation to associated benefits, its magnitude relative to charges for alternative services, or its magnitude relative to income? Finally, it would be most important to know not only the differential effects of participatory payments by income and social class, but also by type and severity of illness.

In seeking answers to these questions we are handicapped by severe limitations in the usual sources of data, and by weaknesses of design in most of the studies that have used the data. Almost all of the information we have comes from the records of insurers, and these data compare persons who have insurance benefits without deductibles or copayments with those whose policies include these features. In some instances the benefits are not completely comparable, as they should be. In other instances, the locales differ, so that we do not know if the observations can be attributed to the features of the benefits or to the more general characteristics of the settings in which the plans operate (110). Even when the plans are in force within the same locale, the populations enrolled are often not fully comparable. The most important reason for this population difference is self-selection in the purchase of insurance. Persons who are likely to use service generally purchase the more complete forms of coverage, while those who do not expect to need care either choose a less generous plan at the start or may selectively drop out of a plan that has extended its benefits. These self-selective tendencies are probably much less powerful in group enrollment, especially when the employer pays all or a major share of the premium, than they are in the individual purchase of insurance. Nevertheless, even large groups may differ from each other in age, sex, income, and other characteristics. It is seldom that the insurer has data that will permit adjustments for the effects of such social and demographic variables. Another limitation in the data possessed by the insurer is that they pertain only to claims made on the insurer. Use of service below the level of a deductible is not recorded. Nor is there complete information about charges for noncovered services or payments made by other insurers. Thus, we have information on the obligations met by the major insurer, but not on the total services received or the charges incurred by the client. To determine the latter it is usually necessary to interview the client directly.

There is, of course, no doubt that deductibles and copayments transfer obligations to the client. Needless to say, the degree to which this transfer occurs depends on the nature of the benefits and the type and magnitude of participatory payments. For example, during January to December 1969, of all charges for services covered under Part B of Medicare, 4 percent did not meet the deductible, 15 percent were paid by the deductible, and 16% were paid through copayment by the client. Thus, deductible and copayment provisions brought about a 35 percent reduction in the obligations of the insurer, before correction for the cost of administering these provisions (111). The magnitude of what we have called the "arithmetic effects" of applying a $50 deductible were estimated by Jesmer and Scharfenberg by excluding both hospital admissions and covered charges below the $50 level from the reported experience of the Federal Employees Health Benefit Program (117). This exclusion would have resulted in a 2.9 percent reduction in hospital admissions and a 0.8 percent reduction in the number of days of care that would have had at least some coverage. Since the admissions that did not generate covered charges exceeding $50 must have been very short, the average length of stay for the remaining admissions would have been increased by 2.1 percent. Costs to the plan would have been reduced almost 15 percent by excluding covered charges incurred by admissions that did not exceed the deductible, and by subtracting $50 from all the remaining admissions that did. Needless to say, this was a purely hypothetical computation which did not include costs of administering the deductible, and assumed that in all other respects utilization of service and prices would remain constant. Under similar assumptions, an earlier study by Sellers reports the effects on insurance payments of excluding the covered charges for 1, 2, 3, etc., days of hospital stay. Sellers also reports the hypothetical arithmetic effects of an unusual form of benefit in which the entire stay is covered, but only if the stay exceeds a specified duration (112).

As we have said, these arithmetic consequences of deductibles and copayments are totally predictable in each particular situation, except that they can be considerably modified by the reactive, behavioral effects that may also occur. Bearing on these latter effects, there is only a small body of literature with imprecisely defined boundaries. Studies of deductibles and copayments are not clearly distinguishable from studies of the extent of services covered and the completeness of the insurer's financial responsibility for these services. In some ways the issue is the same: namely, the less than complete payment by the insurer of charges for medical care. However, in this section we shall deal, in the main, with studies of deductible and copayment features, as narrowly defined. In a later chapter on substitution effects we shall review studies that deal with the effect of covering more or fewer services, either in part or in full. Studies that do not fall neatly into either category will be described in whatever context makes their contribution most meaningful. (For the reader's convenience, the studies that we have reviewed are listed in the bibliography in the order in which they were published [112–124].) Among the studies, the paper by Hall is notable for providing an early assessment of the situation and adding new empirical material (115). Further reviews are to be found in the papers by Williams (116), by Jesmer and Scharfenberg (117), and by Heaney and Riedel (118). The paper by Heaney and Riedel, as well as the paper by Hardwick et al. (120), discuss problems of measurement and research design. The studies by Heaney and Riedel (118), and by Weisbrod and Fiesler (55), are notable for providing before and after comparisons between an "experimental" group that experienced the effect of participatory payments, and a reasonably contemporaneous control group that did not. The most recent study, described by Scitovsky and Snyder (121), and also by Phelps and Newhouse (34), has the distinction of dealing with events in the most highly controlled situation so far described, of using multivariate methods of analysis, and of attempting to elucidate the allocative effects of copayments; however, it lacks a contemporaneous control. Having made these acknowledgements, we shall now attempt to develop certain lines of evidence that bear on our concerns.

The first large-scale study in our series was made by Williams (116), who used data from a 1964 survey of Blue Cross Plans to identify plans each of which offered two forms of coverage—full and participatory payment—and that also provided sufficient information to allow comparisons to be made. Of the five pairs he cites, we have selected four (A, B, C, and D) that had information on age and sex of members. We hope to minimize the effects of self-selection by including only persons enrolled in groups, and by adjusting for age and sex differences between groups that had full coverage and those that had coverage subject to a deductible or copayment.

The plans can be classified into three categories. The first category includes Plans A and B; each of these plans offers both full coverage and deductible coverage, with comparable services covered. The second category includes only Plan C, in which the deductible policy covers more services, so that the presence of the deductible is not the only difference between deductible and full coverage. The third category comprises Plan D, in which both full pay and copayment policies were offered, with comparable coverage. In the first 3 plans (A, B, C), the deductible ranged from $20 to $25 per admission, and in the fourth plan (D) there was a copayment of $4 per day. Unfortunately, we are not told what proportion of daily charges these amounts represent. One suspects that they were relatively small: the deductible may represent approximately the charges for one day, and the copayment about 20 percent of daily charges. Also note that the copayment in Plan D is not a percent of charges but a flat daily sum, a feature that should encourage short, intensive hospital stays.

The key findings from Williams' study are summarized in Table 15. Based on these findings, the following conclusions appear to be reasonable. In Plans A and B, in which we observe the effects of the deductible alone, we find, as expected, fewer admissions and longer stay. The longer stay is attributable partly to the arithmetic effect of excluding from the insurer's data those admissions that did not meet the deductible. One must ask, however, whether the deductible has two additional effects: (1) a rise in the thresh-

TABLE 15. Hospital Utilization and Benefits Paid by Insurer,[a] Four Blue Cross Plans, by Presence of Deductible and Copayment Features, U.S.A., 1964

Measures of Hospital Utilization and Benefits Paid, by Plan	Full	Deductible	Copay	Percent Difference [b]
Admissions per 1000 members				
A	195	171		−12.3
B	184	169		− 8.2
C	116	137		18.1
D	156		136	−12.8
Days per stay				
A	6.2	6.6		6.5
B	6.9	7.6		10.1
C	7.4	7.3		− 1.4
D	8.4		8.3	− 1.2
Patient-days per 1000 members				
A	1,213	1,133		− 6.6
B	1,269	1,289		1.6
C	858	993		15.7
D	1,310		1,129	−13.8
Benefits paid per 1000 members				
A	$27,948	$30,467		9.0
B	26,679	31,615		18.5
C	15,230	27,832		82.7
D	40,667		$33,383	17.9

Source: Reference 116, Tables 1, 2, 5 and 6, pages 32, 33, 37 and 38.
   [a] All data are adjusted to account for differences in age and sex between the two categories of members within each plan.
   [b] "Full" minus "Deductible," or "Copay," as percent of "Full."

old of severity before admission is sought, and (2) a compensatory lengthening of stay to make up, psychologically or financially, for having paid the deductible: a kind of "deductible backlash"! In any event, the longer stays do eat into the reduction in patient-days brought about by the smaller number of covered admissions, to the extent of more than fully neutralizing the reduction in Plan B. Another compensatory phenomenon appears to be that those who have paid the deductible receive more care or more expensive care so that, rather than saving money, the insurer ends up paying more per day and per member. Explanations for this added expense are that those admitted under the deductible plan are more sick or, more probably, that the study design has not fully corrected for differences in population characteristics or in the settings within which patients receive care.

The experience with Plan C is interesting because it suggests that the additional benefits offered under the deductible plan have outweighed the effect of the deductible. Under the deductible plan as compared with the full coverage plan, admissions were more frequent and length of stay was only slightly shorter, so that the total number of patient-days was higher and the benefits much larger in spite of the deductible. There may, however, be other forces at play, since the utilization under both types of coverage in Plan C is so much lower than under the other plans. The experience with Plan D, which has a copayment feature but no deductible, suggests that the copayment not only reduces admissions but also exerts a restraining effect on length of stay. This effect is sufficient to prevent the expected arithmetic increase in length of stay and even to bring about a small decrease. The expectation that care will be more intensive is corroborated by the observation that covered daily charges, including the copayment, are 8 percent higher under the copayment policy (not shown in the table). Nevertheless, because patient days are fewer and the copayment is borne by the client, the insurer does save about 18 percent in payments under this plan as compared to the full-payment alternative. Thus, from the point of view of the insurer, copayment emerges as the more effective device to reduce costs. Needless to say, none of the data include the costs of administering the deductible and copayment features.

We have described Williams' study in some detail because it corresponds in part with our expectations. It suggests: (1) that deductibles and copayments have different effects; (2) that the effect of deductibles is mainly on initiation of care, whereas copayments may inhibit both initiation and continuation; (3) that the initial effect of deductibles may be neutralized by subsequent compensatory reactions; and (4) that the effects of participatory payments must be seen in the context of the total benefit package.

Confirmation of this last hypothesis may be found in a study by Weisbrod and Fiesler that we have described earlier (55). In this study, it was possible to examine changes in the experience of a group who had purchased insurance that reduced the share of the private room fee paid by the client and added complete coverage for diagnostic tests and other ancillary services. The experience of this group was compared with contemporaneous experience in a control group of those who had continued their coverage under the other, less generous plan. Three observations are germane to our current concerns. First, the more generous benefits were followed by a reduction rather than an increase in admissions to the hospital. Only by comparing the greater reduction in the control group can one conclude that the more generous benefits tended to increase admissions to the hospital. The relevance of research design is forcefully confirmed by the necessity of having a contemporary control in addition to the before-and-after comparison for the experimental group. The second observation is that the clients were apparently encouraged to enter hospitals in order to take advantage of the free diagnostic tests and other ancillary services. The third observation was that the reduction of the copayment for the private room charge (from about $8 to $6, out of a total extra charge of about $18 per day) was too small to bring about an appreciable change in the use of private room services. This suggested to the authors that below a certain "threshold," copayments may not have an effect on behavior, but merely represent an arithmetic transfer of obligations between insurer and client (55). However, one must point out that private rooms are often a luxury service, so that a small copayment may be sufficient to inhibit their use.

A more recent study by Heaney and Riedel (118) is relevant to the findings by Williams (116), as well as to the conclusions drawn by Weisbrod and Fiesler (55). Interestingly, the design was very similar to the study by Weisbrod and Fiesler: experience in a sample before and after conversion to full-pay coverage was compared to a reasonably contemporaneous experience in a sample who did not choose coverage under the expanded plan. In this instance, the group with more complete coverage experienced a small but statistically non-significant increase in admissions, a more definite increase in length of stay, and a "markedly significant" increase in patient-days, amounting to about 26 percent.

The findings of Williams (116), of Weisbrod and Fiesler (55), and of Heaney and Riedel (118), all confirm the expectation that copayments depress use of service and that their absence encourages such use, provided the copayments are large enough relative to the benefits. However, there are also unexplained differences, such as the absence of an effect on admissions in the study by Heaney and Riedel and the presence of this effect in the other two studies. Heaney and Riedel believe the lack of an effect of copayment on admissions to be reasonable since, in their opinion, people wouldn't be more likely to enter a hospital simply because daily charges were more fully covered, but would be likely to stay longer if this were the case. As we have said, Weisbrod and Fiesler believe, on the contrary, that people enter the hospital to take advantage of hospital benefits. There was, however, a difference in the two studies in the manner in which benefits were liberalized. In the study by Heaney and Riedel the change was from a fixed daily indemnity payment ($15) to a full payment of the daily charge, but there was no change in coverage of "special services, drugs, x-rays, etc." In the study by Weisbrod and Fiesler the extension of coverage was precisely in these ancillaries, and especially in diagnostic services, which became available without limit. Very tentatively, one might suggest that more complete coverage for the same services could have a different effect from more complete coverage achieved through the inclusion of a new set of services that are available only if a person is admitted to the hospital. It is conceivable, for example, that the availability of payment for diagnostic services in the hospital would encourage admissions and shorten average stay, because admissions for diagnosis tend to be short. On the other hand, more complete coverage of the daily charge might have a smaller enhancing effect on admissions and be more influential in lengthening average stay. We have suggested earlier that copayment expressed as a percent of charges is likely to decrease length of stay as well as other services for which charges are incurred, whereas a copayment expressed as a fixed sum per day might shorten stay but increase the demand for covered services during those fewer days. It is at least a tenable hypothesis that some of the inconsistencies found in studies of the effects of copayments and deductibles originate in details such as these. No doubt even greater differences are brought about by the broader medical care setting under which the plan operates.

The need to view participatory payments in the wider context of a medical care system is well illustrated in a study by Straight (114). The experience reported is that of the Swift Current Medical Plan, which provided the services of physicians to virtually all the residents of the Swift Current Health Region in the southwest corner of Saskatchewan, Canada. It is important to know that, at the same time, hospital services were covered by an independent, Province-wide hospital plan. During the first seven years of the Swift Current Plan, the physicians, who were paid fee-for-service, experienced increasingly high levels of utilization coupled with payment at levels lower than envisaged by the fee schedule—payments were lower because the sum of money available to reimburse physicians fell short of the claims made. Consequently, it was decided to introduce two changes: (1) designate a somewhat larger total sum of money to pay all physicians' fees, and (2) introduce so-called "utilization fees," which were small copayments (ranging from $1-$3) on office, home, and night calls, on the first visit for maternity care, and on minor surgery in the office. These fees were to be collected by the physicians and apparently were added directly to their income, over and above scheduled fee payments by the insurer. Thus, there was an incentive for clients to reduce demand, if they knew that a utilization fee was to be collected. The incentive to the physicians collectively was to reduce service, since this would not reduce total revenue to the physicians as a group, but would raise the fee for each service to bring it closer to the schedule. On the other hand, each physician could increase his own share of the total allocated to physician services by not reducing his services and by collecting the authorized copayments from the patient, at some risk of alienating him. The consequences of this rather complicated set of incentives was a reduction in office and home visits, an increase of physician visits in the hospital, and an increase in minor surgery. The sum of these changes was an increase in the actual fee for each service performed by the physician. However, after a few years, the frequency of home and office visits began to climb towards their previous level, and hospital visits began to decline slowly.

Needless to say, it is not easy to explain these events in the Swift Current Plan. It is possible, as the author suggests, that physicians decided early on not to insist on collecting the copayments, but to reduce office and home visits and substitute hospital care. Presumably this strategy would increase revenue relative to cost and maintain client good will. The author suggests that these effects were attenuated when clients found out that the copayment was seldom exacted. It could also be that the turnover of physicians and the growing supply of physicians in the population, to which the author alludes, reduced adherence to the collective understanding to cut back on services. The effect on minor surgery remains unexplained. Since virtually all residents were covered in this study, self-selection is not a disturbing influence. However, since the number of physicians was small (about 28 at the time the changes were introduced) any alteration in their characteristics would have an appreciable effect on patterns of care.

Unfortunately for those who seek in actual experience clear confirmation of theoretical expectations, not all studies have supported the impression we have gained so far: that deductibles and copayments dimish use of service if they are sufficiently large relative to the cost of service, but that a variety of compensatory or concurrent effects can neutralize the savings expected by the insurer or, even, increase the insurer's costs. On the one hand, we have reports that copayments have been ineffective, and on the other hand, reports that the net effect of deductibles has been to reduce use of service, costs to the insurer, and even the cost of care to the consumer. While findings that do not agree with our expectations can easily be ascribed to limitations in data and in research design, this may not always be the correct explanation. For example, in a reasonably well-designed "retrospective" study, Hardwick et al. compared hospital utilization by subscribers in a group that had a daily $5 copayment for hospital care with utilization by a sample of subscribers from 6 groups with benefits closely comparable to those of the first group but without copayment (120). In this study, there was no evidence that copayment, at the level specified, reduced admissions or shortened stay. The authors acknowledge that not all major factors that influence utilization were controlled in this study. For example, residence was only partially comparable and those in the group with copayment, who were more likely to live in the suburbs, were probably more likely to use suburban hospitals with lower occupancy and smaller charges. However, age and sex, which usually explain a large share of variation in use, were used as control variables in the analysis. Services covered by insurance were also comparable as were employee contributions to the premium. While differences in population characteristics and in medical care settings cannot be excluded as factors in concealing the effect of the copayment, the $5 copayment in this instance appears to have amounted to less than 10 percent of daily benefits, suggesting that it was an even smaller percent of total daily charges. Furthermore, as the author points out, the alternatives that the patient faces are not hospital care versus no care, but hospital care versus office care. Since office care is not covered by insurance, it may be less costly to the patient to be admitted to the hospital and pay a daily $5 fee than to receive care outside the hospital. In this study, male subscribers experienced 400 admissions during 1969. Insurance payments for this group were about $420 per admission, whereas the copayments were only $43 per admission. It is unlikely that anything like the care received in the hospital could be bought outside the hospital for $43, even in a very small proportion of these admissions. Whether patients or physicians make such computations in the selection of alternative forms of care, we do not know for certain. Rosenthal, in a study of the correlates of length of stay in a sample of New England hospitals, found length of stay more closely related to average daily charges than to out-of-pocket charges as a percent of the total charges (38). His conclusions suggest that our assumptions about the possible effects of copayments and deductibles may need to be revised. However, in this instance, the relationships between hospital charges, length of stay, and type of hospital were not examined. It can also be argued that prior knowledge of a participatory payment may have a different effect than an unpredictable and unknown eventual excess of charges over benefits.

Hall has cited several reports in which the introduction of deductibles of the same order of magnitude as those studied by Williams has considerably reduced payments by the insurer (115). In one such study, which we have summarized in Table 16, a $25 deductible was said to have brought about, within one year of its introduction in a fairly stable employee group, a 20 percent reduction in claims per insured, a 15 percent reduction in days per claim, and a 27 percent reduction in payments made by the plan.

TABLE 16.   Insurance Plan Data One Year Before and After Introduction of a $25 Deductible in Employee Group Plan, Place and Date Not Given

Insurance Plan Data	One Year Prior to Deductible	One Year After Deductible	Percent Difference [a]
Average number insured	2,713	2,472	− 9
Number of claims	420	299	
Claims per insured	0.15	0.12	−20
Days in hospital	2,295	1,394	
Hospital days per claim	5.5	4.7	−15
Hospital days per insured	0.84	0.56	−33
Benefits paid	$74,671.16 [b]	$49,450.53	
Benefit per claim	177.79	165.39	
Benefit per insured	27.52	20.00	
Reduction in benefit per insured	—	7.52	

Source: Reference 115, Table 1, p. 259.

[a] "After Deductible" minus "Prior to Deductible" as percent of former.

[b] Source table cites 47,671.16, which appears to be an error.

In this plan, all claims, including those that did not exceed the deductible, were supposed to have been reported. If so, the effects shown are free from arithmetic distortion. Further, if $25 is added to each claim (which overcorrects for the transfers to the client, since not all claims necessarily attain the full amount of the deductible) the cost of care is reduced 25 percent. Assuming this reduction is passed on to the consumer, the premium would be reduced by $7.52 per person insured, which is the trade-off for paying $25 each time an admission occurs, as well as for paying for care by the physician outside the hospital when this is discouraged by the deductible. Assuming hospitalization will be selected if the cost of care outside the hospital exceeds $25, the trade-offs would seem to be an assured gain of $7.52 per person per year, versus the uncertainty of incurring an additional $25 should hospitalization be required, and of incurring up to $25 for a condition that might have required hospitalization. These unusually favorable results were obtained in a very small, highly selected employee group which experienced about 10 percent attrition after the introduction of the deductible. Through no fault of the author, not enough details are available to assess the credibility of the findings in this and the other studies cited by Hall. However, this study has been described in some detail because it illustrates some important considerations in assessment, it contradicts the findings of those who have reported absent or less significant consequences, and it raises a useful degree of doubt in the reader's mind concerning our knowledge about the effects of deductibles.

None of the studies cited so far deals directly with the issue of the differential allocation of services to diseases of different severity or to persons of different income or social class. Concerning the latter, we can make some very tentative inferences from a study, reported by Roemer et al., of the patterns of care under three forms of insurance (52). The three forms studied were "provider-sponsored," "commercial," and "prepaid group practice" plans, all operating in Los Angeles County, California. For each category two plans were selected, one large and one small; each plan had a "reputation of excellence" in its category. Within each plan, enrollee groups were sampled randomly from a frame stratified by group size, followed by a random sample of families and single members within each group. Information was obtained by sending questionnaires through the mail, and by sampling hospital, clinic and office data. The study suffers because the plans were selected for their good reputation, rather than for being representative of their respective categories, and also because almost 50 percent of those to whom questionnaires were mailed did not respond. Furthermore, the members of the different plans were not completely comparable, due to a tendency for the prepaid group practice plans to attract persons with somewhat higher risk and for the commercial plans to attract persons with the lowest risk. Nevertheless, the findings do provide much food for thought; they are used here in a speculative vein, subject to certain assumptions. It is assumed that under prepaid group practice one has the truest estimate of the need for care because there are the fewest financial barriers to care and there are no revenue incentives to the physician to provide care. Under provider-sponsored plans there are usually no deductible or copayment features applicable to hospital care, even though the benefit may not always cover the entire bill. However, because payment to the physician is fee-for-service, there is an incentive to provide care. This is also true for the commercial plans, but these plans generally include financial disincentives to the client in the form of deductibles and copayments, and indemnification rather than service benefits. In this study, the commercial plans typically included a deductible of $100 and a copayment of about 20 percent.

Unfortunately for our purposes, these were not the only differences among plans. Most importantly, the prepaid group practice plans covered care outside the hospitals, while the other plans did not, or did so only to a very small degree. Table 17 shows hospital use by persons in each type of plan, with the persons categorized by social class as determined by Hollingshead's index, which is based on the occupation and education of the family head. Also shown are specified differences between plans. If one takes use of service under group practice as the norm, the addition of fee-for-service incentives to the physician appears to increase admissions and lengthen stay in both social classes (Row D of Table 17). Admissions are particularly affected in the lower class whereas length of stay is influenced to a greater degree in the upper class. Since changes in case mix influence the length of stay, differences in stay are not easy to interpret. However, as a product of the two sets of differences, there is a marked increase in patient-days of hospital care, with a much larger absolute difference in the lower class but a larger relative difference in the upper class. The decided service-enhancing effect of the fee-for-service incentive can be viewed as additional evidence of the importance of the revenue effect. In our next comparison (Row E of Table 17) we attempt to infer the effect of adding financial disincentives to the client, in the form of deductibles, copayments, and less than complete indemnification for hospital charges, while maintaining a fee-for-service incentive to the physician. The effect in the upper class is ambiguous, since the reduction in admissions is more than compensated for by longer stays. In the lower class, though, there is a reduction in admission, little change in length of stay, and a considerable overall reduction in patient days. Thus, participatory payments appear to have a much larger impact in reducing hospital care among the lower class. Since we began by assuming that the use of service in the prepaid group practice plans is the norm, we cannot judge whether the smaller volume of care in the commercial plans is appropriate. For that judgment we have to turn to row F of Table 17 which compares commercial

TABLE 17. Yearly Hospital Admissions and Days per 1000 Persons, Length of Stay per Admission, and Specified Differences in Hospital Use, by Category of Insurance Plans and by Social Class, Los Angeles County, 1967–1968

Categories of Plans and Differences Between Specified Categories	Lower Class			Upper Class		
	Adm.	LOS[a]	Days	Adm.	LOS[a]	Days
A. Prepaid group practice plans	117	7.3	858	80	1.8	148
B. Provider-sponsored plans	196	8.8	1735	90	3.7	335
C. Commercial plans	110	9.2	1119	67	5.7	381
D. "Provider" minus "Group"; attributed to MD incentive	+79 (+68%)	+ 1.5 (+21%)	+877 (+102%)	+10 (+12%)	+ 1.9 (+106%)	+187 (+126%)
E. "Commercial" minus "Provider": attributed to adding client disincentives to MD incentives	−86 (−44%)	+ 0.4 (+ 5%)	−616 (− 36%)	−23 (−26%)	+ 2.0 (+ 54%)	+ 46 (+ 14%)
F. "Commercial" minus "Group": attributed to MD incentives plus client disincentives	− 7 (− 6%)	+ 1.9 (+26%)	+261 (+ 30%)	−13 (−16%)	+ 3.9 (+217%)	+233 (+157%)

Source: Reference 52, pp. 20 and 23.
[a] Length of stay computed from data on admissions and total days.

plans to group practice plans. From this it can be inferred, under our assumptions, that a system that combines financial incentives to the physician with financial disincentives to the client is unable to reduce overall utilization of service to the normative level because whatever reductions are achieved in admissions are more than compensated for by increases in length of stay. These distortions are more marked in the "upper class" where, apparently, there is a greater latitude for discretionary variation.

A more direct test of the differential impact of deductible and coinsurance payments is found in a recent report of experience under Medicare (123). In 1969, all enrollees in the Supplementary Medical Insurance program of Medicare (Part B), were required to pay the first $50 of allowed charges for covered benefits received during a calendar year, plus 20 percent of charges for covered services beyond that amount. It was reasonable to offer the hypothesis that low income persons who had to pay their own deductible and coinsurance charges, would be most inhibited in seeking care, provided the illness that they experienced was not of such severity as to override financial considerations. Accordingly, all persons who had received hospital care during 1969 were assumed to have had severe illness and were excluded from the study. Those who remained were put into one of four mutually exclusive categories, which were chosen to represent a rough order of increasing difficulty in meeting charges out of one's own resources. The categories selected were: (1) Medicare enrollees who received medical care benefits under public assistance programs or who were eligible to have deductible and coinsurance payments made on their behalf through prior arrangement between a state public assistance agency and the Medicare program; (2) enrollees, excluding the above, who had additional coverage for out-of-hospital services, primarily through private health insurance; (3) enrollees who had no coverage for out-of-hospital services additional to that under Medicare, but who were considered to have high income, after adjustment for family size; and (4) enrollees who had "low-to-moderate" family income and had no coverage for out-of-hospital services additional to Medicare. It was expected that persons in the first category would be least likely to be deterred by the deductible and coinsurance features of Medicare from seeking out-of-hospital care, that persons in the fourth category would be most likely to be deterred, and that those in the second and third categories would be intermediate in this respect. A fifth category used in this study cannot be ranked because it includes families that did not belong in the other four categories and did not report annual income.

Data on respondent characteristics, use of service, and charges were obtained through the Current Medicare Survey. This is a continuing household interview survey of a probability sample of Medicare enrollees, each of whom remains in the sample for a period of 15 months. Response rate exceeds 90 percent. Repeated visits to each person, supplemented by memory aids, such as a diary in which the respondent is encouraged to record information concerning use of service and charges, are thought to improve the quality of the data. The key findings obtained in this way are shown in Table 18. In general, they conform to expectations. The propensity to initiate care, the volume of services received, and the charges for such services are all highest for the enrollees in the public medical assistance category and lowest for enrollees from low-income families who have no out-of-hospital coverage additional to Medicare. Enrollees in the remaining two categories occupy an intermediate position. One possible exception to this pattern is the absence of a diminishing gradient in services and visits per person for those who have met the deductible. The investigators interpret this to mean that once the deductible is met, additional care is not appreciably reduced by the coinsurance feature of Medicare Part B benefits. This negligible effect of coinsurance could reflect, in part, the greater severity of illness among those who met the deductible, and, in part, the greater influence of the physician on care subsequent to initiation. The data for charges do not show corresponding gradient differences between all those who have incurred charges and those who have incurred charges exceeding the deductible. However, in this instance, differences in price for comparable services received by enrollees in the four categories could have influenced the findings. The conclusion that the deductible, and possibly the coinsurance, features of Part B benefits can act as a barrier to care is strengthened by the observation that, in the low-to-moderate income group, 30 percent of enrollees reported that they did not see the doctor as often as they thought necessary, and 10% said they did not do so because

TABLE 18. Use of Covered Service, Charges and Unmet Need in Specified Categories of Medicare Enrollees, U.S.A., 1969

Use of Covered Services, Charges and Unmet Need	Categories of Enrollees			
	Public Medical Assistance	Complementary Out-of-Hospital Coverage	High Family Income	Low-to-Moderate Family Income
Percent who incurred charges for services	87	72	76	68
Services and visits per person:				
All who incurred charges	22	12	9	8
Those who met the deductible	34	14	13	13
Charges per person ($)				
All who incurred charges	134	88	95	73
Those who met the deductible	218	145	141	132
Percent who said they did not see the doctor as often as they thought necessary				
For all reasons	34	19	17	30
Because of insufficient money	10	4	4	10

Source: Reference 123, Table 2, page 8, text table on page 18 and Table 10, page 19.

they couldn't afford it. Interestingly enough, equivalent percentages, indicating financial and other impediments to care, were reported for the group of enrollees who, by reason of arrangements under public assistance, should have encountered the least difficulty in overcoming the barrier posed by the deductible and coinsurance features. The difficulties that they apparently did encounter may mean that they had insufficient knowledge of the benefits available under public assistance medical care, or that this program creates barriers all its own.

The interpretation put on the data in Table 18, though plausible, and in keeping with expectations, is subject to a number of cautions, some of which the investigators emphasize. First, the data are subject to sampling variation. Second, the populations in the several groups of enrollees are not comparable with respect to several characteristics that are likely to influence use of service independently of the effect of participatory payments. Most different from the others are the enrollees in the category of "public medical assistance." These are much more likely to be of very advanced age, female, and nonwhite; to have little education and low incomes; and to be impaired in mobility. While enrollees in the remaining three categories are more alike, those in the group with low-to-moderate family income do differ from the other two in having a larger proportion of nonwhites, rural residents, and persons with limited education. These differences lead the investigators to suggest that the category of enrollees under public medical assistance should not be compared with the three others. Another feature that leads to this conclusion is that the data on utilization and charges in this category are inflated by the way in which the category is defined. This is because more than half of the enrollees in this category are included by reason of having received care paid for by public assistance. No wonder, then, that it registers such high levels of utilization. But, in spite of these limitations, the patterns shown by the aggregated data are remarkably stable when examined in detail in population subgroups. The investigators use 12 demographic and other attributes related to health care to classify their study population into 35 subgroups. When the data for each of the 35 subgroups are examined individually, enrollees in the low-to-moderate income category are almost always least likely to incur charges, and almost always show the lowest number of services per person per year. When the two intermediate categories are compared, the dominant pattern is that enrollees who have complementary coverage are less likely to initiate care, but are more likely to receive a larger number of services per person per year. It appears therefore that, excluding enrollees in the public assistance category, those who have high income are least hindered in initiating care, whereas those who have complementary insurance are most likely to receive a larger volume of service. One could speculate that client decisions are responsible for the former effect and physician decisions for the latter. If so, it would have been useful to have data on hospital use, in order to determine the extent to which hospital care was substituted for outpatient visits, even though the deductible and coinsurance provisions of Medicare Part B apply to all care rendered by a physician, including care in a hospital.

Koropecky and Huang have addressed this question, as well as others that we have raised concerning the comparability of the respondents in the four categories of enrollees (124). The data they used are for a subset of the Medicare beneficiaries from the Current Medicare Survey for 1969. The subsample includes only persons who, as part of the survey, were interviewed at least 12 times during 1969, and who, during that period, received at least one physician visit. The latter stipulation was necessary in order to obtain information on the source of payment for the service received. In the survey, each respondent was asked about the source of payment for each bill, whether he had health insurance in addition to Medicare, and the major features of the benefits provided by any additional insurance. With this information, respondents were classified as having full coverage, partial coverage, or no coverage. It is notable that payment for care through welfare was included as insurance coverage and was not distinguished from any other coverage, except that welfare status was included among the variables in the analysis as a respondent characteristic. Persons were considered to have full coverage if, for all visits reported, they invariably indicated that a third party, other than family or friends, would "help pay the part not covered by Medicare" (124, p. 30). Such respondents were assumed to have a coinsurance rate of zero percent. At the other limit of the range of coinsurance payments were respondents who invariably said that only "self or spouse," "family," or "friends" could be expected to help pay their bills, and who did not report health insurance additional to Medicare. These respondents were assumed to have a coinsurance ratio of 20 percent, as specified by Medicare. For all those in between, the coinsurance rate was not known, and had to be estimated using an adaptation of probit analysis. The method of analysis yielded a maximum likelihood estimate of the coinsurance ratio based on the relationship of each of the three insurance coverage categories (full, partial, and none) to a large number of respondent characteristics and interactions among such characteristics.

As to the deductible, the "carry over" provision of Medicare brought about an effective variation, during 1969, ranging from zero to $50. This variation occurs because eligible expenditures during the last quarter of a year can be used to meet the deductible in the same year as well as the deductible during the following year. Unknown to the investigators, the carry-over provisions may have also introduced a bias into ·the data, because persons who had low deductibles in 1969 would have experienced recent illness (in 1968) that could have required continued use of service. This would tend to strengthen the relationship between a lowering of the deductible and a rise in the use of service. In any event, the carry-over provision was the only source of variation in deductibles for persons who had no coverage other than Medicare. For all others, procedures analogous to those used in estimating the coinsurance ratio were used to obtain an estimate of the deductible. Thus, in this study, the coinsurance ratios and the dollar values of the deductibles were not known quantities but maximum probability estimates, based on known respondent characteristics that would influence the probability of being in one of three categories of coverage: full, partial, or none.

Later, many of the respondent characteristics were used in a standardization process to remove extraneous variation in the relation between participatory payments and demand. A set of simultaneous equations had to be employed in order to represent interrelationships between inpatient and outpatient use, and to take account of the tendency that persons who expect to use more service have of buying additional insurance. This tendency introduces a circularity of effects, so that the tendency to use more services "causes" the purchase of insurance which, itself, "causes" the use of more service. This being the case, it was necessary to use a two-stage multiple regression analysis, which was further modified to account for the fact that the coinsurance rate has upper and lower limits of 0 to 20 percent, and that use of service has a lower limit of zero.

When other respondent characteristics were held constant, including the use of hospital services, it became clear that an increase in either the deductible or coinsurance payments, each tested separately, was associated with a reduction in demand for outpatient services, whether measured as charges or as physical units (visits). According to the regression equations used in the analysis, when the coinsurance ratio is held at 18 percent, a change in deductible from $50 to $25 would increase the expected charges for ambulatory services from about $39 to about $46. Similarly, at a deductible level of $50, a change in the coinsurance ratio from 18 to 15 percent would increase the expected charges from about $39 to about $54. The demand for ambulatory services is more responsive to changes in the value of either the coinsurance ratio or the deductible when these values are high rather than when they are low. In fact, when the coinsurance ratio falls as low as 8 percent it has scarcely any effect on demand. The two types of participatory payment have cross effects on each other. When the deductible level is high, demand becomes more responsive to changes in coinsurance, and when coinsurance is high, demand is more responsive to changes in the deductible. From all this, we may conclude that a given level of demand can be achieved by changes in the deductible, in the coinsurance ratio, or in both. The authors provide three curves that show the combinations of deductible and coinsurance levels that are expected to bring about average charges of $75, $50, or $30 per respondent per annum (124, p. 22). All curves are concave to the origin. "This implies that as coinsurance is increased, the reduction in the deductible must be greater and greater to induce or maintain the same level of utilization" (124, p. 26).

In all of the above, other respondent characteristics, including income, were held constant through standardization. When income is allowed to vary, one finds that the effects of deductibles and coinsurance are operative at all income levels, but that the effect is larger at lower incomes than at high incomes. As shown in Figure 7, when the coinsurance ratio is high, increases in income are associated with increases in use of service. As the coinsurance level goes down, the effect of income becomes progressively less marked until at ratios of 10 percent and 8 percent there is a reversal in the direction of the association, so that the visits are more frequent at low incomes than at high incomes. Since these data are standardized for welfare status and for disability status, one may infer that demand is more likely to be congruent with perceived need at low levels of coinsurance than at high. If so, the barrier effects of coinsurance are socially misallocative.

A final interesting observation is that the degree of coverage for

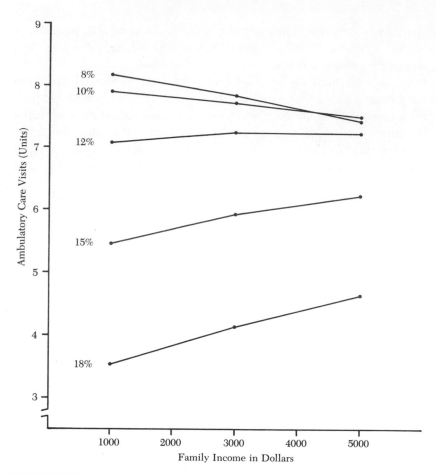

FIGURE 7. Ambulatory services received by a sample of Medicare enrollees, by family income and by effective coinsurance ratio, U.S.A., 1969.

Source: Reference 124, Table 21, p. 19.

physicians' services in the hospital is inversely related to the use of ambulatory services. An increase in coverage for inpatient visits was associated with a decrease in the use of ambulatory visits. This effect was greater at lower incomes and when the regional price for inpatient hospital visits was lower. The relationship to income suggests that the substitution of hospital services for ambulatory services is more attractive to the poor when hospital services are covered. It is not clear what accounts for the relationship to the price of hospital visits.

From these findings we now turn to what is perhaps the most credible study we know of dealing with the effects of copayments (121, 34). The Group Health Plan for Stanford University employees, including faculty, covers care on a prepaid basis at Palo Alto Medical Clinic, and by Palo Alto physicians in the event of hospitalization. Hospital service charges are covered by a contract with a private insurance company. Initially, there were no financial deterrents to service at the clinic. However, because of high utilization the clinic renegotiated the contract at a slightly higher premium rate and with a 25 percent copayment applied to all services across the board. A study reported by Scitovsky and Snyder (121), and also by Phelps and Newhouse (34), examines utilization and costs during the calendar year before the copayment was introduced (1966), and during the first full calendar year after the change (1968). Only persons who were covered during both periods were included, so that population comparability is assured, except for the effect of aging by about one year, which Scitovsky and Snyder correct for in some of their analyses (121). However, an additional attribute that is correlated with aging was not taken into account. This is length of tenure in the plan—a characteristic which, through what we have referred to as seasoning, can bring about systematic changes in use of service when one year is compared with another. As Luft has pointed out, "The 1966 sample includes a number of members who were newly enrolled in the plan; the 1968 sample contains no new members, the most recent enrollees joined in 1965" (122, p. 2). Another event also mars the comparability of the population, through no fault of the investigators. Coincident with the introduction of coinsurance, about 11 percent of the members dropped out, but since the utilization pattern of this group in 1966 was similar to the pattern of those who remained in the plan, the study was probably not significantly damaged (121, p. 20). The data for the study were obtained from "charge slips" kept at the clinic which do not show services received outside the plan. The services of physicians in the hospital are included, but other hospital services and charges are not.

In the setting described above, it is expected that copayment by the client will motivate him to initiate care less frequently, to make fewer visits for situations of comparable severity, and to use fewer ancillary services, taking the nature of illness into account. It is further expected that these effects will be more marked for conditions that are perceived to be less serious, and among persons with lower income. Scitovsky and Snyder are aware of these expectations and set out to look for them in the data. They give much less attention to the presence of incentives to the physician, so that the reviewer must speculate concerning this aspect of the situation. It would seem that if the Group receives a prepayment and the individual physicians within the group are paid a salary, as is likely, then the incentive would be to reduce service in order to redress the adverse financial experience of the previous year, even though the new copayment would contribute an unspecified amount towards redress. If the patient pays the full fee for each service, and, to a lesser extent, if there is part payment in the form of a deductible or copayment, one would expect a reduction in those services in which net revenue is small or negative, and an encouragement of those services, such as laboratory procedures, which usually yield a large net revenue (125). All such revenue effects would be expected to be more marked if the Stanford University group comprised a large share of the case load of the Palo Alto Clinic. Apparently this is not the case, since only 16 percent of income to the clinic comes from prepaid plans, including that for Stanford employees (121, p. 4). As to possible substitution of hospital care for ambulatory care, this is difficult to predict since we have no information on the relative net revenue to the physician, or the relative cost-benefit ratios to the client. Finally, since copayment within the plan must render services outside the plan that much more attractive, or less prohibitive, it is unfortunate that no information is provided concerning this rather frequent occurrence in prepaid group plans (57, pp. 12–14).

Keeping these theoretical expectations in mind, we may now look at the findings which are summarized in Table 19. In general, the changes observed are in the expected direction. To begin with, there is a 24 percent reduction in total physician visits per person. The reduction is largest, relatively, for the very small number of home visits and smallest for hospital visits. The absence of an increase in hospital visits suggests that there was no large substitution of hospital for ambulatory care, although some

TABLE 19. Use of Specified Services One Year Before and One Year After the Institution of a 25 Percent Copayment, Group Health Plan, Stanford University, Palo Alto, 1966 and 1968

Services	Before	After	Difference	Percent Difference
Physician visits per person				
All	5.683	4.315	− 1.368	−24.1
Home	0.064	0.031	− 0.033	−51.6
Office	5.329	4.004	− 1.325	−24.9
Hospital, medical	0.207	0.201	− 0.006	− 2.9
Hospital, surgical	0.083	0.079	− 0.004	− 4.8
Surgical specialty	1.929	1.332	− 0.597	−30.9
Medical specialty	2.760	2.156	− 0.604	−21.9
Percent with no visits				
All	13.4	20.0	+ 6.6	+49.3
Faculty	11.4	15.0	+ 3.6	+31.6
Nonprofessional personnel	14.4	25.5	+11.1	+77.1
Percent with 4 or more visits				
All	54.2	43.4	−10.8	−19.9
Faculty	53.9	46.1	− 7.8	−14.5
Nonprofessional personnel	54.1	40.4	−13.7	−25.3
Annual physicals per person				
All	0.379	0.309	− 0.070	−18.5
Male faculty	0.386	0.294	− 0.092	−23.8
Nonprofessional adult males	0.260	0.127	− 0.133	−51.2
Ancillary services per person	6.026	5.349	− 0.677	−11.2
Ancillary services per visit	1.131	1.336	+ 0.205	+18.1

Source: Reference 121, Tables 4, 9, 10, 11 and 13, pages 7, 11, 12 and 16.

degree of substitution may have been concealed by concurrent changes in the length of stay. As to physician visits in general, there appear to have been effects on both "initiation" and "continuation," since the proportion who made one or most visits was reduced, as was the proportion who made 4 or more visits. The latter reduction suggests fewer visits per episode, although this statistic is not given. Ancillary services (x-rays, laboratory tests, etc.) were also decreased, but less than visits, so that the number of ancillary services per visit increased. This may indicate, as the authors suggest, that the visits were for more severe episodes of illness, or that the client had less influence in the reduction of procedures recommended by the physician than on visits that the client initiated or controlled to a greater extent. It may also be that laboratory investigations substitute, in part, for visits, or that the revenue they generate because of the copayment encourages their use by the physician. In favor of the last hypothesis, it was observed that, during the period under study, the clinic as a whole experienced an even larger increase in the use of ancillary procedures than the Stanford University Group did.

There is another evidence of differential effects, possibly related to actual or perceived severity of need. As we have said, hospital visits, which are presumably for more serious illness, were hardly reduced at all. The percent reduction was somewhat less for therapeutic than for preventive services. In adults, annual physical examinations appeared to be especially vulnerable to reduction. On the basis of information in the clinic record, an attempt was made to categorize the reason for visits as "possibly minor" and "other." The possibly minor complaints were warts, headaches, earache, colds, acute pharyngitis, acute tonsillitis, acute upper respiratory infection of multiple or unspecified sites, hay fever, indigestion, constipation, back pain and back ache, dizziness, palpitation, cough, and fatigue. The reduction in visits for these "possibly minor" complaints was somewhat greater than the reduction for all other cases: 22.5 versus 16.4 percent, respectively. Unfortunately, there is no direct assessment of the appropriateness of the visits or of the care provided during visits, for minor or other complaints, so that we can only speculate about the significance of the changes in the volume and pattern of care.

The authors seem to believe that some of the reduction represents reduced frequency of unnecessary services, whereas some of the reduction, especially in annual physical examinations, represents a reduction in necessary care. There are, of course, those who would question the value of annual examinations for all adults and, therefore, would be more prepared to view the changes described as tending towards more appropriate adjustment of use to need.

The other aspect of allocation is the differential effect by income or social class. Here the findings suggest that the barrier effects tend to be more marked among personnel of lower education and income and in their families. For example, nonprofessional personnel, compared to faculty, become even less likely to initiate care or to receive care of long duration. Most striking is the much greater reduction in annual examinations among adult male nonprofessional employees of the University as compared to male faculty. This does not appear to be due to differences in age. Although these allocations by social class may represent different responses to the perceived utility of these services, they could be construed as socially misallocative.

In summary, the introduction of a coinsurance feature in the Stanford plan was associated with less, but more intensive, ambulatory care and no reduction in hospital care. There were, in addition, important reallocative effects, so that the volume of services was reduced to a greater extent for preventive services as compared to therapeutic services, for therapeutic services for minor illness as compared to more serious illness, and for persons of lower socioeconomic status as compared to higher. Most adversely affected were annual physical examinations for nonprofessional adult male employees. All these findings are pleasingly in line with theoretical expectations and could be taken as confirmation of such theory, if it were not for the several limitations in study design that we have pointed out. Luft has argued that several of the findings could have occurred without the institution of coinsurance, if it is assumed that persons who stay longer in the plan use fewer services, that turnover is greatest among nonprofessional personnel, that an initial health assessment is required as a condition of employment or is encouraged by the plan, and that such an assessment is likely to reveal minor abnormalities that require attention (122). While all these assumptions are plausible, and the greater turnover among nonprofessional personnel is known to be a fact (121), the consequences, as far as biasing the findings, are likely to be small.* In searching for factors, additional to the barrier effect of the copayment, which may have influenced the results, we are more inclined to emphasize the need for a closer examination of the more general context of the health care system, with particular emphasis on incentives to physicians.

From our review of the empirical findings we must conclude

* In an unpublished communication, Scitovsky presents data which suggest that, in the population studied, new enrollees do not have appreciably higher utilization rates, and that, even if they did, the effect would be too small to alter significantly the findings and conclusions of the study.

that deductibles and copayments always have an arithmetic effect. In addition, if they are large enough in absolute terms, or relative to income, to total charges, or to the costs of alternative types of care, they will have a depressing effect on use of the services to which they apply. Deductibles are most likely to have an effect on the initiation of care, and they may to some extent, though not invariably, be compensated for by higher utilization subsequent to initiation. Copayment appears to have an effect on initiation as well as continuation of care. All deterrent payments are likely to have differential effects according to type of condition and social class or income. The differential effect by type of condition is likely to be socially useful since it tends to depress use for less serious and less urgent conditions to a greater extent than for conditions that are more serious or more urgent. However, when this allocation is made through fiscal deterrents it can easily go wrong. To the extent that the client's perception of need for care is not medically accurate, preventive services may be foregone, access to proper professional evaluation may be inhibited, or care for severe, long-lasting illness may be curtailed. The differential effect by social class would be considered to be misallocative unless the barrier payments were graduated to income. All of these effects occur if all other things are equal. But this assumption of equality is seldom true. We must emphasize, once again, that the effects described could be enhanced, attenuated, or even negated by other forces in the medical care setting, and among these forces incentives to the physician are the most salient.

Whatever the behavioral consequences of participatory payments may be, they cannot be achieved without cost to the insurer. It is unfortunate that there are no data, at least none that we have found, that tell us what these administrative costs are. Thus we have to rely on the impressions of administrators, as cited in a national poll of Blue Cross and Blue Shield Plans, from which we quote:

Another point raised in the Blue Cross and Blue Shield poll was what was described as the introduction of an 'administrative nightmare' by the use of coinsurance, deductibles or copayment. . . . Including a deductible and/or coinsurance clause immediately introduces extra steps in the administration of the program—one of which is computation. With coinsurance, it can be a fairly simple step since often the carrier just looks at the bill, computes its share and pays it. But a deductible introduces more steps. The carrier must examine each bill and match it against its records. It must determine how much of the deductible the patient has already paid. If part of it has been paid, the carrier must note how much more the patient has to pay before it assumes payment. The carrier also must give this information to the patient. It must tell the patient how much more of the deductible he has to pay before the carrier's coverage will then take over.

About the time the patient begins to understand the deductible, he receives a statement from the carrier and finds he still owes money because of coinsurance. By this time, the patient is usually confused because the idea of deductibles and coinsurance is not easily understood, particularly in combination. Another problem that is raised is who is billed for these features when several physicians treat a patient. . . .

Who, among these physicians, should be paid in full for his services and who should receive partial payment from the insurer and the remainder from the patient? . . .

So when contracts call for deductibles or coinsurance, a carrier must, among other things, keep track of which contracts have these provisions, how much they are and how much of the bill the patient pays and how much the carrier pays. And, it should be noted, the computation of the deductible and coinsurance must be done each contract year. At the beginning of next year, the process begins once again. [119, p. 10]

Substitution of Services

Introduction

In our discussion of the context for benefit design, we emphasized the complex interactions of the medical care process and the services it generates. We concluded that medical care benefits cannot be viewed as an assemblage of independent items, but must be seen as a system of subtly interactive parts. Some services are prerequisite to other services; some services depend on others for their effectiveness or safety; and some services may be substituted for others with consequences for quality and costs. In this section we shall deal at somewhat greater length with substitution, and with its implications for benefit design. As we have said earlier, this discussion of substitution will overlap our preceding discussion of the effects that are produced when benefits are limited through the imposition of participatory payments. As we shall see, the implications of substitution also derive from what we have already said about the general and benefit-specific effects of insurance, and of the graded effects of the scope and depth of coverage. Recognizing these antecedents, we shall focus in this section on the consequences of providing coverage for specific services with the intent not only of influencing the use of *these* services, but also of influencing the use of *other* services, so that care becomes generally more appropriate to need and less costly.

Theoretical Considerations

A succinct and reasonably systematic analysis of the more general effects of providing specified benefits requires a framework and a nomenclature, which we have attempted to provide in Table 20. Under the heading of "Incentives" we have indicated, in sum-

TABLE 20. A Proposed Framework for Understanding the Localized and Extended Effects of the Provision of Benefits for Specified Services

Incentives	Localization of Effect	Mechanisms for Bringing About of Extended Effects	Effects on Use of Other Services
Client initiative and compliance	Localized or specific		
Price effect	Extended or generalized (to other services than the one specified by the benefit)	Substitution Arithmetic Reactive	Decreased
Income effect			
Changes in preferences, expectations, etc.		Functional complementarity Scrutiny, discovery Exposure to intervention	Increased
Physician initiative			
Price and income consequences to client			
Net revenue to physician			
Net revenue to institutional affiliate or employee			
Professional norms of appropriateness, quality, etc.			

mary form, the factors that influence changes in use of service in response to the provision of benefits. These factors have been discussed in an earlier section. Our interest now focuses on the distinction between the localized effects that are specific to the benefit under consideration and the extended effects that go beyond that benefit so as to influence other services. These effects are indicated in the second column of Table 20. From our general discussion of the effects of insurance, one would expect an increase in the use of any covered service. Whether there is a more generalized or extended effect, and what that effect may be, is harder to predict. Forces come into play that can work in contrary directions. To the extent that a covered service can replace other services, legitimately or otherwise, the use of those other services will be reduced. In Table 20 we continue to make the distinction between arithmetic and reactive consequences that we introduced in our discussion of participatory payments. However, the distinction may not be as useful for classifying the effects of substitution. We should also note that "substitution" does not necessarily mean replacement by a less appropriate or less desirable service. The value judgment is an additional, though obviously important, aspect of the substitution. Needless to say, substitution leads to a decrease in the use of a service for which a substitution has been made. However, there are forces that can indirectly increase the use of other services, at the same time that the direct effect increases the use of covered services. Once again, this more generalized increase may be intended, legitimate, and useful; or it may be none of these. The increased use of a service may come about in a variety of ways; one mechanism is the functional complementarity among services. For example, insurance for hospital services may increase the demand for the services of the physician because the latter are necessary for the former. Additional services may also be generated because certain services permit observation and investigation of patients, leading to the discovery of new illnesses for which additional services are then provided. This appears to be a perfectly legitimate and desirable consequence, unless care becomes trivialized because it is so easy to get. A third category, "exposure to intervention," has been added to our table because exposure to physicians can lead to the generation of services of dubious value. Whether the provision of these services derives from the physicians' general preference for "doing something" (126), or from greed, is immaterial at this point. We merely wish to indicate that exposure to some providers in some settings can be a hazardous undertaking.

The resultant of these contrary forces is difficult to predict. The relative potency of the service-reducing and service-generating forces would vary according to the constellation of benefits and services under consideration, the characteristics of the beneficiary population, and the characteristics of the physicians and of the settings in which they practice. Perhaps the key variable, in most instances, is the nature of the incentives to the provider. Where the incentives are predominantly professional, the extended, service-reducing effect of substitution can become evident if it is more powerful than the concurrent, service-enhancing effects of complementarity or discovery. In some situations the backlog of unmet or undiscovered need may cause the substitution effect to become apparent only later. However, in situations in which revenue incentives are dominant, it is likely that whatever substitution effects occur will be more than counteracted by increases in use, some legitimate and others not.

Empirical Observations

Many of the studies we have described earlier have a bearing on substitution of services. Now we will consider a selection of studies that deal specifically with attempts to rationalize medical care and reduce costs by providing a broader range of benefits so that less costly services can be substituted for more costly ones without reducing quality. Since hospital care is both very expensive and differentially favored by the traditional forms of health insurance, almost all the studies we will cite have examined the hospital-sparing effect of providing benefits for specified services outside the hospital. We shall begin our presentation by dealing with the effects of providing a progressively broader range of presumably hospital-sparing benefits in settings that do not alter the traditional fee-for-service incentives. We will then consider the effects of providing such benefits within settings that are more bureaucratized and that alter the financial incentives to the physician.

Outpatient Diagnostic Services and Hospital Use
in Unorganized Settings

There is a general presumption, in our opinion well-founded, that hospital services are often improperly used (1, pp. 363–380). It is reasonable to assume that part of this abuse arises from the desire to take advantage of diagnostic services covered under hospital insurance but not available as a benefit outside the hospital. It is not surprising, therefore, to find a reasonably early preoccupation with the possible hospital-sparing effects of adding outpatient diagnostic benefits to plans that already cover in-hospital care. In 1965, Steep and Tilley reviewed the experience of three such plans, all under the auspices of Blue Cross and Blue Shield (127). The findings are difficult to interpret because of deficiencies in the data and in study design. For example, when those who had outpatient diagnostic coverage were compared with those who did not, it was not possible to establish comparability of population characteristics or to correct for differences in these. Where employee groups were compared before and after the introduction of outpatient diagnostic benefits, there were no contemporaneous controls. In some instances, even the number of persons at risk was not precisely known, and had to be estimated. Finally, in all instances clients had exercised a choice to purchase more liberal insurance, so that self-selection must remain an issue, even though insurance was purchased on a group basis and through employer-employee negotiation. If the findings are taken at face value, one can find, in the data assembled by Steep and Tilley, subgroups in which the introduction of outpatient diagnostic benefits was associated with a reduction in admission to the hospital, with some compensatory increase in average length of stay, but an overall net reduction in patient-days. However, taken as a whole, the hospital-sparing effects were neither sufficiently consistent nor sufficiently large to exceed the cost of the diagnostic benefit itself. In some instances there was an actual increase in total cost to the insurer. Even more disappointing results were reported in an earlier study by Kelly (128). In this case, the Blue Cross and Blue Shield organizations of Maryland had instituted a plan for steelworkers that covered diagnostic x-rays, encephalograms, electrocardiograms, and basal metabolism determinations, whether performed in the inpatient or outpatient services of the hospital or in the office of a physician; a yearly limit of $75 per person was placed on tests done in a doctor's office. Unfortunately for the study, at the same time those employees who were paid by salary, about 15 percent of the total, had hospital medical benefits added to the basic surgical coverage possessed by all workers. These combined changes appeared to result in roughly a 5 percent increase in admissions during each of three successive years, with the average length of stay remaining comparatively unchanged. Thus, one finds no savings in the use of the hospital while there is the added cost of outpatient diagnostic services, which increased to a remarkable degree. However, once again, one must view the findings with caution, since more than one change was introduced in the benefits and there was no contemporaneous control to correct for the possible presence of more pervasive secular trends in hospital use. In a subsequent paper Kelly both lengthens the period of observation by an additional 5 years and provides one reasonably but not fully satisfactory comparison group (129). From this, it becomes immediately apparent that the trend toward increased admissions was not confined to the group with outpatient diagnostic benefits, though it is somewhat steeper in that group. It also appears that after the first 3 years there was no appreciable further increase.

The pattern of increased hospital use in association with the introduction of outpatient benefits was observed, once again in Maryland, when an even broader range of outpatient diagnostic benefits was offered to selected groups. Added to the benefits already mentioned were "pathology and laboratory work," but with dollar limits and 20 percent coinsurance imposed on the entire package. During the next two years, the groups with these benefits showed a 40 percent increase in admissions, a 14 percent decrease in length of stay, and a 21 percent increase in total patient days per 1000 enrollees. The groups without these benefits experienced a 6 percent increase in admissions and almost no change in length of stay, with a resultant 7 percent increase in patient days. However, once again, lack of comparability of populations remains an issue, because of possible self-selection in purchasing more liberal insurance. Kelly concluded that the availability of outpatient diagnostic benefits is likely to cause an increase in net hospital use over the first three years, followed by stabilization at a higher rate. In addition to this larger cost for hospitalization, the insurer (and the consumer) had to bear the cost of the diagnostic benefit, which was widely used by physicians. Kelly attributes the greater use of hospital services to the increased likelihood that illness will be diagnosed as a result of the more frequent use of outpatient diagnostic services. Accordingly, he hopes that the increased costs are offset by better care and improved health. However, he also provides anecdotal evidence of the abuse of office x-ray services, especially by general practitioners, and describes administrative controls on such services (129, p. 35).

An additional example of the effect of outpatient diagnostic services on hospital use is cited by Fogel (130), who also reports from Maryland, where the subject appears to have been a continuing preoccupation. But in this instance the benefit was more circumscribed, being confined to the performance of certain diagnostic investigations outside the hospital, preparatory to the patient being admitted for elective surgery. The author reports that a survey preceding the institution of the benefit had shown that "an average of 1.04 inpatient days could be saved for each elective surgical admission" with a range from 1 to 4 days per patient (130, p. 42). He documents the large number of tests performed prior to hospitalization, and maintains, without citing the evidence, that "the implementation of presurgical scheduling . . . allowed the hospital to maintain a high standard of patient care and utilize its facilities more efficiently. The patient days 'saved' prior to surgery, allowed inpatient facilities to be used by other patients. Furthermore, the problem of canceled operations the night prior to the procedure has been somewhat alleviated" (130, p. 59). Although the report by Fogel concerns only one hospital, and does not document the impact on hospital use, it has been cited because it illustrates several points to which we want to draw attention. First, the performance of tests before, rather than after, admission in cases already slated for surgery approximates our category of "arithmetic" substitutive transfers. It is to be noted, however, that even this kind of transfer could have important consequences to the efficiency of the surgical service; for example, by reducing uncertainty as to whether the patient is ready for the operation. The second issue is the question of what happens to the beds released through substitution. If these are filled by other patients who also carry insurance, there may be no savings to the insurer. The nature of the financial or other benefits to the community depends on whether the released beds are appropriately used. Finally, Fogel raises the question of cost savings to the insurer versus those to the hospital. The insurer and, indirectly, the client, pay less for each episode of surgical care, because the savings from a reduced hospital stay more than offset the cost of pre-hospital diagnostic tests. On the other hand, the hospital could lose revenue if the cost of such tests is not included in the computation of its per-diem reimbursement formula by such programs as Medicare and Medicaid. Thus, "the hospital is not fully reimbursed and, in essence, is financially penalized for being efficient in the delivery of health care" (130, p. 54).

So far, we have dealt with the possible effects that the introduction of outpatient diagnostic benefits can have on hospital use and on the costs of medical care, in situations where hospital services are, to some degree, already covered by insurance, and where the fee-for-service incentive to the physician remains intact. The conclusion, from the admittedly inconclusive studies that we have reviewed, seems to be that, except for the rather unusual situation where tests that were already slated to be performed in the hospital are performed ahead of admission, the provision of outpatient diagnostic benefits adds the cost of these benefits without a comparable reduction, and possibly with an increase, in hospital use. The hoped-for reward is said to be earlier discovery of disease rather than lower costs, although we suspect that diagnostic tests may be wastefully used either to bring revenue to the physician, or to help reassure or impress the patient. Even when diagnostic tests lead to the discovery of illness, the hospital may be wastefully used if a broader range of outpatient services is not available as a benefit; this problem brings us to a selection of studies that examine the effect on hospital use of providing a broader range of services, including care by a physician in his office and in the patients' home.

Outpatient Physician Care and Hospital Use
in Unorganized Settings

Health planners have long been beguiled by the attractive prospect that if hospital insurance were extended to include home and office care hospital care could be reduced sufficiently to at least offset the costs of the extended benefits, and that this could be done without any alteration in the fee-for-service system of medical care. In the Canadian province of Saskatchewan, Roemer believed he found a natural laboratory where this expectation might be put to the test (131). Since 1947, the entire population had been covered by statutory hospital insurance virtually without limitation on benefits. In addition, in several areas of the Province there were certain plans that provided non-hospital services, including physicians' services in the office and home. The range of benefits varied from plan to plan; and so did the method of payment to physicians, being fee-for-service in some plans and salary in others. Data for hospital use during 1954 were available by geographic area, making it possible to compare areas according to the presence or absence of a plan that covered all or a majority of the residents for non-hospital services. When allowance was made for size and rurality of communities, it was clear that use of the hospital was lowest where there was no coverage for non-hospital services, whereas it was highest where coverage for non-hospital services was most generous and where physicians were paid fee-for-service. An intermediate level of hospital use was encountered in areas where there was less than universal coverage of residents, or where coverage was universal but the range of non-hospital benefits was somewhat restricted and physicians were paid a salary rather than fee-for-service. Furthermore, the more generous fee-for-service plans appeared to increase not only admissions to the hospital but, frequently, length of stay as well. According to Roemer, these effects could not be attributed to differences in age or sex composition, and were not likely to be explained by differences in education. On the contrary, they were more likely to be explained by three factors: the discovery of illness through more frequent access to physicians, use of the hospital by the physician in order to help him cope with increased demand, and the fee-for-service incentive to provide more care irrespective of site. But none of this, apparently, dismayed Roemer, who saw in his observations "a free expression of health need," and an overall improvement in efficiency, since more care was provided at lower cost per unit through substitution of at least some outpatient for some inpatient care.

The next piece of evidence, in chronological order, comes in a study by Shipman et al. of experience under the Medical Service Corporations in the state of Washington, in a county not too far from the Canadian border (132). Here, the King County Medical Service Corporation, an instrumentality of the county's physicians, offered contracts to employee groups that included the services of physicians in the home and office, usually without a deductible. In addition, the Boeing Airplane Company purchased similar benefits for its hourly employees. Data on use of service were compiled for two samples: one of families of Boeing employees, from which single-member families were excluded, and another of employees of other firms. Workers employed by Boeing had coverage for hospital care and for home and office care for themselves and members of their families, the latter subject to a first-visit deductible. Other workers had coverage for hospital care for themselves and for family members, as well as coverage, without a deductible, for home and office care for themselves only. In order to test the effect of the extended benefits, which included nonhospital services, data were compared separately for males and females, after an adjustment was made for differences in age between those who only had the hospital benefit and those who had the extended benefit. It should be pointed out, however, that this adjustment does not alter the large proportion of employed heads of households among males who had extended benefits.

The findings are summarized in Table 21. As expected, there was greater use of home and office services in the group that had coverage for such services; this is the specific or localized effect of the benefit in question. As to the more generalized or extended effects, one finds more frequent, rather than less frequent, use of the hospital, especially for surgery. However, hospital stays are very markedly shorter in length, so that the overall effect is a large reduction in patient-days of hospital care. As to total charges, the net effect appears to be a slightly higher level of charges per person, the best estimate for which is 8 percent. For a more representative population—one equivalent to the general public in age, sex, and income class—the increase would be nearer 5 percent (132, pp. 91–92). Once again, the cost of the added benefit is not fully offset by reductions in hospital use, but a broader range of choices has become available in the delivery of care. Whether this greater flexibility has been used to the best advantage cannot, un-

TABLE 21. Utilization [a] of Specified Services and Total Charges for Medical Care for Persons Having Insurance for Home and Office Care, Expressed as Percent Greater or Less Than Utilization and Charges for Persons Covered for Hospital Care Only, King County Medical Service Corporation, Washington, 1956

| | Percent Difference | |
Services and Charges	Male	Female
Home and office calls	+ 12	+ 40
Hospital admissions	+ 7	+ 12
Hospital admissions for surgery	+ 15	+ 31
Hospital admissions for other reasons	− 6	+ 9
Days per admission [b]	− 67	− 34
Hospital days	− 65	− 26
Number of hospitalized surgical procedures	+ 22	+100
Total charges per person		
All persons	− 16	+ 17
Persons with family income above $3,500 [c]	+ 5	+ 26
Persons with family income below $3,500 [c]	−129	− 69

Source: Reference 132, Tables 16, 25, 26, 27, 28, 29, 40 and 42 pages 68, 76–79, 88 and 90.

[a] Adjusted for age.

[b] Hospital days ÷ hospital admissions.

[c] Computed from data in source.

fortunately, be documented. The large increase in surgical procedures, which we encountered repeatedly as a correlate of expanded benefits, raises a serious question of possible abuse.

An additional interesting feature of the findings is that the consequences of extended benefits may vary by sex, age and income. In Table 21 one observes that females respond more to the service-enhancing effect of extended benefits. This occurs even though females are more likely to be dependents and to be subject to the first-call deductible from which employed subscribers are exempt. The data (not cited in Table 21) also show differences in response by age, although these are so variable as to be difficult to summarize. However, females 65 and over in the extended benefit group regularly received less home, office and hospital care than their counterparts who had hospital benefits only. As to differential response by income, data are available only for charges. When family income was above $3,500, both males and females in the group with extended coverage incurred more charges than their counterparts who had hospital benefits only, and the relative excess was larger for females than for males. When family income was below $3,500, the findings were quite different. Males and females with extended coverage incurred smaller charges per person than their counterparts who had more limited coverage, although the difference was relatively not as great for females as for males.

There is no easy explanation for these differential effects. The numbers of low income persons and of old females in the sample were rather small, and the authors wondered whether there was "some non-random factor involved in selecting more sickly persons from old age and low income groups into in-hospital than into extended coverage" (132, p. 91). As to the greater responsiveness of females to the use-generating effects of benefit extensions, this appears to be a phenomenon that has been repeatedly observed, though not well understood (87). Weisbrod and Fiesler, among others, suggest that the explanation lies in the lower opportunity costs of care for women (55). It may also be that unemployed women, relative to male breadwinners, have to put up with a larger amount of unmet need until the extension of benefits permits them to express that need. In this study, interpretation is made somewhat more difficult by the nature of the analysis, which compares persons rather than family units. This type of comparison was made because there were two sets of families with two different types of coverage. In one set (those employed by Boeing), almost all members had extended coverage, whereas in the other set (those not employed by Boeing) only the employee, usually a male, had extended coverage. Thus, familial patterns of behavior, which presumably affect all members of a family, could have been confounded with the intrafamilial distinction of whether a family member has more or less insurance. However, the authors do provide data for the two sets of families as well. An examination of these data suggests that members of Boeing families, who have extended coverage for virtually all members, are more likely to see a physician at least once during the year, suggesting a greater propensity to initiate such contacts. The number of calls per person, which represents physician as well as client initiative, also favors the Boeing families, but not to the same degree, nor as consistently. Family income, as well as the importance of the illness, as judged by the type and amount of care required, appear to play a role that bears on the allocative effects of benefits. Boeing families, who have extended benefits, show smaller differences by income in the number of home and office calls per person, and appear to use more of these services for minor illness than do members of families in which only the breadwinner has extended benefits. Table 22 shows the effects of income and importance of illness in female members, who have been singled out to sharpen the comparison between the two forms of coverage, since all the females in the Boeing group have extended coverage, either as employees or dependents of employees, whereas in the non-Boeing group only the relatively few women employees have extended coverage. It is clear that the specific service-enhancing effect of the extended benefit is restricted to minor illness and, moreover, fails to equalize use of ser-

TABLE 22.   Home and Office Calls Per Person, by Type of Coverage, Type of Illness, and Family Income, Female Members Only, King County Medical Service Corporation, Washington, 1956

| Family Income and Type of Illness [b] | Type of Coverage [a] | | Boeing as Percent of Non-Boeing |
	Boeing	Non-Boeing	
Under $3,500			
Major illness	4.8	5.4	89
Minor illness	2.9	1.6	181
Both	7.7	7.0	110
$7,500 and over			
Major illness	2.7	2.7	100
Minor illness	2.4	1.4	171
Both	5.1	4.1	124

Source: Reference 132, Table 10, page 62.

[a] Workers employed by the Boeing Airplane Company had coverage for hospital care and for home and office care for themselves and for members of their families, the latter subject to a first-call deductible. Other workers had coverage for hospital care for themselves and for family members, as well as coverage for home and office calls for themselves only.

[b] Major illnesses were those requiring one or more nights in the hospital, a charge of fifty dollars or more, seeing a doctor five or more times during the year, or regular treatment of a chronic condition. Illnesses requiring less attention were defined as minor. Physicians' calls for minor illnesses were collected for the last six months of the survey year and doubled.

vice for major illness in the lower income group. To the extent
that this is true, the effect of the extended benefit is misallocative.
However, this effect is somewhat counterbalanced by the larger
increment of use for minor illness in the lower income group, as
compared to the higher, an effect that would be considered socially desirable, especially if it could be shown to have contributed to the small volume of care for major illness in the low income group. As one notes these mixed effects, one should
remember that they pertain only to the specific or "localized" effect of the extended benefit on home and office calls. Comparable
data for the more generalized effect on hospital use are, unfortunately, not available.

More information concerning the effects of adding home and office benefits to hospital insurance, but without change in the organization of care, comes in a report by Avnet of experience under
Group Health Insurance (133). Under the auspices of this organization, employee groups who lived in the New York-New Jersey
Metropolitan Area could select a "limited plan" that covered
mainly the services of physicians in the hospital (133, p. 39), or a
"comprehensive plan" that covered physician services in office,
home, and hospital, out-of-hospital x-rays and laboratory services,
as well as other auxiliary services such as radiotherapy, ambulance
services, and home nursing visits. Care was received from physicians in the community, who were paid fee-for-service according
to a schedule. There were no deductibles or copayments, but
"nonparticipating" physicians were free to charge fees additional
to those specified in the schedule. The data reported are for services provided under the insurance plan to a random sample of
subscribers and their dependents during 1964. Since the data
come from insurance records, there is no information about use of
home and office services by persons covered by the limited plan.
The specific or "localized" effect of the extended benefit cannot,
therefore, be measured. The more generalized effects on hospital
care can, however, be examined, and are shown in Table 23.
When adjustments were made for age and sex, persons with comprehensive benefits were a little more likely to be admitted, but
had somewhat shorter stays, so that patient-days per person were
lower by about 5 percent in the group with comprehensive benefits. When age-adjusted data were examined separately for males

TABLE 23. Hospital Use by Sex and by Type of Benefit [a], Group Health Insurance Plan, 1964

Hospital Use	Both Sexes [b]			Male [c]			Female [c]		
	Comprehensive	Limited	Percent [d] Difference	Comprehensive	Limited	Percent [d] Difference	Comprehensive	Limited	Percent [d] Difference
Admissions per 1000	127.7	122.3	+ 4	96.3	103.3	− 7	152.0	140.0	+9
Days per admission	7.8	8.7	−10	8.4	9.3	−10	7.7	8.3	−7
Patient-days per 1000	1001	1058	− 5	809	960	−16	1163	1162	0

Source: Reference 133, Tables 136 and 137, pages 374 and 375.

[a] Persons with "limited" benefits had coverage for the services of physicians in the hospital. Persons with "comprehensive" benefits had coverage for services of physicians in office, home and hospital as well as coverage for certain diagnostic and auxiliary services outside the hospital.

[b] Adjusted for age and sex.

[c] Adjusted for age.

[d] Use under comprehensive benefits compared to use under limited benefits.

and females, only the former showed a moderate hospital sparing effect that could be attributed to having comprehensive benefits. Men with comprehensive benefits had 7 percent fewer admissions and a 10 percent shorter length of stay, on the average, resulting in 16 percent fewer patient-days of hospital care. By contrast, females with comprehensive coverage entered the hospital more frequently than their counterparts who had limited coverage, but stayed fewer days per admission, so that the patient-days of care used were essentially identical in the two groups of female enrollees. In sum, Avnet points out that while the savings in hospital use were "substantial", they were "only a fraction of the additional premium for comprehensive coverage" (133, p. 376). Thus, the experience reported by Avnet is generally comparable to the earlier findings of Shipman et al. under roughly similar circumstances, except that the effect of the extended benefit on hospital use were "substantial," they were "only a fraction of the addi-

The studies we have described in this section have varied a great deal in sophistication of design and in their ability to achieve comparability between those who have extended benefits and those who do not; but all of these studies, without exception, have suffered from the defect of self-selection in the populations they have studied. For this reason, one views with great interest a truly experimental study which has been reported by Hill and Veney (134) and, independently, by Lewis and Keairnes (135). For this study, groups of subscribers to Blue Cross and Blue Shield in Sedgwick County, Kansas (which includes the city of Wichita) were sampled in a manner that yielded three study groups, one experimental and two control, which were comparable with respect to the proportion of single to family contracts, payments to single and family contracts, and use of hospital services. The employee groups in the experimental sample were actually given, at no cost to themselves, a set of out-of-hospital benefits that included the services of physicians, laboratory services, drugs that could not be self-administered, and psychiatric evaluations and treatment. The choice of benefits was calculated to reduce the need for inpatient hospital services, and the object was to see whether hospital use would, indeed, be reduced. To this end, a variety of means were used to inform both physicians and subscribers in the experimental group of the availability of the extended benefits. Insurance records were used to obtain information about hospital use for each of the experimental and control groups during an eight month period of the year preceding the introduction of the benefit, and during the corresponding eight calendar months immediately following. In this way, the effect of seasonality was held constant, even though the experiment did not run a full year, as had been planned, because costs proved to be higher than expected. Towards the end of the experimental period, a household survey was conducted to obtain additional information not found in insurance records. The data on hospital use permitted a comparison of experience before and after the introduction of the extended benefits for the experimental and control groups. The conclusion was that there had been no significant difference either in use of hospital services or in costs during this period. However, further analysis suggested, but by no means conclusively, that there may have been a reduction in admissions of short duration and an increase in admissions of long duration—contrary effects that balanced out in the aggregate. Presumably the reduction in admissions of short duration was due to the substitution effect of the extended benefit, whereas the increase in admissions of longer duration was due to the discovery of illness. Hill and Veney argue that in a short-term experiment such as this the two effects might balance each other, but that in the longer run the substitution effect would predominate.

So much for the effect on hospital use. For data on the use of non-hospital services we must turn to the paper by Lewis and Keairnes (135). For this study information was obtained by telephone from small subsamples of the experimental and control groups. The information pertains only to the final month of the experimental period and the month following the end of the period. No significant differences were revealed. The two groups were equally likely to contact a physician, either on their own or at the suggestion of the physician; for both groups, the physician contacted was equally likely to be a general practitioner; and for both groups the visit to the physician was equally likely to involve a physical examination, a prescription, an injection, an x-ray film, a urine or blood specimen, or an arrangement for a laboratory test to be made. The only important difference was the presence of a significant negative association between the frequency of physician contacts and social class in the control group, in contrast to the absence of such a relationship in the group with extended benefits. To the authors, "this finding suggests that the special benefits may have elimintaed a financial barrier to physician utilization for lower-income subscribers," even though this increased access to a physician was not associated with any decrease in hospitalization (135, p. 1410).

Even this one positive finding should, however, be viewed with caution. It appears that the experimental and control groups, though comparable with respect to hospital use prior to the institution of the extended benefit (and, as it turned out, after that), were not really alike after all. A little over 85 percent of the experimental population were in three employee groups: public school teachers, university employees, and city employees. Public school teachers alone constituted about three-fifths of the contracts in the experimental group. Since we do not know how social class was defined, and we suspect it was based on income alone, it could very well be that occupational and educational attributes of the social classes within the experimental group, rather than the extended benefit, may have been responsible for the lack of relationship between social class and physician contacts in that group.

In order to determine whether the extended benefits had an effect on the use of services outside the hospital, information is needed, for both experimental and control groups, about the utilization of these services before and after the institution of the extended benefits, and, preferably, following their termination. In the absence of this sequence, one can only speculate about the apparent lack of a difference in the use of out-of-hospital services between the experimental and control groups. But here another factor intervenes: an astounding lack of knowledge about the availability of the new benefits by the experimental population and by their physicians. Of 30 physicians interviewed, more than half did not know the extent of hospital and non-hospital benefits available to their patients. Only 41 percent of the subsample of the experimental group knew that there had been a recent change in their benefits, and only 52 percent knew that they had coverage for home and office care. To make the distinction between the groups even less sharp, 23 percent of the control group also thought there had been a recent change in their benefits, and 30 percent thought they had coverage for home and office care. It is not possible to say whether the findings in the control group indicate a natural state of misinformation, or whether they represent an unintended spread of information beyond the experimental group. If the latter, it is interesting to note that this "halo" effect occurred even though the sampling of employed groups, rather than of subscribers within the same groups, was designed to prevent it. For these reasons, and because the experiment was of short duration, the finding that extended benefits appear to have little or no effect, whether localized or generalized, must remain open to serious doubt. This study does, however, point out that there may be serious problems in communicating accurate information about the availability of benefits and their precise features. This is a problem that has been noted in other contexts, and is a matter of considerable importance in the administration of medical care programs (136–139).

The resort to large scale experimentation in order to answer critical questions about the effects of health insurance finds more recent expression in a project of almost breath-taking audacity proposed by Newhouse and his associates at the Rand Corporation (140). At an estimated cost of $32 million (as of 1973) the investigators plan to offer one of 16 different health insurance plans to carefully chosen samples of families in four different geographic locations, and to study both their health care behavior and their health over a period of three or five years, as compared to families that will serve as controls. As a consequence, the investigators hope to determine the effect providing coverage for certain services has on the consumption of other services, with particular attention to the substitution of ambulatory care for hospital services. But this is only a small element in a much larger set of objectives. Perhaps the most important objective is to elucidate the effect of carefully graduated reductions in price on use of service, and how this relationship is further influenced by factors such as severity of illness, income, total expenditures, the workload of physicians in the several study sites, and the delivery of care through several variants of health maintenance organizations. The graduations in price will be achieved by designing the insurance plans offered to the study population so that there are several combinations of stepwise variations in the coinsurance percentages for inpatient and outpatient services and in the maximum out-of-pocket dollar expenditure expressed as a percent of income (140, Table 1, p. 13).

Not content with studying in awesome detail the effect of price on use of service, the investigators bravely grasp what is possibly the thorniest thistle in health care policy: the effect that various levels of use of service have on health status itself. Accordingly, they propose to perform an initial and terminal assessment on each beneficiary that will include a medical history, a physical examination, laboratory and other diagnostic tests, an inventory of current and recent symptoms, and a subjective assessment of the beneficiaries' own health and the health of their children. Further information on health status and the utilization of health services will be obtained at quarterly interviews and, possibly, through a weekly "postcard survey" (141).

Needless to say, all this effort is intended to yield answers to fundamental questions that would illuminate and guide policy in the formulation of a national health plan (142). Some critics have argued that the study will fail to achieve this purpose because of key weaknesses in design. To begin with, much too large a burden of analytic objectives is placed upon too small a sample of families. There will be only about 2,000 families in the study group, distributed among four geographic sites and 16 health insurance plans. By contrast, the number of variables under study is very large indeed. There are also doubts about the extent to which the process of observation itself, especially the repeated inquiries into health behavior and health status, will alter behavior so that it ceases to be generalizable. Most fundamentally, changes in the behavior of a small number of families at any one site, over a relatively short period of time, will not bring about those systemic responses in service capacity, price, technological change, and statutory regulation that are key elements in assessing the impact of a scheme of national magnitude (143). Since the study is already under progress, little will be gained from a more detailed critique. There will be many opportunities to point the finger should the study fail, or join the bandwagon of celebrants should it succeed. In the meantime, we can freely admire the conceptual sophistication, the skill, and the enterprise of the investigators, if not their wisdom.

Outpatient Physician Care and Hospital Use in Organized Settings

So far, in our description and evaluation of empirical studies that have dealt with the substitutive effect of benefits, we have examined situations in which different kinds of benefits were offered, but the manner in which medical care was provided remained unaltered. The general context was the private practice of medicine on a fee-for-service basis, occasionally modified by a fee schedule, which was not always binding. Under these circumstances, the substitutive effects of benefits could sometimes be seen under an overlay, as it were, of other effects that brought about an increase in use; an overall reduction in the cost of care was seldom, if ever, encountered. It was even arguable whether quality had always improved, since it was suspected that greater access to care was counteracted, to an undetermined extent, by unjustified use of the more generous benefits.

In the light of this experience, it is important to ask what would happen if an extended range of benefits were offered within the context of a system that weakened the effect of financial incentives to individual physicians and strengthened professional influences and controls. Experience under prepaid group practice immediately comes to mind, and is frequently cited, to support the view that coverage for services outside the hospital will have a profound hospital-sparing effect. In order to interpret this experience it is necessary to consider the associated variables that may influence use of service. These are shown schematically in Figure 8. For want of a better terminology, we include under the heading of "organized care" the set of arrangements that are thought to alter incentives for physicians, and which are presumed to be characteristic of prepaid group practice and other formalized schemes for the provision of care. It is appropriate to think of "organized care" in this vague manner, since our understanding of the relevant attributes is incomplete, at best. The other variable is much more specific and has to do with the presence or absence of coverage for services outside the hospital, generally understood to mean therapeutic and diagnostic services in the doctor's office or in an ambulatory care facility.

Four categories result from the two-by-two classification de-

| | Coverage for Services Outside the Hospital [a] | |
Organized Care	Yes	No
Yes	A	B
No	C	D

FIGURE 8. Classification of arrangements for the provision of care by type of benefit

[a] All plans are assumed to have coverage for hospital care.

picted in Figure 8. There are no empirical examples of Type B: organized care without extended benefits. The three remaining categories yield three comparisons between categories. These are A to C, A to D, and C to D. We have already dealt with comparisons of the last kind, which attempt to identify the effects of extended benefits under fee-for-service private practice. What remains for us to do is to compare Type A (which stands for prepaid group practice or any comparable arrangement) first with D (which stands for limited benefits under fee-for-service private practice), and then with C, which sands for extended benefits under fee-for-service private practice. The object of this exposition, and of these comparisons, is to determine whether it is the extended nature of the benfits or the different form of organization that is responsible for lowered hospital use in "organized" settings. We have already skirmished with this question in our section on revenue effects, where we referred to the extensive literature dealing with the subject (32, 49-52, 56-74). Here we will take another look at some selected studies, with special emphasis on the possible effects of the extended nature of the benefits.

The studies we have selected all come from the New York City area. Although this area is a large and diverse conglomerate of subparts, it may also contain pervasive influences that lead to similiarities in patterns of care, although this is very difficult to substantiate. The prepaid group practice studied is, in all cases, the Health Insurance Plan of Greater New York (HIP). In this organization, care was provided by full-time or part-time salaried physicians affiliated with groups that were reimbursed on a per-capita basis. Thus, there were no fee-for-service incentives either to the physicians individually or to the collectivity of physicians within each group. Very few groups were based in a hospital, and coverage for hospital services was through a separate arrangement with Blue Cross and Blue Shield. As a result, there was no direct incentive to cut down on hospital care. In fact, it could be argued that admitting a patient to the hospital would reduce certain expenditures to the group, notably for diagnostic investigation (71). On the other hand, this tendency to hospitalize patients may have been counteracted by difficulties encountered by some groups in obtaining hospital affiliations (73), by the time physicians would waste attending patients in several hospitals, by the absence of a financial incentive to provide care in any setting, and by the presence of professional incentives to avoid unnecessary care. In these studies, experience under HIP is compared with experience under Blue Cross-Blue Shield or under Group Health Insurance (GHI). As is well known, the "Blues" mainly cover hospital services and care provided by physicians in the hospital. Group Health Insurance differed little from Blue Cross-Blue Shield, except that it offered the large majority of its enrollees non-hospital benefits reasonably comparable to those offered by HIP. Neither Blue Cross-Blue Shield nor GHI interfered with the private practice of medicine beyond using fee schedules, which were binding only on "participating" physicians, and then often only for enrollees below a specified income level. Thus, physicians were paid fee-for-service and were often able to demand and receive fees larger than those specified in the fee schedule.

Having this general context in mind, we can now examine the several studies whose findings are summarized in Table 24. These findings are arranged in the configuration indicated in Figure 8. Unfortunately, information on ambulatory services is very incomplete, so that usually we can only deal with hospital care, not knowing what compensatory changes, if any, have taken place in services received outside the hospital. The first comparison, A_1-D_1, contrasts the hospital experience of a 20 percent sample of HIP members employed by the City of New York (many of whom were teachers, a category suspected to have high levels of utiliza-

TABLE 24. Use of Hospital Services Under Specified Conditions, New York City Area, Time Periods Within 1955–1964, Inclusive [a]

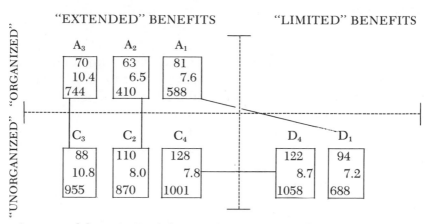

Sources and dates: A₁–D₁, Reference 62, 1955; A₂–C₂, Reference 49, 1956–1957; A₃–C₃, Reference 60, July 1, 1956, through June 30, 1957; C₄–D₄, Reference 133, 1964.

[a] "Extended benefits" mean coverage for home and office care in addition to hospital care. "Limited benefits" mean coverage for hospital care only. "Organized" stands for prepaid group practice and "Unorganized" stands for fee-for-service, private practice. The hospital data listed in each box, reading from top to bottom, are admissions per 1000 per year, days per stay, and patient-days per year. Data in comparison A₂–C₂ are for matched samples. All other data are adjusted at least for age and sex. Comparisons other than the ones indicated cannot be made.

tion) with the hospital experience of a sample of Blue Cross-Blue Shield enrollees from groups whose members were not exclusively employed in manufacturing. Reading from top to bottom in the boxes labeled A₁ and D₁, it is clear that, after correcting for age and sex, those enrolled in HIP had fewer admissions (81 versus 94 per 1,000 per year), slightly longer stays (7.6 versus 7.2 days) and a 13 percent saving in patient days (588 versus 688). The credibility of these findings is somewhat reduced by the fact that 37 percent of non-HIP members were hospitalized outside New York City proper, whereas only 5 percent of HIP enrollees were hospitalized outside the City. Since there could be more beds per capita outside the city, and since the availability of hospital beds is an important influence on the use of hospitals (144–150), this difference could be an important, uncorrected factor that would explain why Blue Cross members used the hospital more. However, the findings have been duplicated so often in other settings that one can accept them as valid without much danger of being wrong (58). In other words, we may safely conclude that extended benefits coupled with an organized mode for the delivery of care are associated with a significant hospital-sparing effect. It is not clear, however, whether it is the more comprehensive nature of the benefits, the "organized" nature of the program, or the confluence of both features that is responsible for the effect observed.

To help find the cause of this effect, we move on to two studies in which the extended nature of the benefits is held constant, but the formal organization of care is varied. The findings are shown in the pairs A_2-C_2 and A_3-C_3 in Table 24. The first of these pairings is a study of the members of three unions who were offered a choice of HIP or GHI. Samples, matched for age, sex and size of family, were drawn from each of these self-selected enrollee populations. The A_2 sample was drawn from enrollees who selected HIP coverage, and the C_2 sample from those who chose GHI. Although the samples were matched on three variables, the C_2 sample had a slightly higher level of education, fewer persons of Puerto Rican and other West Indian nationality, and fewer blacks. However, if persons who expect a greater need for service are apt to select group practice (139), this tendency in the A_2 sample may balance the greater propensity of the better educated whites in C_2 to seek care; but this surmise must remain doubtful in this study. Fortunately, the differences between A_2 and C_2, as shown in Table 24, are very striking indeed. Although both plans included ambulatory care benefits, the A_2 sample, enrolled in HIP, used less than half as many hospital days as the C_2 sample, who were enrolled in GHI. Even the length of stay was 19 percent less under HIP, in spite of the difference in case mix that must have been brought about by 43 percent fewer admissions for HIP enrollees.

Information is also supplied about visits to a physician. Unfortunately, the figures cited are for nonobstetrical, nonsurgical physician visits in home, office, and hospital. However, if one visit is counted for each hospital day of care, one can conclude that enrollees in HIP and GHI consume equal amounts of physician services, but that HIP enrollees make about 20 percent more office and home visits, in exchange for which they receive approximately 50 percent fewer days of hospital care. It should be pointed out, however, that while these very approximate magnitudes of substitution hold for this pair of matched samples, they cannot be generalized to other population groups.

Similar differences in hospital use, though not quite as large, were found in another study (A_3-C_3) which compared members of three locals of the International Ladies Garment Workers Union who also had a choice of selecting HIP or GHI. The main feature of these samples is the preponderance of adult females, a population suspected to be particularly responsive to benefit extensions, except that, in this instance, we are dealing with wage earners for whom the opportunity costs of seeking care could be high. This characteristic notwithstanding, extended benefits in an organized program were associated with markedly reduced hospital use, as compared to experience under a plan that offered similar benefits under the fee-for-service system of providing care. We must conclude, therefore, that the features associated with "organized" care, as we have described it, can by themselves bring about a reduction in hospital use.

This conclusion acquires even greater significance when we examine the final comparison, C_4-D_4, in Table 24. This comparison, which we have already described in some detail, is between GHI enrollees who have comprehensive benefits and GHI enrollees who have limited benefits. It is clear that the comprehensive benefit is associated with a higher rate of admissions, a shorter stay, and only a slightly lower number of patient days. Accordingly, we must conclude that extension of benefits without restructuring of incentives to the physician is associated with little reduction in hospital use, whereas restructuring incentives in the manner of HIP seems to have a strong effect in reducing hospital use. However, it is not known whether this effect can occur independently of an association with extended benefits. The final piece of evidence that would permit us to answer this question is missing. As the reader can see, there is a blank field in the upper right hand corner of Table 24. Until that hiatus in our figure, and in our argument, is filled by appropriate research, the weight of evidence can be taken to support the conclusion that a mode of organization that reduces fee-for-service incentives and strengthens professional concerns is necessary in order to attain the reductions in hospital care that are made possible by offering comprehensive benefits.

Of late, studies from "neighborhood health centers" have suggested that under these auspices also the availability of ambulatory care that is associated with a particular, though not completely specified, configuration of professional incentives will bring about a reduction in hospital use. For example, Alpert et al. have compared use of service by two similar groups of low-income families before and after one of the two groups was enrolled in a program of "comprehensive, family-focused pediatric care" based at the Children's Hospital Medical Center in Boston (96). Data on use of service were obtained from experimental and control groups through household interviews at 6 month intervals, supplemented by daily logs kept by the mother for 28 days out of each 6-month period. The provision of ambulatory care to the experimental group, in a setting that encouraged health maintenance and ready access to care in the event of illness, brought about a slightly larger number of visits to physicians. The striking difference between groups, however, was in the relative frequency of visits for health maintenance as compared to visits for the care of illness. In the experimental group there was an increase in the former and a decrease in the latter, relative to the experience of the control group as well as relative to the experience of the experimental group itself prior to enrollment in the program. There was an associated reduction in the use of the hospital by the experimental group. The only exception was during the first 6 months, when hospitalization rates in the experimental group were unusually high, presumably because a backlog of unmet need was being detected and cared for. During this period, there was also an unusually high incidence of preventive visits to the physician, presumably for the same reason. Thus, this small, but well-controlled, study illustrates with reasonable clarity both the substitutive and the discovery effects of a comprehensive program of benefits under organized auspices.

Equally interesting, though not so well-controlled, is a study of the effects of the establishment of a neighborhood health center in a geographically isolated, low-income, public housing development in South Boston (97). A household survey prior to the establishment of the Center had shown that 3 out of 5 hospital admissions from this population were to Boston City Hospital. Consequently, the records of this hospital were checked to determine hospital use 12 months prior to, and 18 months after, the advent of the Health Center, by a sample of 209 families with 980 members, excluding those who were 65 and over. For this population, there was a reduction in hospital admissions of 41 percent during the first year, and a further reduction of 73 percent during the second year, which amounted to a total reduction of 84 percent during two years. In spite of these striking changes, the average length of stay was not much altered. The authors considered the possibility that these enormous reductions represented, at least to some extent, a shift in the site of hospitalization from Boston City Hospital to other hospitals. To test this possibility, data on all hospital care were obtained from welfare records for a subset of 61 households, comprising 269 persons under 65, who had been on welfare during this entire period. For this subset the reduction in hospital use, though not quite as large, was within a comparable order of magnitude. Over a period of two years, admissions were reduced by 69 percent, average length of stay by 35 percent, and patient-days by 80 percent. Unfortunately, there are no data on ambulatory care before and after the institution of the Health Center, so we have no measure of the substitution of office for hospital care.

By contrast to the study reported by Alpert et al., no discovery effect is evident, possibly because data are not given for periods shorter than a year. In addition to the limitations in data and design already mentioned, including the absence of contemporaneous controls, the values for the second six months of the second year were not obtained directly, but computed by extrapolating from the experience of the first year, thus assuring that the relative decline during the second six months of the second year would be as large as the relative decline during the second six months of the first year. A more interesting feature of a panel study such as this, in which a group is observed for a relatively long time without additions to the group, is the absence of independence between events during successive years. For example, as we pointed out in a previous chapter, some procedures, such as tonsillectomies, appendectomies, and cholecystectomies, cannot usually occur more than once, and must decline with time merely through attrition (94). We do not know what the temporal sequence of risk is for other health care events in a panel population, when the effect of aging can be excluded. In the study we have just described, there was a reduction of 86 percent in obstetrical admissions to Boston City Hospital in the two years during which the original sample of 209 families was under observation. The authors, who seem to be as puzzled as we are by this finding, comment as follows: "Although a family-planning service was made available in this community, its effects, obviously, could hardly be felt until the second year. A more likely explanation for the drop in births during the first year is the nature of the panel-study design: as an aging cohort, it is subject to diminishing fertility" (97, p. 810). In addition to biological aging, it is likely that women who have recently had one or more children will decide not to have more children for some time to come. This kind of attrition, plus the large random variation likely to occur in a sample of this small size, may adequately explain some of the aberrant findings in this study. In any event, these irregularities do not alter the more general conclusion that providing out-of-hospital services through a variety of organized ambulatory care programs can reduce the volume of inpatient hospital care, provided physicians are not paid fee-for-service.

Home Care and Hospital Use in Organized Settings

In our discussion of the substitutive effects of benefits we dealt first with the possible impact of providing diagnostic services outside the hospital, and then of extending these benefits to include care by the physician in the office and the home. The emphasis has been on the provision of care for the ambulatory patient in the hope of preventing the need for confinement to the hospital. In this context, organized home care may be seen as yet another extension of benefits, this time designed to care for the bed-ridden or house-bound patient in order to reduce the necessity for admission to the hospital or to hasten the discharge if the patient has already been admitted. Home care may have other advantages, psychological or social, to the patient and his family, as well as some drawbacks. Here we are concerned only with the impact on use of service, with particular attention to the hospital-sparing effect. In this respect, many claims have been made that home care reduces hospital use and lowers costs, but those claims have not usually been substantiated by valid evidence (151). Accordingly, we shall only review the very few reasonably well-controlled studies that have attempted to examine these claims.

The first of these studies is a little classic reported by Bakst and Marra in 1955 (152). For this study, patients with cardiac disease, classified III-C or of greater severity at the time of admission, were randomly assigned to an experimental or control group at the time of their discharge from Boston City Hospital. In addition to satisfying the requirements of the clinical classification signifying serious heart disease, patients were included in the study only if they had not been under the care of a private physician and were being discharged to their homes. In this manner, 55 patients were included in the experimental group and 35 in the control group. The published report does not explain this inequality in numbers, but it does show that the two groups were comparable by age, sex, and marital status, as well as with respect to cardiac diagnosis. However, we are given no information about comparability with respect to associated medical conditions at the time the sample was selected. There must have been a fair amount of other illness, since this was a group of elderly people, and poor. The median age for both groups was 64; 31 percent of the control group received care in the home by a visiting nurse, and were seen at home or in the clinic by second-and third-year residents supervised by a qualified cardiologist or internist. The control group was left to its own devices, receiving care in the ordinary manner, which in this instance, by design, did not usually include the services of a private physician. Data concerning the experimental group were generated by the service program itself. Unfortunately, there was no comparable source of information for the control group. Data on the control group had to be collected and pieced together from many sources, including reviews of hospital and outpatient records, reports of the Visiting Nurse Association, and records of the vital statistics division of the health department. For this reason, it would not be surprising if there were some underreporting for the control group in this study. This should be kept in mind when examining the findings which are shown in Table 25.

As expected, the experimental group received many more services in the home, and fewer services in the hospital outpatient department. In addition to the services by the physician and the nurse, which are shown in the table, the social worker made many visits to patients in the experimental group, and, in some instances, care had to be extended to other family members as well.

TABLE 25. Utilization of Specified Services and Mortality Rates for Two Groups of Cardiac Patients, One Provided with Home Care Services and the Other Left Undisturbed, Boston, 1954

Sample, Use of Services and Mortality	Received Home Care	Did Not Receive Home Care
Number of Patients	55	35
Patient-days of observation	14,393	10,253
Utilization/1,000 patient-days [a]		
Physician visits to the home	105.3	3.4 [b]
Outpatient department visits	5.6	22.5
Visiting-nurse visits	71.6	29.6
All hospital admissions	3.5	3.8
All hospital days	59.5	42.3 [c]
Cardiac hospital admissions	0.7	2.6
Cardiac hospital days	14.1	23.3
Non-cardiac hospital admissions	2.8	1.2
Non-cardiac hospital days	45.4	21.0
Deaths/1,000 patient-days	0.90	0.98

Source: Reference 152, Tables 2 and 3, page 447.

[a] Recomputed from data in the source so as to correct for difference in length of observation of the two groups.

[b] Approximate

[c] In the original data, component hospital days do not add to total days. For the recomputed data the sum would be 44.3 days.

By contrast, hospital care was comparable for both groups, although the reasons for using the hospital were different. The experimental group was admitted relatively more frequently for non-cardiac conditions, whereas the control group was admitted more frequently for cardiac illness. If it is assumed that health status was comparable in the two groups, this finding suggests that home care was successful in managing the patients' heart disease at home, and was also instrumental in uncovering additional illness for which hospital care was necessary. Thus, the substitutive effects of the home care benefit were more than offset by the "discovery effect" of these same benefits, at least in this group of elderly and seriously ill patients. Once again, we find confirmation of the aphorism that "a little medical care breeds more medical care."

As to cost, although data are not cited, it is obvious, as the authors also conclude, that overall costs were considerably increased rather than decreased. The justification for the home care program must, therefore, rest not on the reduction in the costs of care, but the improvement in health. Unfortunately, information concerning this matter is very meager. According to the authors, "The careful interpretation of the illness situation to the patient and the family resulted in improved acceptance of the problem and considerable relief of emotional stresses" (152, p. 449). But we have no information about improvement in the ability to function, whereas mortality rates in the two groups were reasonably alike. We must, therefore, remain in doubt about the cost-to-benefit relationship in this kind of program for this kind of population.

Essentially similar conclusions may be drawn from a more recent study by Hanchett and Torrens of the impact of a home nursing program for patients with heart disease (153). In this study, 239 patients with chronic congestive heart failure, who attended the outpatient clinics of St. Luke's Hospital in New York City, were randomly divided into two groups. The control group continued to receive care in the outpatient department, as before. Patients in the experimental group were visited at home by a public health nurse, who also worked with the patient and the physician in the clinic. The two groups were comparable by age, sex, ethnic origin, type of heart disease, and functional classification. Both groups consisted mainly of elderly women who were limited in their physical activity but were not confined to bed. During observation for a period of 2½ years, patients in the experimental group were admitted to the hospital, more frequently, and used about 20 percent more hospital days than did the control group. There was, however, as in the study by Bakst and Marra, a difference in the reasons for hospital use. The experimental group used the hospital less (by almost a third) only for congestive heart failure, the diagnosis which was the criterion for inclusion of patients in the study. The experimental group used the hospital more for cardiac diagnoses other than congestive heart failure (by more than two-thirds), and for all non-cardiac diagnoses (by almost a half). The authors attribute this pattern to "intensive observation of the study group patients" (153, p. 685). Unfortunately, we are not told how the patients' health was affected by this intensive observation and the additional care that it engendered.

In a small number of studies attention has been given to the fundamental issue of health outcomes consequent to the institution of home care services. Stone et al. have published a brief report on a study comparing a group of non-indigent persons who were referred for home care to a partially matched sample of persons who were eligible for home care but were not referred (154). The degree of progress towards recovery from illness, as judged by the physician attending each case, was comparable for the two groups, but the cost of care was much lower in the group that had home care. Unfortunately, this study is so carelessly reported that the meaning and validity of its findings cannot be properly assessed. It is cited here mainly because it suggests that the substitutive effect is dominant when home care of relatively short duration is offered as a substitute for hospital care, for a variety of reasonably self-limiting conditions. This is quite a different situation from the provision of home care for the long-term management of old and chronically ill patients, where closer observation results in more rather than less care, and where it is necessary to decide whether the additional care provided is justified by its impact on health.

For a closer look at the effects of home care on health we turn to two elegantly designed and executed studies reported by Sidney Katz and his associates (155, 156). In the first study, 20 patients who had well established, severe rheumatoid arthritis were assigned to each of two groups. Both the experimental and control groups continued to receive care at the arthritis clinic of the University Hospitals of Cleveland, but the experimental group were also visited in the home by a public health nurse who met in conference with the clinic staff in order to coordinate care for her patients. The two samples were comparable with respect to demographic characteristics, type of illness and functional ability. Although the patients ranged in age from 16 to 75, many were elderly, with an average age of 52.5 years, and severely handicapped. It is fair to say, therefore, that while the demands on the care-providing system were likely to be great, the rewards were likely to be small. It transpired, in fact, that during a 12-month period of observation there were no significant differences between experimental and control groups in occupational therapy visits, social service visits, podiatry clinic visits, or eye clinic visits. By contrast, the experimental group used a great deal of home care: approximately 3.6 visits per person per month. This was more than 11 times as many visits as were received by persons in the control group. In addition, the experimental group made 30 percent more clinic visits and 144 percent more outpatient therapy visits, and used 143 percent more hospital days. Thus, a larger amount of outpatient and home care was associated with more, rather than less, care in the hospital. In this study a great effort was made to measure outcomes in as precise and valid a fashion as possible, with several instruments being used for the purpose. The additional amount of care lavished on the experimental group had no effect on the degree of confinement to the home, on the time the patient took to walk 50 feet, or on the time the patient took to climb 8 steps. There was, however, a significant advantage with respect to some other measures of outcome. A scale that measured the activity of the disease process and its impact on the patients' joints and muscles showed a little less deterioration and somewhat greater improvement in the experimental group. Patients in the experimental group were also less likely to deteriorate in their capacity to perform the activities of daily living, and they were less likely to suffer economic dependence. Whether this degree of improvement or lack of deterioration is worth the additional cost of care cannot be answered, since no single unit was used to measure both costs and benefits. One cannot escape the impression, however, that the yield was small.

The second study reported by Katz et al. was even more ambitious. The patients who were studied were at least 50 years old and had been discharged to their homes from a chronic disease rehabilitation hospital, where they had been for at least one week. The patients were divided into two groups of 150 each, one experimental and one control. Each of these groups was further subdivided into two sub-groups; one group was assessed every three months, and the other group was assessed only at intake and at termination, two years later. The factorial design was adopted to permit identification of the effects of the assessment procedures themselves, either alone or in conjunction with the treatment procedures. Patients were assigned to the four sub-groups in the study by a random process that assured equal probability of being assigned to any sub-group. This produced subgroups that were highly comparable in several characteristics that were thought to be important to the observations. Steps were also taken to control bias in the assessment of patient status. Those who assessed the patients were kept separate from those who provided care. The assessors were assigned to patients at intake in a random manner. For the terminal assessment, each patient was assigned, also in random fashion, to an assessor who was different from the one for the intake and subsequent observations. All patients in the experimental group were referred to the local visiting nurse agency and became eligible for the services that were part of the agency's program, except that some small modifications were introduced to meet the needs of the research study. The object was to determine what the effects of home nursing care would be on an elderly group of patients, who were suffering largely from strokes and other diseases of the nervous system, fractures, arthritis, and chronic vascular disease, and who had been discharged from a chronic disease rehabilitation hospital to which they had been admitted because they were "disabled and judged to have a potential for rehabilitation" (156, p. 83).

By design, the experimental group received much more home nursing care than the control group: a total of 5,667 visits for the former, versus 834 for the latter, which is almost a seven-fold difference. Only 23 percent of the control group received any home nursing, while 97 percent of the experimental group did. The likelihood of being hospitalized during two years was high for both groups, but higher for the experimental group (63 percent) than the control group (51 percent). By contrast, patients in the experimental group were less likely to be admitted to nursing homes, although the precise figure is not given. Nor are we given information on length of stay either in hospital or nursing homes. Use of service was increased in the experimental group, "especially for persons who were older, more disabled and more severely ill. Among these people, quantitative estimates of increased use of physicians and hospitals varied from 17 to 48 percent, generally being 25 percent or greater" (156, p. 92). As to the outcomes of care, no differences in "function, injury and mortality" were demonstrable when experimental and control groups were compared as a whole. However, certain subgroups, usually of persons who were less seriously disabled, seemed to have benefited from home nursing. There were also some persons who appeared to have reacted by reducing their social interaction with persons other than the nurse. It would seem, therefore, that home nursing is a modality of care that needs to be selectively applied, and that its effect, at least in the range of conditions represented in the sample, is to arrest or retard deterioration in physical and mental function, rather than to bring about improvement. Also, like other modalities of care, it may have undesirable side effects in certain situations, as evidenced by the reduction in social interaction in a subset of patients who had poor mental function and cardiovascular-renal abnormalities. Interestingly enough, the process of assessment itself had some effects, namely, reducing admissions to the hospital and "reducing decreases" in social interaction. There were also joint effects in the group that received nursing care and was also assessed at three-monthly intervals. These effects were "fewer returns to employment, more physician services, and less non-nurse attendant care," as if the nursing and assessment "tended to reinforce the sick role, as defined by Parsons" (156, pp. 84–85). All in all, in this experiment, the inputs of care were large and the rewards appear to have been small, although a precise calculus of costs and benefits was not made. Some believe this calculus cannot, or even should not, be made.

The conclusion to be drawn from controlled studies of the effects of home care is that the net effect is an increase rather than a decrease in hospital use, and that the costs of care go up rather than down. The true function of the home care benefit, therefore, is to add another choice to the modalities available to the physician, so that care can be matched more precisely to need. The assumption is that, in this way, the most cost-effective mix of services will be chosen. However, not a great deal is known about the relationship between costs and effects, and physicians are either averse to, or unskilled in, assessing this relationship. As we have said before, the conclusion that home care increases costs and hospital use does not mean that there is no substitutive effect to the home care benefit, but merely that the sustained supervision made possible by home care reveals new needs as these develop. It is also necessary to point out that these conclusions are derived from studies of a certain category of patients: those who are old, chronically ill, and often poor. There is almost certainly a category of patients who suffer from relatively short-term illness, or acute exacerbations of chronic illness, in whom the hospital-sparing effect of home care would be dominant. Unfortunately, this effect has been so poorly documented that one must defer judgment on its reality, although one hopes that it is there.

Extended Care and Hospital Use in Organized Settings

Those committed to the rightness, as well as the feasibility, of providing comprehensive benefits have also hoped to reduce hospital use by offering nursing home care as an alternative. A demonstration project was designed with the express purpose of testing this expectation; of the several accounts that describe the project, we have chosen the final report as the basis for our assessment (157–159).

On June 28, 1967, the Kaiser-Permanente Health Plan of Portland Oregon, with support from the U.S. Public Health Service, initiated a program that added home care and extended care facility services to an already established hospital-based prepaid group practice. The services provided were roughly analogous to those envisaged under Medicare, but were available to all plan enrollees irrespective of age. A major objective of the demonstration project was to determine the need for such services, as well as their capacity to reduce hospital use and overall costs.

For several reasons, the setting chosen was considered particularly suitable for this purpose. There was an identifiable enrolled population which could be presumed not to have a significant backlog of unmet need. The physicians in the prepaid group had no apparent incentive to use unnecessary and expensive services, and could be counted upon to accept and use new additions to the range of services already at hand. Finally, there was a well established data system that could provide information on use of service and costs over a period of years. A portion of this information is shown in Table 26. The data cited are for 1966, which was the last full year preceding the project; for 1968, during which the program was in continuous operation; and for 1969, immediately after it was terminated (in December 1968). In all instances except one, utilization data for the first 6 months of the year are doubled in order to arrive at a yearly figure.

Since the proportion of enrollees eligible for Medicare differs a little from year to year, it is best to examine the data separately for

TABLE 26. Data Relevant to Use of the Hospital and Extended Care Facility, Kaiser-Permanente Health Plan, Portland, Oregon; by Type of Patient, Specified Years

Population, Beds, Use, and Costs	1966	1968	1969
Hospital discharges per 1,000			
Total	97	90	91
Non-Medicare	88	79	81
Medicare	247	223	221
Hospital average stay in days [a]			
Total	5.6	4.9	5.7
Non-Medicare	5.0	4.6	5.2
Medicare	8.9	6.2	8.2
Hospital patient-days per 1,000			
Total	541	442	522
Non-Medicare	437	363	421
Medicare	2,198	1,373	1,802
ECF days per 1,000 [b]			
Total	—	149	—
Non-Medicare	—	75	—
Medicare	—	1,043	—
Hospital plus ECF days per 1,000			
Total	541	591	522
Non-Medicare	437	438	421
Medicare	2,198	2,416	1,802
Total population	82,229	108,203	124,450
Total beds [c]	141	230	230
Total beds per 1,000	1.7	2.1	1.8
Total unduplicated discharges per 1,000 [d]	97	91	91
Average stay in days [a]	5.6	6.2	5.7
Total days per 1,000	541	591	522
Total occupancy rate (computed) [e]	85%	76%	76%

Source: Reference 159, Tables 32, 36 and 37, pages 76 and 81–83.

[a] Patient-days ÷ discharges.

[b] Extended Care Facility days for entire year (see text).

[c] For this and subsequent items the total inpatient facility (hospital plus extended care segments) is considered to be one undifferentiated unit.

[d] There were only 194 direct admissions to the ECF during 1968.

[e] (Hospital + ECF days) ÷ (Total beds × 365) (100).

the non-Medicare and Medicare categories. Under examination, a reasonably clear pattern emerges. During the year of the project there was a definite reduction in the hospital discharge rate, and this rate was not restored to its previous level when the project terminated. While there was also a reduction in the average length of stay, this reduction was confined to the project year. The joint effect of these two factors was an almost 40 percent reduction in hospital days per 1,000 enrollees during the year of the project, with partial restoration to the previous level during the six months following its termination. It appears, therefore, that there was a significantly lower use of hospital services during the project year. But, needless to say, there was also a counterbalancing use of the services of the extended care facility, so that the rate for total inpatient days of care, including hospital days as well as days in the extended care facility, was highest during the project year and lowest during the six months immediately following.

Several aspects of these findings require further analysis and interpretations. We may begin by asking how much of the observed pattern of hospital utilization can be attributed to the institution and termination of the project, and did the home care component make a separate, identifiable contribution? The answer to the second part of this question appears to be "no." Most admissions to the home care program were from the ambulatory care service or from the extended care facility, with relatively few direct admissions from the hospital. In addition, a review of a sample of home care patients by their attending physicians led to the judgment that very few hospital days were saved through the use of home care. The investigators conclude, apparently with good reason, that the hospital-sparing effect of the home care program was negligible. They also conclude that the extended care service did result in a saving in hospital days; however, this conclusion requires much closer examination. First, it is necessary to determine whether the changes in hospital utilization could have come about, at least in part, through the influence of other, concurrent events. Second, it is necessary to evaluate the degree to which the peculiarities of this prepaid group practice reduce the confidence with which one may generalize from the findings to other situations. Both of these considerations lead us to an examination of the factors that influence the choice of the site of care: the hospital, the extended care facility, or some alternative. We have already excluded the home care program as a significant alternative in this setting, because its hospital-sparing effect was negligible. The choice of ambulatory care cannot, unfortunately, be examined directly, because no data are provided; but ambulatory care remains implicitly the dominant alternative selected when neither the hospital nor the extended care facility are chosen as the site of care.

Among the factors that influence the choice of the site of care, perhaps the most important is the supply of hospital beds in relation to need or demand. In this instance need, as well as client-generated demand, are probably well represented by the size of the enrolled population and its composition. Although clients do have a preference for specific sites of care, it is likely that the major factors in this prepaid group practice plan are the incentives that influence the physicians individually, the physicians as an organized group, and the hospital and extended care facility as separate accounting units. The investigators make a point of emphasizing that when physicians are not paid on a fee-for-service basis, there is no incentive for them to provide unnecessary, expensive services, such as hospital care, in preference to less expensive alternatives. However, it is not clear how much physicians as a group might benefit financially from transferring a share of their work to the hospital, or how much the hospital might benefit by resisting this tendency or by transferring a share of its case load to the extended care facility. In this case, we are not given the information about detailed financial arrangements which might reveal these incentives.

But incentives are not only financial. When physicians are overworked it is likely that they are influenced to transfer a greater share of their work to an inpatient facility, especially if it is conveniently located (160). At the beginning of the project there were 85 physicians and 89,672 enrollees in the Kaiser-Permanente Plan in Portland, a ratio of one physician to 1,055 enrollees (159, pp. 5 and 38). Whether this is too few or too many is hard to say, since so many factors influence the productivity of physicians and the demand for care (1, pp. 509–634). We do know, however, that the extended care facility was physically and organizationally a part of the hospital, an arrangement that was convenient to the physicians and conducive to the movement of patients between the two segments of inpatient care. When patients were transferred, the attending physician retained responsibility for care, a feature that under most, though not necessarily all, circumstances, would facilitate the transfer. In addition, there was considerable effort to inform the physician, and to persuade him to use the program, an influence that must have reinforced whatever incentives there may have been to use the extended facility—because of financial advantage to the group of physicians or the hospital, because of large physician work loads, because of the proximity of the facility, and because admission to the facility did not entail a break in the patient-physician relationship.

Demand was also generated by members of the project staff, who constantly reviewed the status of patients in the hospital and informed the attending physician of cases who would be suitable for transfer to the extended care facility. The patients themselves seldom raised an objection to the move. In fact, "the great majority of patients" were unaware that a "significant change" had occurred in the nature of the care they were receiving when transferred to the extended care area of the inpatient service (159, p. 17). In this new location, care continued at a level of intensity not very different from that experienced, towards the end of the stay, in the hospital area, and the duration of stay was generally short, being about 10 days on the average (159, p. 57 ff.).

Essentially then, this study reports experience in a hospital that was organized to provide both the intensive and intermediate care components of the "progressive patient care" spectrum, rather than where there was a clear distinction between the hospital and a separate extended care facility (161). It is no wonder then, that under the circumstances described, admission of Medicare beneficiaries to the extended care segment was four times as frequent as for the U.S. as a whole, while the average stay was less than a fourth as long. As the investigators clearly recognize, we have here "two very different concepts of extended care utilization" (159, p. 56).

Another consideration that must be taken into account in interpreting the findings is the supply of inpatient beds relative to potential need and demand. At the beginning of the project, the hospital had 144 beds, of which 141 were apparently operational (159, pp. 4, 127). The ratio of 1.7 operational beds per 1,000 persons, is considerably lower than the more usual 4 or 5 per 1,000, even when corrected for the lower proportion of aged persons among the members of this plan. The relative tightness of the bed supply is reflected in the high occupancy rate, which appears to have exceeded 90 percent, as well as in the remarkably low rate of hospital use, which was perhaps from one-half to one-third less than experienced under comparable circumstances outside prepaid group practice (159, p. 5). The suspicion that the supply of hospital beds was not merely a comfortable adjustment to this low level of demand is reinforced by frequent reference to determined efforts to keep hospital use under control, and validated by the opening, in March 1967, of an additional unit of 110 beds designed and equipped to be used either for "acute" or for "extended" care (159, p. 4). It is likely that the availability of these beds was an important stimulus to the initiation of the extended care project. In any event, the new beds were allocated in a manner that gave the hospital a total of 160 beds and the extended care facility 70 beds, for a total of 230 operational beds and, presumably, 24 beds held in reserve (159, p. 127). But, in the interval, there occurred a large increase in the enrolled population (possibly related to the availability of additional inpatient facilities) as well as a small increase in the proportion of aged persons among the enrollees. In 1968, the project year, there was a total of 2.1 inpatient beds per 1,000 enrollees, a small improvement over the ratio of 1.7 per 1,000 in 1966. But, by the beginning of 1969, the ratio was 1.8 per 1,000, and beds were nearly as scarce, relative to pop ulation, as they had been in 1966.

These observations on bed supply have a number of implications. To begin with, the relative scarcity of hospital beds, the low level of hospital utilization, and the active efforts of the utilization review apparatus, suggest that relatively few patients remained in the hospital beyond the point of necessity, so that there was limited room for substitution by the extended care facility. This suggests that the extended care facility should not have helped a great deal in reducing hospital use. The investigators report that this was indeed the case prior to the institution of the project, when a "distant" extended care facility was available for Medicare patients (159, p. 6). The key event in the history of this project, as we see it, may not have been the project itself, but the expansion of the inpatient bed capacity from 141 to 230 operational beds. That some of the additional beds were set apart for less intensive care than were others, may have been a relatively less important, though still significant, feature. The data relevant to this hypothesis are in the bottom half of Table 26, where the total inpatient facility is considered as one undifferentiated unit. Examination of these data shows that the increase in beds per 1,000 enrollees during 1968 was accompanied, as expected, by longer average stays and a higher number of patient-days per 1,000 than were found during 1966 or 1969, when the bed ratios were lower. This made it possible to maintain a reasonably high occupancy rate throughout the period of observation.

The only markedly aberrant observation is the relative nonresponsiveness of the admission rate. This may be due, in part, to the determined efforts to control hospital use that were made throughout this period. We know, for example, that during the period 1966–1968, the department of surgery "was attempting to provide as many surgical procedures as possible on an outpatient basis," apparently with considerable success (159, p. 85). More important, perhaps, was the degree of separation of the hospital and extended care segments of the inpatient service, so that admissions took place almost exclusively to the more crowded hospital segment. The median monthly occupancy rate in the hospital segment was approximately 88 percent, while the rate was 63 percent in the extended care area (159, p. 127). In considering the possible role played by bed supply, the investigators contend that "the project never operated under the constraint of a bed shortage that might have artificially limited the use of either the hospital or of the ECF" (159, p. 57). They also point out that "the monthly fluctuations in number of admissions and in average stay in the extended care facility and in the hospital did not appear to be correlated. Although various measures were tested to determine whether the fluctuations were interrelated or related to some constant factor, no regular patterns could be discerned" (159, pp. 57–58). Our own interpretation is that the smaller supply of beds in the hospital segment of the inpatient service in 1968 than in 1966 (1.5 beds per 1,000 versus 1.7 per 1,000) plus the efforts to control hospital use, account for the reduction in the admission rate observed in 1968. However, during 1968 additional efforts were made to generate use of the extended care segment, partly by reducing the length of hospital stay by substituting an equal number of days in the extended care facility, and partly by lengthening care somewhat beyond that, because the lower oc-

cupancy of the extended care facility allowed, and perhaps encouraged, this further lengthening in the stay. By 1969, the
enrolled population had grown sufficiently to permit termination
of the distinction between hospital and extended care beds, with
only a small increase in bed supply per 1,000 enrollees over the
1966 level. Accordingly, hospital use remained under control. If
this interpretation is correct, the compartmentalization of the hospital into intensive care and intermediate care areas served to curb
hospital admissions during a period of relatively higher total bed
supply, even though these reductions were more than offset by
longer stays in the inpatient facility as a whole. However, because
care in the extended care segment is less costly, it is necessary to
consider the effect of these changes on the total cost of care.

The data pertaining to an estimation of relative costs are summarized in Table 27, with more detailed information by Medicare
eligibility for the years 1966 and 1968. Comparisons are made
under two alternative assumptions. The first assumption is that
discharge rates and average lengths of stay for each age group
should have been the same in 1968 as they were in 1066, had it
not been for the institution of the extended care program. When
the expected number of patient days of hospital care are computed
under this assumption one finds a "saving" of 7,722 days of hospital stay at $72.62 per day. Against these savings, there are 16,554
days of extended care at $39.08 per day. The result is a net excess
cost of $86,158, which amounts to an additional $0.77 per enrollee.

Under the second assumption, only the reduction in length of
hospital stay, and not the reduction in discharge rate, is attributed
to the operation of the extended care program. If so, the savings in
hospital days are fewer and the increment in total cost is larger.
One must conclude that the institution of the extended care program did not reduce the costs of care, even under the first, more favorable, assumptions: that the changes in admission rate and in
length of stay were completely attributable to the institution of the
extended care program, and that the cost of the days of care saved
was equal to the average daily hospital cost. These assumptions
are overly generous, since the days of hospital care that are saved
are near the tail end of hospital stay and are, therefore, less intensive in care and correspondingly less costly. It follows that the

TABLE 27. Use and Costs of Inpatient Care before (1966) and after (1968) Opening an Extended Care Facility, by Type of Patient, Kaiser-Permanente Health Plan, Portland, Oregon

Use and Costs	Total	Non-Medicare	Medicare
Observed hospital days			
1966	41,664	31,757	9,907
1968	47,662	36,316	11,346
Expected hospital days for 1968 [a]			
First assumption	55,384	41,707	15,443
Second assumption	53,077	38,748	15,553
Hospital days "saved" [b]			
First assumption	−7,722	−5,391	−4,097
Second assumption	−5,415	−2,432	−4,207
ECF days, 1968	16,554	7,706	8,848
Cost of ECF days 1968 (dollars) [c]	646,930	301,150	345,780
Cost of hospital days "saved" (dollars) [d]			
First assumption	−560,772	−391,494	−297,524
Second assumption	−393,237	−176,612	−305,512
Net costs (dollars)			
First assumption	86,158	−90,344	48,256
Second assumption	253,693	124,538	40,268
Net costs per enrollee (dollars)			
First assumption	0.77	−0.88	5.69
Second assumption	2.28	1.21	4.75

Source: Reference 159, Table 36, pages 81–82.

[a] The first assumption is that discharge rates and lengths of stay in 1966 remain unchanged. The second assumption is that discharge rates change, but the 1966 lengths of stay remain unchanged. Computations are based on age specific rates for 3 groups in the Non-Medicare and 2 groups in the Medicare categories. Totals do not equal the sum of the parts due to rounding.

[b] A negative sign means 1968 value is less, i.e. there is a saving in days or costs.

[c] At $39.08 per day.

[d] At $72.62 per day.

savings from the substitution of extended care for hospital care are significantly smaller than cited, and the net increment in cost is correspondingly greater.

One could further argue, with some justification, that there can be no important savings in total cost unless there are savings in total patient days used, because, assuming the entire inpatient stay is necessary, the hospital adjusts its staffing patterns and other inputs to the lower average severity of illness in its case load. The onus of proof is on those who contend that separation of the hospital into segments of progressively less intensive care produces an aggregate reduction in these inputs (162, 163). They could counter the arguments against extended care facilities by asserting that even if costs are no less, the care and the health of the patients is improved. In this particular instance, the investigators cite evidence of patient improvement under extended care (159, pp. 77–99). Unfortunately, there is no way of knowing whether the degree of improvement would have been less if care had continued in the ordinary way, in the hospital rather than in the extended care facility.

Outpatient Psychiatric Care and Other Care in Organized Settings

In our examination of the effects of ambulatory, home, and extended care benefits we have focused on the hospital-sparing effect because the high cost of hospital care has been generally regarded as a problem. Needless to say, the substitutive effect of benefits should have an influence beyond hospital-sparing, and its effects in other contexts are worthy of study. To illustrate this, we now turn to two studies of the possible effects of the availability of outpatient psychiatric services on the utilization of other ambulatory care services in prepaid group practice.

Since in prepaid group practice the financial barrier to the receipt of office care has been reduced, the "abuse" of such services by at least some enrollees may be costly to the plan and demoralizing to the medical staff. Even more important, though sometimes overlooked, is the possibility that the patient continues to demand and to receive services which are not the ones that he truly needs, so that he remains both exigent and distressed. Goldberg et al. addressed themselves to this problem in a study of a sample of enrollees in the Group Health Association of Washington, D.C. The enrollees had been referred to a psychiatrist, who then determined whether they were eligible for further treatment under the terms of a psychiatric care benefit offered by the group practice plan (164). At the time, utilization of ambulatory services in the plan generally was level or rising, but in the sample referred for psychiatric care the number of persons who made other clinic visits was reduced by 14 percent, the number of persons who used x-ray or laboratory services was reduced by 16 percent, the number of physician services was reduced by 31 percent, and the number of x-ray and laboratory services by 30 percent. These differences, which were not likely to have occurred by chance, were found in subgroups distinguished by age, race, sex, and psychiatric diagnosis. Only 25 percent of those referred made more visits during the year beginning three months subsequent to referral as compared to the year prior to referral, while 60 percent made fewer visits. Persons who had made the greatest use of ambulatory care services prior to referral were those who experienced the greatest reductions in use following referral. On the other hand, the number of psychiatric services given appeared to be unrelated to the degree of reduction. Persons who were referred to the screening psychiatrist, but did not receive further service, experienced about as much reduction in the use of other ambulatory care services as did those who received a good deal of psychiatric care. Unfortunately, we are not told to what extent psychiatric services substituted for non-psychiatric services, so the net effect on clinic use cannot be assessed. Nor do we know whether the psychiatric services had an impact on hospital use.

For more complete information we must go to an earlier study by Follette et al. which was both better conceived and better executed than Goldberg's study (165). During the period of this study, 1959–1964, outpatient psychiatric services were available at reduced cost to some subscribers to the Kaiser Health Plan in the San Francisco area. Patients could seek this care on their own or could be referred by their physician. The experimental sample included every fifth psychiatric patient whose initial interview took place between January 1 and December 31, 1960. There were 152 such patients, each of whom was matched with a patient from the "records of high medical utilizers," who had not received psychiatric care at the clinic. The variables used for matching were age, sex, socioeconomic status, medical utilization in 1959, and a weighted index of psychological distress as revealed by entries on the medical record. To be included in the study all patients had to have remained in the health plan for three successive years,

1959–1961. Thus, for the year before and the two years after patients in the experimental group began to receive psychiatric care, there were 152 patients in both experimental and control groups. Subsequently both groups decreased in size by a process of attrition, but at about the same rate, so that at the end of an additional three years there were only 95 experimental and 98 control patients. For purposes of analysis, patients in the experimental group were further subdivided according to the number of psychiatric sessions they had received during their first year. These subgroups were comprised of patients who had had: (1) one session; (2) "brief therapy," which meant 2 to 8 sessions; and (3) "long term therapy," which meant 9 sessions or more. Data on use of service were obtained from plan records. This means that there was no information about use of service outside the plan, a deficiency which was also true of the study by Goldberg et al. (164). Data are available on hospital days and on units of outpatient services, one unit being counted for each contact with any outpatient facility and for each laboratory or x-ray report, irrespective of the number of tests in each report.

During the six years of observation, the control group was found to maintain a reasonably uniform level of outpatient and hospital use. By contrast, all three experimental groups showed roughly comparable yearly reductions in outpatient and hospital services. However, most of the decline in utilization occurred during the first two years of psychiatric care. When the number of psychiatric visits were added to non-psychiatric service units, it was concluded that patients in the "long term therapy" group had merely replaced one form of care by another. However, for the patients who received less psychiatric care, there appeared to be a net saving in services provided by the plan. If it is assumed that, in the absence of psychiatric care, the experimental group would have experienced the same level of use of service as the control group during each of 5 years, one can derive from the published data estimates of the services saved. Each person in the experimental group received an average of 10.2 psychiatric services during 5 years. The corresponding savings would be 25.9 units of outpatient care and 6.34 hospital days. For the subgroup that received only one psychiatric visit during the first year, the comparisons are much more favorable. In return for 1.08 psychiatric visits there would be a saving of 27.5 units of outpatient care and 7.35 hospital days per person.

Unfortunately we do not know what costs are associated with each type of service, so that the net savings cannot be computed as a single value. Furthermore, the study design is such that we cannot tell what proportion of patients enrolled in the prepaid group practice plan may be expected to experience a net reduction in the costs of care, and how much, in response to the institution of psychiatric care. The authors, aware of this and other limitations in the study, instituted a prospective study to further explore the matter (166). Meanwhile, they remind us, quite correctly, that the benefits of psychiatric care go far beyond the savings in cost of service, to include improvement in the performance of the patient, in the performance of other family members and, through interrupting the transmission of acquired behaviors, even in the mental health of future generations. But all this is something that we accept on faith, and that goes beyond our present, rather narrow, concern with the substitutive effects of program benefits.

The major purpose of the prospective study initiated by Cummings and Follette was to obtain a less biased estimate of the utility of psychiatric care in reducing use of other services, by eliminating the effect of self selection in seeking psychiatric help (166). Accordingly, they began with a sample of persons who had voluntarily participated in the multiphasic program of the San Francisco Kaiser-Permanente plan. It was possible, through a series of questions that form part of the screening procedure, to identify a population, comprising 36 percent of the whole, who were considered to be at risk. This was further reduced to a number equal to 8 percent of the whole, by a chart review which identified those patients who scored high on a scale of psychological distress. It was found that this residual group, in addition to having a variety of psychiatric disorders, exhibited a high level of utilization of both outpatient and inpatient services. However, when the physicians in the Plan were requested to consider referring a subset of this high risk group for psychiatric care, only half were referred and, of those referred, a negligible number reported for care. It was, therefore, not possible to generate a study population, and the investigation had to be abandoned. This suggests that although the provision of psychiatric services to selected members of a health care plan may result in reductions in the use of other services, the institution of a routine procedure that would fully exploit this property is likely to be thwarted by a lack of cooperation by physicians and patients. Not everything we know, or think we know, is capable of implementation, which may sometimes be fortunate!

Summary of Findings and Policy Implications

It is now time to ask ourselves what we have learned from attempts to extend the scope of benefits, and what guidelines to policy and action we can derive from the effects we think we have observed. A certain amount of risk is inherent to what we are about to do because our empirical observations have been so few and so poorly conducted, and our theory so tenuous and weak. Nevertheless, one must come to some conclusion, no matter how tentative, at least as a step towards further testing. With these words of caution, it is safe to say that the specific or localized effect of an added benefit is to encourage the use of that benefit so that there is an increase in service, as well as allocative effects, such as we have described in our section on use of service. The generalized or extended effect is more complex, being the resultant of several forces, including the "discovery" and "exposure" effects, which increase use of other services, and the substitution effect, which reduces use of other services. These different influences, and their net effect, are no doubt responsive to all the factors that influence use of service in general. The studies we have reviewed throw some light on a subset of these, to which we shall restrict ourselves. The first of these factors is the nature of the additional benefit itself. By this we mean the place it occupies or the function it performs in the medical care process, and its relationship to other benefits in the plan or program. The second factor is the nature of the patient's need, and his propensity to seek care. The third factor is the nature of the context within which the physician performs his work and the configuration of incentives which motivate him. These categories obviously cover large numbers of variables, but our information concerns only a small subset of these.

When we consider the set of studies that describe extensions of benefits without altering the prevailing organizational context of care, we are brought almost to a halt by the observation that the only truly experimental study, in which extended benefits were not selected by clients but conferred by the insurer, failed to reveal any notable effects, either specific or generalized (134, 135). However, our confidence in this finding is shaken by the observation that many subscribers and physicians had wrong information about the availability of benefits, and by the possibility that the substitution effects were neutralized by the service-enhancing effects in an experiment of such short duration.

The other studies that we have reviewed throw light on the relevance of the three kinds of factors. We note, first, the role played by the nature of the benefit itself. I believe the data justify the hypothesis that the provision of outpatient diagnostic benefits alone, without the concurrent provision for care by the physician outside the hospital, handicaps the full realization of the hospital-sparing effect of the outpatient benefit, so that it is superseded by the effects of discovery and of possible overuse. The relevance of patient characteristics is evidenced in the observation that females, for reasons that are not well understood, are more likely to respond to the service-enhancing generalized effect than are males. The effect of the organizational context becomes apparent when the studies in which benefits have simply been extended are compared with those in which there has been not only an extension of benefits but also a greater degree of formal organization that, among other things, reduces the financial incentive to provide service and strengthens professional incentives. From the comparison of these data it is not unreasonable to propose that the usual forms of private practice have some property, probably the revenue incentive, which greatly attenuates the substitutive effect of added benefits. By contrast, the substitutive effects are strengthened under "organized" care. However, it is not known what property of "organized" care is mainly responsible for the difference. In particular, we do not know whether it is the absence of the fee-for-service incentive, the presence of professional incentives, or both, that are responsible. Furthermore, we have no studies of prepaid group practice without extended benefits that could help us decide whether the "organization of care" in the absence of benefit extension will also have a hospital-sparing effect, and to what extent. However, we do know from other studies, mainly of teaching hospitals as compared to non-teaching hospitals, that a hospital-sparing effect is to be expected even in the absence of extended benefits (1, pp. 104–116; 167; 168).

Studies of benefit extensions under organized auspices have revealed the relevance of two further variables to the effects of benefit extensions. One is the backlog of unmet need, which may create an initial rise in use of the substituted service, to be followed by a reduction later. The second variable is the chronicity of illness when associated with old age. Need for care is being continually generated, so that any extension of benefits that increases the likelihood of close, continuing supervision will so augment the discovery effect that all kinds of services are consumed in larger amounts. Under these circumstances a new type of "abuse" or "misallocation" may come to the foreground, unless controlled by some property of the system. This misallocation is the tendency to provide amounts of care out of proportion to the benefits the care can produce.

We conclude that a wider range of benefits enlarges the choices that the physician, in consultation with the patient, can make in the management of health and illness. This creates the opportunity for the selection of the most cost-effective configuration of care. However, whether this opportunity is grasped, or fully exploited, depends on many other factors. In fact, the extension of benefits not only offers opportunities for improving quality and reducing costs, but also opportunities for excessive use and misallocation. Thus, comprehensive benefits probably require a greater degree of organization in the delivery of care, rather than less. What organizational structures are devised, and what administrative procedures are adopted, depends on an understanding of who bears the costs and who derives the benefits when patterns of care are altered by the extension of benefits. In a later section we will discuss who pays for the costs and who uses the services. Here we will merely point out that the calculus of costs and benefits depends in part, on what happens to the surplus capacity released by the reduction in demand, for example, for hospital care. If hospital beds are retired and new hospital building postponed, there are obviously savings to all concerned, including the insurer, the consumer and the community at large. However, if released capacity, either in hospital beds or in physician time, is occupied by other persons who carry insurance, there may be no net savings to anyone. If those other persons have a lower priority in need, there may be misallocation as well. If hospital beds are not used, but the hospital is run at lower occupancy without reduction in staff, there will be loss of efficiency and higher costs to the hospital which may, to a varying extent and in varying ways, be passed on to the insurer and the consumer. Presumably this is a temporary effect which is offset by the postponement in the need to build a new hospital plant. All this reinforces our earlier statement that the provision of comprehensive care seems to bring with it the need to take a more comprehensive view of the health service system, so that the favorable consequences are enhanced and the undesired effects mitigated.

4

Prices

Theoretical Considerations

We have seen that the provision of benefits means a reduction in out-of-pocket payments and, therefore, a reduction in price at the time services are received. In our previous expositions this effect on price has been used to explain, at least in part, changes in the quantity and mix of services used. These changes, in turn, can have an additional important influence on price, with further effects on use of service. This round of events, which so closely resembles a dog chasing its tail, cannot be described without some repetition of what we have already discussed. Nevertheless, the need remains for a more complete and unified account of how prices respond to the expansion of program benefits, of the factors that influence this response, and of some of the consequences.

Varieties of Price

First, we need to arrive at some common understanding of what varieties of prices there are, and what to call them. The large category of indirect prices or costs will be excluded at the outset. Thus, we will not be concerned with expenditures for travel or the value of alternative uses of the time that has been used to receive care, although we may mention such considerations as they become relevant to our understanding of other prices. We will be concerned with direct prices, which represent monetary payments to the producers of a service by the consumers themselves or, on their behalf, by a third party such as a private insurance company or a public program. The routing of the payment, whether directly to the provider of care, or through the intermediacy of the consumer, will not concern us here.

Accordingly, we will distinguish only four categories of price: "reported," "actual," "average," and "net." The reported price is that which physicians and other providers say they ordinarily charge for any specified service. The actual price for each specified service is the one in fact paid by, or on behalf of, consumers. Strictly speaking, average and net prices are variants of actual price, the first representing total actual outlays per unit of service, and the second including only out-of-pocket payments per unit of service. Since net prices are also average prices it would be more precise to speak of "average gross" and "average net" prices, rather than simply of "average" and "net," as seems to be the practice in the literature we shall describe.

The reported price is represented by the medical care categories and items in the consumer price index of the Bureau of Labor Statistics. Although these prices are reported by providers as their "customary" or "representative" prices, and have been used as such in analyses of the effects of insurance (150, 169), we feel that a name that is both precisely descriptive and vaguely skeptical would be more appropriate. This is because the construction of the price index for medical care goods and services is fraught with so many ambiguities that the precise meaning of the index is hard to specify. Without attempting to fully document this assertion, it may be useful to indicate some of the limitations of the index and, by the same token, prepare the reader to be cautious in interpreting the data that we will present in a later section.

The consumer price index is based on the purchasing patterns of city wage-earner and clerical worker families, and on the prices they pay. This base is used because the index was originally intended for use in the adjustment of wages to the expenditures necessary to sustain a given standard of living. Thus, while urban areas are well represented in the index, rural areas are not. To construct the index, periodic population surveys are conducted to establish the purchasing habits of consumers; and retail outlets (including the providers of medical care) are continually surveyed in order to obtain information about customary prices. Needless to say, only a few of the many items of goods and services that are consumed are selected for pricing. Those selected are presumed to represent the whole. In a field like medical care, where technology changes rapidly, the periodic surveys of purchasing habits tend to lag behind current patterns, and the few items selected for pricing tend to become unrepresentative of their categories. For example, until 1960 only three prescribed drugs were used to represent the entire armamentarium of pharmacotherapy; and one of these, penicillin, stood for all antibiotics. Similarly, until 1964, the daily room charge alone stood for the panoply of hospital services, and was presumed to reflect the remarkable changes that had occurred in hospital care during preceding decades (171). Even now, the gamut of surgery is represented by herniorrhaphy for adults, plus tonsillectomy and adenoidectomy for all ages.

It is true, of course, that the index has undergone periodic revisions, so that new and more representative items are added from time to time. While this improves the validity of the index, it also raises the problem of assuring comparability between time periods, particularly in dealing with changes in the quality of goods and services (172, pp. 159–162). Corrections for quality, including the ability of medical care goods and services to generate health, are a particularly vexing issue. If no corrections are made, price increases may be unduly emphasized, since no account is taken of improved amenities or of superior ability to bring about improvements in health. If corrections for quality are made, we fail to take note of the increasing financial burden on the consumer. Scitovsky contends that those who seek medical care often do not have the option to buy lower quality at a lower price, but must pay the going price for services prescribed by others. If so, adjustments for quality are inappropriate in the price index, and the proper unit for pricing is the bundle of goods and services that collectively constitute the usual care for a given health situation (173, 174). It is likely that there is no single best answer to the question of whether to adjust for quality, since the issue depends so heavily on the use to which the price index is to be put. If the index is to be used to specify the wages necessary to maintain a given standard of living, the changes in price reflected in the index should be only those that remain after corrections have been made for any concurrent increase in quality, provided items equivalent in quality to those available prior to the price change are still available for purchase, or one can get the same results with a smaller quantity of the newer, higher quality item. Since the defining of a standard of living is the prime purpose of the consumer price index, the difference in price is ignored when a new item replaces an old item in the index, by a process which is referred to as "linking." "Linking treats the entire difference in prices as a quality difference, though part of it may be a real price change. This price change is not reflected in the index" (171, p. 15). It follows that the price index tends to underestimate the rise in prices in at least two ways: first, by failing to reflect soon enough the coming into vogue of new and more expensive patterns of care and, second, by introducing new items in a manner that ascribes the higher price of the new substitutes entirely to their qualitative superiority. However, Klarman has pointed out that the lag in introducing new items may also fail to reflect the fall in price of some items, notably drugs, as their use becomes more prevalent (172, p. 156).

Another source of error in the price index is the validity of the information on the prices themselves. The few providers who are chosen to report prices may not adequately represent the whole. Moreover, the definitions of the units of service, and the manner in which charges are assigned to those units, can change so as to make the prices used for the construction of the index either more or less representative of the actual charges that consumers pay. The onset of Medicare and Medicaid has been said to have altered prices in this way. For example, Klarman et al., on the basis of information in the *Annual Report on Medicare* (175), refer to "the tendency by some physicians to fractionate the bill for an office visit and to charge separately for laboratory services and vaccinations," so that the price of the visit as reported in the index is an underestimate of what the patient pays in connection with the visit (176, p. 14). On the other hand, it is believed that hospital daily room-and-board charges now reflect more closely the actual cost of this element in hospital care than they did in the past (171, p. 21). While it is difficult to arrive at an estimate of the net effect of all these limitations on the validity of the price index, it is fair to say that, for our purposes, the index must be viewed only as a very rough indicator of changes in one kind of price: the price reported by the providers of services and goods.

The actual price, as we define it, is the price paid by the consumer, or by a third party on his behalf, for each of the items included in the consumer price index. The reported price and the actual price are different because the same price is not charged to everyone for equivalent services. This is particularly true of the services of the physician, who has traditionally adjusted his charges to the ability of the consumer to pay. In theory, this adjustment has not been accompanied by any change in the characteristics of the service itself, but, in practice, this constancy would be difficult to substantiate. Hence, actual price becomes a rather artificial construct, although it does have conceptual utility. Average price is more firmly rooted in reality; it reflects not only differences in actual price for identical services, but also differences in one or more attributes of the services themselves, and in the mix of services that constitute a given bundle of care. Thus, the average price of the physicians' visit would reflect, among other things, the mix of visits in the office, the home, and the hospital, the extent to which the service is provided by a generalist or a specialist, and any adjustment of the price to the ability to pay. Reported price, actual price, and average price all reflect what the provider of care receives from whoever pays him. "Net price" differs from the others in referring to direct, out-of-pocket payments by the consumer. It excludes third party payments made through voluntary or compulsory insurance, or through other private or public programs.

A simple example may help clarify the distinctions being made. When a physician says that he charges $20 for the first office visit, we understand this to be his reported price. When a patient says that the same physician charged him $15 for the first office visit we understand this to be the actual price in this instance. When the patient says that the physician saw him five times and charged $150, of which the patient paid $25 and his insurance plan paid $125, we understand the average gross price to have been $30 per visit and the average net price to have been $5 per visit, without specification of the content of these visits.

Effects of Benefits on Prices

Prices are influenced by the provision of benefits and, in turn, influence the behavior of consumers and providers. It can be postulated that the provision of benefits increases actual prices, and therefore average prices too, because the provider preceives the consumer's eligibility for benefits as an enhanced ability to pay. The provider is also more likely to collect from clients who may have otherwise been delinquent in meeting their obligations. Thus, as third party payments become more prevalent, physicians regard more patients as similar in their ability to pay, and the gap between actual prices and reported prices narrows. Even more important, the net price to the consumer is lowered, both in absolute terms, and relative to other goods and services. As we have described in earlier sections, the reduction in the net price of insured services relative to the net price of uninsured services is expected to lead to an increase in the consumption of the former relative to the latter; and the reduction in the net price of medical care goods and services relative to the prices of goods and services in general, is expected to lead to a rise in medical care consumption as a whole. As a result of the reduction in net prices, clients with benefits have a greater readiness to accept the recommendations of the physician. The physician is also expected to alter his behavior, acting partly in response to the preferences of patients, partly in the interest of the patient as the physician perceives it, and partly in response to his own interests and preferences, monetary as well as non-monetary.

As we have described in detail earlier, the overall effect of the reduced net price is to increase demand for service and to change the mix of services consumed. But, as Martin Feldstein has emphasized, an equally important effect, during a period when medical technology is growing more elaborate, is to change the nature of the service itself, so that it becomes more costly (170, pp. 32–35). In this way, "insurance can increase the demand for expensive care for affluent families with substantial assets as much as for families with lower incomes and small savings" (170, p. 76). The rise in prices is further encouraged to the extent that the supply of services lags behind the rising pressures of demand.

The provision of benefits increases prices by reducing the disparity between actual and reported prices and, also, by raising the reported or customary prices themselves. This means that part of the earlier reduction in net prices to the consumer may be wiped out. Whether the consumer incurs this loss, and to what extent, depends on what proportion of charges must be paid by the consumer rather than the plan: the larger this proportion, the greater the loss in protection. The loss in protection sets in motion a new chain of events. As insurance purchases are renegotiated by the larger employee groups, and as public programs come up for legislative review, pressures are generated to adapt these plans and programs to the increased demand and the higher prices which they have helped generate themselves. A new cycle begins in the upward spiral that seems to lead to ever-increasing prices.

Factors Influencing Price Response

A number of factors play such a significant role in the progression we have described that they deserve some further elaboration. The first factor is technology. It has long been recognized that technological change has a number of sometimes antithetical effects on the medical care system and on health. On the one hand, it improves the ability to maintain or restore health, thus improving productivity and reducing further demands on the system. On the other hand, it can also generate new needs and demands, and can even reduce the yield in health relative to amount of care. The adverse effects occur because disease can be discovered earlier; because persons can survive to an older age while suffering from an existing illness or developing now illnesses, which may be incurable, but must continue to receive attention; and because a more complex technology can be elaborated without an increased capacity to improve health (1, pp. 150 ff.).

Recently, particular attention has been paid to the balance between the complexity of the technology and its effectiveness in generating health. This balance is an important factor in determining prices, use of services, and the overall costs of medical care. Feldstein has distinguished "technical change without scientific progress" from "technical progress." The former raises prices and costs; the latter has the potential, at least, to reduce these (170, pp. 42–51). Fuchs and Kramer have distinguished technical advances that are "physician-using" from those that are "physician-saving," and have suggested that at certain times the balance tends to be towards one or the other of the two, with profound consequences to productivity, prices, and overall costs (150, pp. 13–15). In a similar vein, Thomas recognizes three levels of technology: "high technology," "halfway technology," and "non-technology." The last of these comprises the traditional, supportive care that is all that medicine can offer when the causes of disease are obscure and its consequences irremediable. The second consists of the often highly elaborate techniques, such as the artificial kidney or heart surgery, that deal with the results of diseases rather than their underlying mechanisms. Only the first, high technology, which enables us to prevent illness or to deal successfully with its causes, has proven effective in reducing the cost of care. The other technologies only offer the prospect of an ever-rising burden in costs with relatively meager returns in health (177).

The second factor that influences prices is the precise response of supply to demand. The general presumption is that rising demand will prompt producers to ask for higher prices, and consumers to pay them, which in turn will stimulate supply to a point where a new balance is established. In the short run, physicians are capable of working longer hours, of altering the pace of their work or of otherwise changing the manner in which they produce care. Hospitals can run at higher occupancy and change their pace or manner of operation (1, pp. 321–402). In the long run, more physicians can be trained and more hospitals built. Whether these things will happen, and to what extent, depends on what motivates physicians and hospitals, and what constraints they are subject to. Many students of the field have emphasized that hospitals, and perhaps even physicians, do not simply seek profit, and that the market for medical care is not like other markets (172, pp. 10–19). Feldstein has proposed that "the physician is an individual who determines his quantity and price to maximize utility and not profit," and that utility includes the ability to select interesting cases, to discharge ethical obligations, and to enjoy a greater amount of leisure (169, p. 122).

From these postulates about the relationships between demand, price, and supply, as modified by the peculiarities of the medical care market, it is difficult to predict the net response of physicians to a situation that would permit their prices to rise. A rise in prices would enable physicians to earn more for the same amount of work, or to enjoy more leisure without a reduction in their customary level of income. If the physicians choose either of these alternatives, the rise in prices would, paradoxically, fail to evoke the expected immediate increase in supply. Another peculiarity of the

medical care market may intervene to impede the expected progression from increased demand to higher prices and, from there,
to greater short-run supply: it has been suggested that although
prices do rise in response to demand, physicians are restrained by
ethical considerations from charging what the traffic will bear
(178, pp. 14–16). If this is true, the capacity of higher demand to
evoke a proportionate rise in the short-run supply of physicians'
services is weakened, first, by a less than proportionate rise in
prices, because of ethical constraints, and, second, by a smaller
rise in supply relative to the higher prices, because some physicians will prefer leisure to higher income. The attractiveness of
more leisure is greatly enhanced if, as is true of many physicians,
current work loads are close to the limits of endurance. The short-
term response of supply to higher prices is further handicapped by
the unwillingness of physicians to change traditional modes of
practice, and by legal and other restrictions on their ability to do
so. The disparity between demand and supply, and the attendant
upward pressure on prices, becomes established if the training of
new personnel is not, or cannot be, sufficiently accelerated; this is
true of physicians (1, pp. 403–419). The upshot is a peculiar situation in which the rise in prices is neither sufficient to smother
demand nor fully effective in calling forth the necessary supply, so
that a recalcitrant shortage persists.

While this picture may represent the situation in general terms,
it is reasonable to expect that individual physicians will differ in
their response to the rise in demand. We are not, of course, concerned with idiosyncratic differences that may be included under
the rubric of personal preferences, but with shared regularities in
behavior. In the absence of information on this subject, we may
speculate that prices will increase more steeply: (1) when physicians are already fully occupied, or believe they are; (2) when the
services they provide tend to require a great deal of personal attention that cannot be readily delegated to others; (3) when the
services are highly technical in nature and, therefore, offer a readily acceptable rationale for the rise in price; and (4) when the
social and interpersonal nexus of practice is "cosmopolitan," uni-
versalistic, and technical, rather than local, particularistic, and af-
fectual (179). It might be thought that prices would rise when the
services provided are more likely to be critical to survival or are

perceived to be. However, this is precisely the kind of situation that accentuates the conflict between business and professional values, so that the outcome becomes difficult to predict. It could be that in certain situations, where interpersonal and social obligations are strongly operative, the critical nature of the illness retards rather than enhances the rise in prices. In the absence of such restraints, a rise may occur.

If these speculations have any validity, consultants will be more likely to raise their prices than primary physicians, and surgeons than internists. All other things being equal, prices are more likely to rise in urban areas than in rural areas; but prices may not rise as much in larger cities because it is suspected that they have a more plentiful supply of physicians than the smaller towns. It is difficult to predict which services will experience a larger increase in prices: office visits or visits in the hospital. While the hospital locale is more impersonal, hospitalized illness is generally more severe and hospital care more technical, and these are hypothesized to be factors that enhance the capacity to raise prices. The hospital also offers many opportunities for the delegation of care to others than the private physician, a factor that we have said would tend to moderate the increase in the charge made by the physician.

The market for hospitals is peculiar, being largely, though not exclusively, nonprofit in nature. Accordingly, in response to rising demand, hospitals do not raise prices in order to increase profit, although they are certain to seek a somewhat more favorable balance of revenue against costs than is usually possible. Similarly, patients are unable to offer higher prices when there is excess demand; prices do rise, and dramatically at that, but for different reasons altogether. While it is not clear what motivates a complex, non-profit community agency such as a hospital, it may be inferred, from the work of Feldstein and of others, that those responsible for hospital policy must keep in balance three major concerns: (1) a perceived level of quality, below which care should not be permitted to fall; (2) the ability to respond to demand for care; and (3) the need to break even financially, in the end. The happiest way to balance these concerns is by operating the hospital at a level of occupancy that signals a comfortable but satisfyingly efficient pace. The level of occupancy and the pace of operations may not, necessarily, be those that are technically the most efficient, since a large number of considerations, including the access of physicians to beds, play a role in determining what is desirable.

Unhappily for those who seek equilibrium, when new demand is generated by the provision of benefits, constant pressure is put on the hospital to provide more and better care. The key element is the demand by physicians and their clients for a new product, increasingly richer in amenities and in technological content. According to Feldstein it is this demand, and no other, which accounts for the major share of the rise in hospital prices (170). Nevertheless, there will also be an increase in the volume of care supplied, with attendant consequences to price. We have said that in the short run hospitals have some capacity to operate at a more rapid pace and at higher occupancy. The effects of this response are likely to vary. In hospitals that had previously run much below capacity, the larger demand may improve efficiency and should lower prices rather than raise them. But other hospitals may become overloaded, with a consequent reduction in the efficiency of operations, and a disproportionate rise in costs, which must be passed on as higher prices to the consumer (1, pp. 350–357). In the longer run, the building of hospital beds is probably more responsive to demand than the training of physicians, but a too ready response may have a paradoxical effect. An over-abundance of hospital beds that are run at low occupancy is inefficient and contributes to rising prices, as well as to the generation of additional demand. Feldstein suggests that the hospital can use additional revenue either to expand capacity or to provide more sophisticated care (149). However, since so much of the hospitals' capital funds come from outside sources, it is possible that the decision to provide better care will also be the correct strategy for attracting funds for expansion. In any event, variation among hospitals in the way they alter prices in response to rising demand may be expected to depend, among other things, on the hospitals' financial position at the outset, on the initial occupancy ratio relative to capacity, on the constituency to which it looks for capital funds, on its perceived role and objectives relative to technological leadership, and on its need to compete with other hospitals for scarce personnel or community support.

A third important factor that influences the response of prices to benefits is the method by which the insurance plan or government program pays for the services of physicians and hospitals. It is generally believed that when hospitals are paid on the basis of justified costs, there are few restraints on the refinement, enrichment, or elaboration of care, and few incentives for efficient operation. Payment to physicians on the basis of fee schedules does constitute some restraint on prices, although the scheduled fees go up as a result of frequent renegotiation. Payment according to "customary and prevailing" fees, by contrast, encourages physicians to raise their prices as a group, and virtually requires every physician to apply his higher prices to the majority of his patients. Thus, the customary and prevailing fee becomes a positive inducement to inflation. Price inflation is likely to become easier, under any method, when the providers are highly organized and when the organizations they negotiate with are to a large degree controlled by themselves, as has been true of Blue Cross and Blue Shield. The use of these organizations as carriers or intermediaries in the Medicare program may have assured that the interpretation of governmental regulations was most favorable to the providers. By contrast, it is likely that when consumers are required to make out-of-pocket payments there will be restraints not only on use of service but also on increases in price.

Empirical Observations

We must now examine experience in recent decades to see how well it accords with expectation. In particular, we are interested in finding out whether the several varieties of price have responded as we have predicted to the greater prevalence of third party payments, how consumers have reacted to these changes, and how the providers of care have both contributed to the price changes and responded to them. The literature concerning the possible effects of insurance on use of service has already been reviewed. Here we are more explicitly concerned with the price variable itself.

Recent Trends in Prices

A great deal of the evidence concerning the relationship between the provision of benefits and the prices of medical care can

TABLE 28.   Index Numbers (1967 = 100) for Percent of Specified Personal Health Expenditures Met by All Third Party Payments [a] for Selected Items in the Consumer Price Index, U.S.A., Selected Years, 1950–1970

Third Party Payments and Prices	1950	1955	1960	1965	1970	1970 Minus 1950
Third party payments as percent of total						
Personal health expenditures	56.6	73.2	79.8	84.8	108.9	52.3
Hospital care	77.1	89.5	95.3	95.4	100.1	23.0
Physicians' services	31.3	59.3	70.0	75.7	122.8	91.5
Consumer price index						
All items	72.1	80.2	88.7	94.5	116.3	44.2
All services	58.7	70.9	83.5	92.2	121.6	62.9
All medical care services	49.2	60.4	74.9	87.3	124.2	75.0
Semiprivate room	30.3	42.3	57.3	75.9	145.4	115.1
General physician office visit	54.9	65.4	75.9	87.3	122.6	67.7
Tonsillectomy and adenoidectomy	60.7	69.0	80.3	91.0	117.1	56.4
Dentists' fees	63.9	73.0	82.1	92.2	119.4	55.5

Source: Data on price are from Reference 181, Table 3, page 13. Information on third party payments in Table 7 of Reference 182 was used to compute percentages for 1967 which were then used to derive index numbers using data in Reference 183 pp. 83–85.

[a] Includes private insurance as well as governmental programs.

be considered circumstantial, since it is based on the occurrence of parallel trends during recent decades. It is possible to review only a few of the many studies that have described the changes in the components of the consumer price index and have attempted to explain the trends of those changes. The recent work of Rice and Horowitz is a good example (171, 180). Table 28 summarizes the findings for the years 1950 to 1970. Keeping in mind the limitations in the consumer price index, which we mentioned in a previous section, one observes that prices for medical services increased faster than the prices for all services, and even faster than the prices for all items in the index. Among the items that are included in the index for medical care services, it is clear that, during this time span, professional services increased at a rate reasonably close to all services, whereas hospital services increased at such a remarkably high rate that they must be held responsible for the major share of the excess increase in medical care prices over the prices of services generally. During this time there was also an increase, as shown in Table 28, in the proportion of personal health expenditures paid through private insurance, governmental programs, and other sources. In view of our theoretical expectations, it is tempting to see the increase in third party payments as the cause of the price rise. Unfortunately, a closer examination of the rates of change shows a lack of precise correspondence. As shown in Figure 9, the proportion of personal health expenditures paid by third parties rose at a higher rate for the services of physicians than of hospitals. This occurred partly because there was much more room to expand the coverage for physicians' services, so the relative change was much greater for these services. For example, between 1950 and 1965 (the year preceding Medicare) the percent of personal expenditures paid by third parties increased from 65.8 percent to 81.5 percent for hospital services, and from 15.2 percent to 36.8 percent for physician services. The absolute difference was 15.7 percentage points for hospital services and 26.6 percentage points for physician services, whereas the relative changes, as shown by the index numbers cited in Table 28, were 18.3 and 44.4 percentage points, respectively. Perhaps even more important, during this time period (1950–1965), one observes a marked and progressive slackening in the expansion of third party payments, which occurred in parallel fashion for both hospital care and physician services. By contrast to this reduced increase in third party payments the prices for hospital care increased at a faster rate than the charges for office visits to general physicians, and the rate of increase in hospital prices tended to accelerate rather than to slacken from one five-year period to the next. A further observation, which is shown in the table but not in the figure, for the sake of simplicity, is that dentists' fees and the prices of a tonsillectomy and adenoidectomy increased in a degree and manner that followed the trend line for the price of a visit to a general physician's office. In fact, the price index for all services followed a not too different course.

It is difficult from these observations to infer a causal rela-

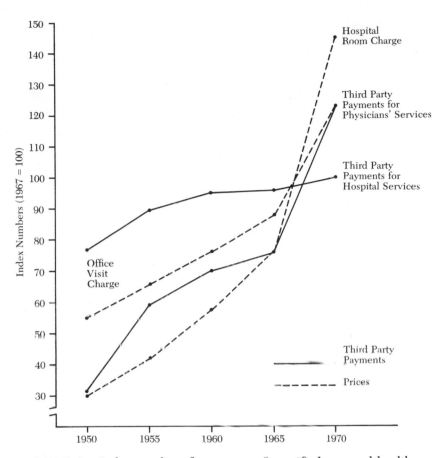

FIGURE 9. Index numbers for percent of specified personal health expenditures met by third party payments,[a] and for the hospital semiprivate room charge and a general physician office visit, U.S.A., selected years, 1950 to 1970.

Source: See sources for Table 28.
[a] Includes private insurance as well as governmental programs.

tionship between third party payments and prices. But a case could be made for a causal relationship by making some assumptions. The disparity between the rates of increase in coverage and in reported prices could be explained on the basis of a nonlinear relationship between the two, such that equal increments of coverage bring about larger increases in price when coverage is initially high than they do when it is low.

This could occur if resources that were already strained by demand were subjected to further demand, even if relatively small. However, this would not explain why dental services, for which there is very little insurance, have experienced price increases not too unlike those of physicians' services. This suggests that factors other than third party payments must have a dominant effect, unless one assumes that dentists acknowledge and follow the price leadership of physicians. But the rise in the prices of all services suggests that one must look outside the medical care system itself for an explanation of the major share of the price increases between 1950 and 1965 in the services of physicians and dentists. The subsequent period, between 1965 and 1970, is so closely associated with large-scale governmental involvement in the financing of personal health services that we shall have to examine it separately and in detail in a later section. But before we do so, we need to review the findings of some studies that have used more precise methods of analysis to examine the trends we have described merely by inspection. These studies are: (1) a time series analysis of national data for physicians between 1948 and 1966 by Feldstein (169), between 1948 and 1968 by Fuchs and Kramer (150), and between 1952 and 1969 by Huang and Koropecky (184); (2) a cross-sectional analysis of state data for physicians for 1966 by Fuchs and Kramer (150); and (3) an analysis of combined longitudinal and cross-sectional state data on hospitals, for 1958 to 1967, by Feldstein (149).

One important feature of several of these studies is that they distinguish three varieties of price: customary, average, and net, along the lines that we have described, our approach being based on their work (see Appendix A). Feldstein began this line of inquiry by postulating that physicians charge insured persons the customary prices that are reported in the price index, and that those who are not insured pay a lower price, presumably for the same services. The national survey reported by Andersen and Anderson gives information on use of physicians' services, and on the expenditures incurred for those services, by persons who have medical and surgical insurance and by those who do not. Expenditures for physician services by the uninsured are reported to be 0.51 of those by the insured (20, p. 139). In an undisclosed manner, Feldstein estimated that use of physician services by the uninsured was 0.76 that of the insured. It follows, if it is assumed that services are comparable in kind, that the uninsured must pay 0.67 the price paid by the insured (0.51/0.76 = 0.67). Unfortunately, it was not possible for Feldstein to compute the two ratios, representing relative use of service and price, for each year in his series. Consequently, he had to assume that these ratios had remained unchanged between 1948 and 1966. According to this assumption, changes in average price from year to year would only depend on changes in customary (reported) price and on the proportion of persons who had medical and surgical insurance in each year. The other two factors that could influence the computation of the average price—the use of service and the expenditures of the uninsured relative to the insured—would be assumed to have remained unchanged. The average price in each year is determined by adding the expenditures incurred by the insured and the uninsured, and dividing this total by the services used by both. For the uninsured, net price is by definition the same as actual price. For those who have insurance, actual price is assumed to be the same as customary or reported price, and the ratio of net price to actual price is equal to the ratio of out-of-pocket expenditures to total expenditures.

The relationship among the several prices for 1963, under the assumptions made by Feldstein, are shown in Table 29. The sources of information and the computations used to arrive at the relative prices are shown in Appendix A. The major conclusions are that, in 1963, the average actual price for the services of physicians was 0.91 of the customary price reported in the Consumer Price Index and that, as a result of insurance, the average net price was reduced to 0.68 of the customary price. It should be noted, however, that the net price for the insured was not much different from the net price for the uninsured. If one accepts the data and the assumptions used, one must conclude that the higher utilization rate of the insured could not be attributed to a lowering in price alone, but to a lowering in price relative to certain attributes of the insured, including their income.

Fuchs and Kramer adopted Feldstein's approach for determining relative prices, but introduced certain modifications in the basic assumptions as well as in the methods of computation (150, pp. 47–51). They retained the basic assumption that the insured

TABLE 29. Relative Prices for Services of Physicians Paid by The Insured,[a] The Uninsured, and The Total Population, Under Specified Observed Experience and Assumptions, U.S.A., 1963

Experience, Assumptions, and Prices Concerning Physicians' Services	Insured	Uninsured	All
Observed experience			
Proportion of population	0.66	0.34	1.00
Use of service per person	1.00	0.76	—
Expenditures per person	1.00	0.51	—
Proportion of expenditures not covered by insurance	0.68	1.00	0.75
Assumptions			
Actual price as proportion of customary price	1.00	—	—
Computed relative prices			
Actual price	1.00	0.67	0.91
Net price	0.68	0.67	0.68

Sources: For use of service per person see Reference 169, p. 123. Other information is from Tables in Reference 20 as follows: for population covered p. 76, for expenditures, p. 139, and for expenditures covered, p. 92.
[a] Surgical and medical insurance.

pay the reported customary price, but applied it to insured services only. For uninsured services, the insured were assumed to pay a price midway between the reported price and the price paid by the uninsured. Accordingly, there were three actual relative prices, rather than two. If the price paid by insured persons for insured services is 1.000, the price paid by insured persons for uninsured services is 0.835. As was true in the work of Feldstein, these relative prices were determined on the basis of data available for 1963, and were assumed to be constant in all other years. The reader will recall that Feldstein assumed that the ratio of use of physician services by the uninsured to use by the insured also remained constant at 0.76, which was the value observed in 1963. Fuchs and Kramer do not adopt this convention. They account for the effect of a widening scope of benefits by allowing the ratio of utilization by the uninsured to utilization by the insured to vary inversely as a function of the real dollar value of benefits. Moreover, relative utilization is determined in a manner that takes account of the mix of services and the relative cost of services. Data from national household surveys were used to compare the insured to the uninsured as to their relative use of "outpatient," "inhospital surgical," and "inhospital other" services in 1963. The mix of these three types of services, and their prices relative to each other, were obtained from the survey of Medicare enrollees for January-December 1968. The relationships between the services and prices were assumed to remain constant during all years, even though the utilization ratio of all services (weighted and combined) was made to vary according to the real dollar value of benefits during each year, as already mentioned. Using these assumptions and sources of information, both of which are partly different from those in Table 29, we can arrive at an alternative set of relative price estimates for 1963. Table 30 shows the alternative data, assumptions, and estimates, and Table 31 compares the two sets of relative prices. The major difference is that in the estimate based on the data and assumptions used by Fuchs and Kramer (Table 30), the net price for the insured is lower than that for the uninsured, even though the latter are assumed to pay reduced prices. Presumably, this reduction in net price goes some way toward explaining the higher rate of utilization by the insured.

To reiterate, the relationships shown are only provisionally valid, and only for 1963. They are only valid for 1963 because as the scope of benefits broadens, the disparity in average net prices paid by the insured and the uninsured will widen, and as the proportion of the population with insurance increases, the difference between average net price and average actual price will also increase. The findings are only provisionally valid because they depend so heavily on the accuracy of the data used and the validity of the assumptions adopted. Two of these assumptions are particularly critical. The first is that the insured pay the customary price, as reported in the consumer price index, either for all services or for insured services only, depending on the specific assumption. While this may be a reasonable assumption when governmental and voluntary insurance programs pay the customary and prevailing fee, it is not clear what the situation was when commercial insurance was more likely to make specified indemnity payments, and Blue Shield was more likely to exercise control over fees by using schedules and requiring that participating

TABLE 30. Relative Prices for Services of Physicians Paid by The Insured, The Uninsured, and The Total Population, Under Specified Observed Experience and Assumptions, U.S.A., 1963

Experience, Assumptions and Prices Concerning Physicians' Services	Insured	Uninsured	All
Observed experience			
Proportion of population	0.722	0.278	—
Use of service per person	1.000	0.651	—
Expenditures per person	1.000	0.481	—
Proportion of expenditures not covered by insurance	0.573	1.000	0.640
Assumptions			
Actual price as proportion of customary price,			
for insured services	1.000	—	—
for uninsured services	0.835 [a]	—	—
Computed relative prices			
Actual price	0.91	0.67	0.86
Net price	0.57	0.67	0.59

Source: Reference 150, pp. 47–51.

[a] The assumption is that if the actual price for the uninsured is 0.67, the price of uninsured services purchased by the insured is $(1 + 0.67)/2$.

TABLE 31. Specified Relative Prices for The Insured, Uninsured, and the Total Population, Under Two Sets of Observations and Assumptions, U.S.A., 1963

Prices by Population Group	Observations and Assumptions as Shown in:	
	Table 29	Table 30
Reported price [a]	1.00	1.00
Actual price		
Insured	1.00	0.91
Uninsured	0.67	0.67
All	0.91	0.86
Net price		
Insured	0.68	0.57
Uninsured	0.67	0.67
All	0.68	0.59

Source: See Tables 29 and 30.

[a] Consumer Price Index

physicians make no additional charges except to families exceeding specified income limits. Fortunately, the precise relationship between actual fees and the fees reported for the price index is subject to empirical verification.

The second assumption is perhaps more disturbing and more difficult to verify. It holds that any difference between the expenditures of the insured and the uninsured, if it is not accounted for by a difference in the volume and mix of care, is due to a difference in price. It could very well be that part of the difference is in the content and the quality of care. If so, the difference in price for items of equal quality is not as large as the relative prices suggest. As to the absolute level of prices, we have presented the data showing how they have risen in recent years. Needless to say, as reported prices rise, all the other prices will follow suit. As our next order of business we will examine these time trends in greater detail; we will try and understand their causes, with particular reference to the role of third party payments; and we will explore their consequences.

Using national data, and the assumptions and methods already described, Feldstein found that during the period between 1948 and 1966 the customary—or reported—price index rose 3.2 percent per year, the average actual price 4.1 percent per year, and the average net price 2.1 percent per year. A one percent increase in the proportion of expenditures covered by insurance was associated with a rise of 0.36 percent in average price and a decrease of 0.64 percent in net price. "Thus more than a third of the increased coverage is diluted by induced price increases; physicians receive this major share of the gains from increased insurance. . . . Society is thus indirectly forced by the market to pay physicians a high price for the risk-pooling advantages of health insurance" (169, p. 129). In addition to the dissipation of part of the benefits of insurance through increases in price, the price rise itself has the paradoxical effect of reducing the quantity of services supplied, measured as the ratio of personal expenditures for physicians' services to the average price of these services. The conclusion is that "when insurance increases, physicians raise average price and lower quantity" (169, footnote p. 130). The effect on demand of changes in average prices and net prices could not be determined because the relationships revealed by the regression equation were unreasonable. For example, average price was insignificantly related to demand, whereas more insurance appeared to reduce demand and higher net prices to increase it. Since none of the alternative economic models tested by Feldstein were successful in explaining the trend in demand, he concluded that physicians have not allowed prices to rise as much as they could, and they have, as a result, created a situation of excess demand, which gives physicians considerable discretion over both their prices and the quantity of care they will provide. However, the several findings are so much a consequence of the assumed relationship between insurance and price, that they must be accepted as suggestive rather than conclusive.

In an examination of national trends during virtually the same period, 1948–1968, Fuchs and Kramer have more carefully documented and emphasized the limitations in their data and in their assumptions (150). Their analytic tool is to divide this period into three component periods and to look for correspondences between the three periods in the rate of change of variables for insurance, price, demand, and supply. The major findings are summarized in Table 32. The period between 1966 and 1968 will be discussed in a subsequent section on the possible impact of Medicare and Medicaid. The focus now will be on a comparison of the two other time periods, 1948–1956 and 1956–1966.

The object of the comparison is to determine whether differences in the rates of change in the independent variables, which are third party coverage and physicians per person, can explain differences in the rates of change in the dependent variables, which are prices and demand. The changes in the independent variables were as follows: during 1956–66, the rate of growth in third party payments per capita was much slower than in 1948–56, while the rate of growth in physicians per capita accelerated, in contrast to the slowing down that took place during 1948–56. Both of these developments should have reduced the rate of growth in reported prices in 1956–66 as compared to 1948–56. In fact, the rate of growth in reported prices remained unchanged. Average actual prices grew at a lower rate in 1956–66 than in the preceding period, and the average net prices grew at a higher rate. This is in line with the less rapid growth in third party payments during 1956–66, but this correspondence is built into the data by the way these prices are defined and computed. Ex-

TABLE 32. Rate of Change in Income and in Specified Aspects of The Services of Physicians, U.S.A., Specified Periods 1948–1968

Income, Third Party Payments, and Attributes of Services of Physicians	Percent per Annum Continuously Compounded			
	1948–1956	1956–1966	1966–1968	1948–1968
Income and Insurance				
Real disposable income per capita	2.2	2.4	2.6	2.2
Third party payments per capita	17.7	9.4	24.2	12.5
Prices				
Consumer Price Index				
All items	1.8	1.5	3.5	1.7
Services of physicians	3.0	3.0	6.1	3.2
Average (actual) price	4.4	3.6	8.1	4.2
(Average) net price	1.1	1.9	−6.8	1.3
Demand				
Expenditures per capita	4.1	6.6	9.1	3.2
Quantity per capita	−0.4	3.0	0.9	2.1
Supply				
Private practice physicians per Capita [a]				
Unweighted	−1.3	0.5	—	−0.3
Weighted [b]	−1.1	0.9	—	0.0
Visits per physician	—	—	—	−0.7
Quantity per physician	—	—	—	2.1

Source: Reference 150, Tables 2, 4, 6, 7, 13 and 14, pages 7–17.

[a] The data are for 1949–57, 1957–67 and 1949–67.

[b] Specialist = 1.2 generalists

penditures per person and quantity of service per person (quantity being defined as the ratio of expenditures to average price) grew much more rapidly in 1956–66 than in 1948–56. This is out of line with the less rapid growth in third party payments during this time period, and the associated less rapid increase in average prices. Part of the acceleration in quantity and expenditures may have been generated by the increasing supply of physicians. However, Fuchs and Kramer believe that it is mainly the consequence of the increasingly elaborate technology which developed during 1955–1966, without corresponding increases in the ability to improve health. This is held to be in contrast to technological developments during 1948–1956, which included introduction of several antibiotic and chemotherapeutic agents. Thus, while advances during 1948–1956 tended to be physician-saving, those between 1956 and 1966 tended to be physician-using. There is some internal support for this hypothesis in that visits per physician decreased during 1948–1968, while quantity of service per physician increased, suggesting larger inputs per visit. The authors believe that their hypothesis is supported by external evidence such as the deceleration of the reduction in crude death rates, and the reversal of the declining trend in the length of hospital stay. Thus, Kramer and Fuchs agree with Feldstein that changes in demand are not adequately explained by changes in insurance and in price. However, they propose that the explanation is to be found in the characteristics of the technology rather than in the generation of excess demand by physicians.

Huang and Koropecky have also studied the secular trend for physicians' fees during the period before and immediately after Medicare was introduced (184). However, they confined their attention to fees as reported in the consumer price index. Also, unlike the studies we have just reviewed, they had no reason to call upon the properties of the technology, or a paradoxical response of supply to price in order to explain the observed trend. For the period 1952–1969, the annual percentage change in physicians' fees was related to a number of independent variables, using multiple least-squares regression. An equation using only three dependent variables was able to reproduce with considerable accuracy the observed trend line for reported prices during this period. These variables were: (1) the rate of change in third party payments, including government programs; (2) the rate of change in the Consumer Price Index for all goods and services; and (3) a dummy variable that distinguished the period before Medicare from the period after (184, p. 9).

Relationships of Price to State Characteristics

Fuchs and Kramer supplemented their time-series analysis of national data on physicians' services with a cross-sectional analysis employing data for each of the 33 states where expenditure data were available during 1966. Since medical technology can be assumed to be reasonably equal in all states, it ceases to be a disturbing factor in the analysis, and the influence of other variables is easier to discern. Since many of these variables are not independent of each other, regression analysis was done in two stages. In the first stage a predicted value was obtained for each endogenous variable by regressing it on all exogenous variables. In the second stage, the actual value of an endogenous variable was regressed on relevant exogenous and endogenous variables, using predicted values for the latter. Furthermore, since a large number of variables could, a priori, be expected to play a role, the two-stage process described above was repeated, so that variables without explanatory power could be dropped. In this way, the 25 endogenous and exogenous variables in the preliminary model were stripped down to eleven: 6 endogenous and 5 exogenous. Among the exogenous variables eliminated because they were shown to be non-contributory were "median years of education, persons 25 and over," "percent black," and "percent 65 and over." Among the variables retained, the quantity of care that was produced or consumed was measured as hospital days plus home and office visits, with weighting of the components so that hospital visits represented 1.71 times as much care as did office or home visits, and office or home visits by specialists represented 1.93 times as much care as visits by generalists. Expenditure data were based on income tax returns by physicians, which showed relatively large unexplained variations from year to year, raising questions about their accuracy over short periods of time. Average price was defined as the ratio of expenditures to quantity. This means that price is determined in a reasonably direct manner without assumptions concerning the relationships between reported prices and the prices paid by insured and uninsured persons. Net price was presumably determined by excluding insurance benefits from expenditures. Unfortunately, benefit data were not available by state, but had to be derived from the number of persons in each state who carry surgical insurance, and from benefit data for the nation as a whole, as reported by the Health Insurance Institute. Needless to say, the assumptions and limitations implicit in these measurements, as well as others which the authors describe in detail, must be kept in mind in interpreting their findings.

Using their method of analysis, the investigators find that where the average or net prices are higher, the quantity of care consumed is smaller, but that the effect of price is very small. The elasticities for average actual price range from −0.104 to −0.356, and for average net price from −0.059 to −0.201. The effect, though small, is in the expected direction. By contrast, the effect of price on the quantity of care produced per physician appears to be either equivocal or paradoxical. At best, it might be concluded that where average prices are higher, physicians tend to produce fewer services rather than more. The effect of insurance on the productivity of physicians was not tested in the final model. Since price appears to have such a small effect on quantity consumed, it is not surprising to find that the prevalence of insurance, measured as benefits per capita, has an equally small effect on quantity consumed. However, the effect of insurance could not be measured accurately because insurance was included in the net price variable and was highly correlated with disposable personal income per capita. Presumably, the effect of insurance was due to the reduction in net price, which is a consequence that is established by definition. By contrast, the relationship found between average price and the prevalence of insurance is totally unexpected. In the states with higher average prices, insurance benefits per capita are lower rather than higher. This finding cannot be reconciled with assumptions that insured persons pay higher actual prices, unless it is also assumed that where insurance is more prevalent the customary or reported prices are markedly lower; but this latter assumption runs counter to what is believed concerning the inflationary effects of insurance.

In summary, the cross-sectional analysis of state data suggests that prices, and therefore health insurance, are not important in explaining the differences between states in use of service. Perhaps the most significant single variable is the number of physicians in private practice per unit population; this in turn, is positively related to the number of hospital beds per 1,000, the average price of physicians' services, and per capita disposable personal income. The explanation appears to be that physicians settle in states where conditions are professionally, and otherwise, favorable, and where the physicians are able to generate the need for their own services. However, the quantity of services is not as large as would be expected from the prevalence of physicians alone, since in the states where there are more physicians, fewer services are produced per physician.

The effects of insurance, price, and other factors on hospital services have been examined by Feldstein, who also used states as the units and multiple regression as the tool for analysis (149). There were a total of 470 observations, one for each state during each of the years from 1958 to 1967. The prevalence of insurance was defined, in a manner similar to that of Fuchs and Kramer, as the percent of expenditures covered by insurance. However, since this ratio is available only for the nation as a whole, it had to be derived for each state in an indirect manner. For each year, the percent of persons who have hospital insurance in each state is known with reasonable accuracy. National survey data for 1963 (20) were used to estimate that the uninsured consume 83 percent as many hospital days as the insured and pay 42 percent of the gross price of hospital care, which the insured are assumed to pay in full.

If these relationships are assumed to remain unchanged, and if it is also assumed that the percent of expenditures paid yearly by insurance for the insured at the national level applies to each of the states, it is possible to compute the percent of expenditures covered by insurance in each state, each year. Obviously, this method allows for the expansion over time of insurance benefits per person insured but does not allow for variation in the scope of benefits among states at any given time. As we have already indicated, the percent of expenditures not covered by insurance is a measure of average net price relative to gross price. The value for gross price was obtained not from the consumer price index but from data on hospital cost per day as reported by the American Hospital Association. But the price that was considered important in determining use of services was "relative net price," defined as the ratio of average net price of hospital services to the consumer price index for all goods and services, the latter being assumed to apply to all states during a given year. The relative net price was, indeed, found to be a very important predictor of hospital use. Among several variables tested, per capita disposable income and hospital beds per person were also found to be important. The relative net price variable can itself be viewed as the product of two ratios: the ratio of average net price to the gross price of hospital services, and the ratio of the gross price to the consumer price index of all goods and services. In the regression equation that holds per capita disposable income as constant, but does not include the hospital supply variable, Feldstein found that a one percent increase in the relative net price or either of its two component ratios was associated with about 1 percent decrease in hospital use, brought about equally by reductions in admissions and in length of stay. This is quite in contrast to the rather feeble effect of price and insurance on the use of physician services, as reported by Fuchs and Kramer (150). However, when the supply of hospital beds and physicians are added as variables to the regression equation, it transpires that the insurance variable is not significantly related to use of service, whereas the ratio of gross price to the consumer price index is, but at a reduced level of association.

The prevalence of hospital beds clearly has an important effect on use of services, so that a one percent increase in beds per person is roughly associated with a half percent increase in patient-days. Part of this is due to what Feldstein calls a "pure availability effect" and part due to an association with lower gross prices. But it is not clear why, when these effects are held constant, the insurance variable ceases to have a significant association with use of hospital services, whereas the relative gross price does. Feldstein wonders whether this is due to a "statistical artifact." He also speculates that in the decision to admit persons to the hospital the relative gross price is more important than the relative net price, and the net price is either not important, or important only to length of stay. The findings jibe with this interpretation, and the interpretation is in agreement with the report by Rosenthal that, in New England hospitals, gross rather than net charges appear to be more closely related to length of stay (38). But if these speculations are sustained, the result would be a serious blow to our hypotheses concerning the effects of insurance. For this reason we must once again draw attention to limitations the accuracy of the data and the validity of the assumptions in this set of studies. These are well recognized by the investigators concerned, especially by Fuchs and Kramer, who are careful to present their findings as suggestive and provisional rather than definitive or final. The degree of confidence placed in the findings is also conditional upon one's view of what inferences may legitimately be drawn from studies that use spatially defined areas as units of analysis.

Needless to say, the cross-sectional analyses by state indicate the degree to which certain specified state characteristics explain some other state characteristics. However, unless the data satisfy certain requirements, it would be hazardous to extrapolate from such "ecological correlations" to statements concerning how individuals or families would behave relative to influences such as insurance or price (17, 185, 186). For example, Fuchs and Kramer report that education, age and color were characteristics of state populations, in the aggregate, that were not useful in explaining differences among states. It is hard to reconcile this finding with what is known about the relationships between these factors and use of service by individuals and families, and, in particular, with the increasing relative prominence of color and education as determinants of health behavior (6, 7).

What, then, does all this mean? It is useless to pretend that the answer is clear, or that the findings fully support our hypotheses about the effects of insurance on price, and of price on use of service. Particularly discordant are the findings by Fuchs and Kramer that the states with more insurance had lower average actual prices rather than higher, and that neither insurance nor price were important predictors of the quantity of service used. Similarly incongruous is the finding by Feldstein that when per capita disposable income and hospital beds per person were held constant, use of hospital services was related to relative gross price rather than to relative net price. However, it is possible to reconcile the substance of the empirical observations with our hypotheses by using a certain interpretation of the findings. The reader will recall that the trends in price and in third party payments between 1950 and 1965 had two features that required explanation. One was that a deceleration in the growth of third party payments was accompanied by an acceleration in the rise in prices for both physician and hospital services. The second was that the more rapid growth in third party payments for physicians than for hospitals was accompanied by a more rapid rise in the prices of hospital care than of medical services.

The first of these observations can be explained by coincidental changes in technology: first, its almost geometric growth and elaboration, and second, a change in its character, so that it is more likely to generate services and costs rather than to reduce need through controlling illness. A contributory factor, in the case of physicians, is that they appear to respond to a rise in prices by producing less rather than more. They respond in a similar way to an increase in their numbers relative to population. In this way, increments of demand for physician services can produce a disproportionately low response in supply and a disproportionately high increment in price. It can be postulated, therefore, that although the rate of growth of insurance had slowed down, physicians had reached a point where they were exchanging more leisure for greater income.

The second observation, that the growth of hospital prices was greater than the growth of physicians' prices even though the growth of insurance for the latter was more rapid than for the former, can be due, in part, to the much larger technological content of hospital care. This disparity may have been further accentuated by a continuing transfer to the hospital of technical functions that physicians could well have performed in their offices. In part, the disparity may have arisen because physicians have not increased their prices as much as they could have, but instead have generated, as Feldstein and others have proposed, an established state of excess demand. The implication is that without this restraint, the social machinery for which is not understood, the rate of increase in the charges of physicians would have been much closer to that of hospitals. The contribution of third party payments is that they generate the demand which enables the consumer to buy, and the producer to sell, a greatly enriched variety of care. Third party payments, then, are part of the fuel that powers the engine that runs the complex apparatus of hospital and physician responses that we have described. The reader already knows the empirical basis for this interpretation, and can judge for himself how much of it is fact and how much is only speculation subject to further testing.

Possible Effects of Medicare and Medicaid

The introduction of Medicare and Medicaid in 1966 provides us with an almost experimental situation in which to examine more closely the effects of a rapid expansion in third party payments on the prices of medical care.

Trends in Hospital Prices and Physicians' Fees. The temporal relationship between the rise in prices and the growth in third party payments brought about by Medicare and Medicaid has already been shown in Table 28 and Figure 9. Table 33 gives more detailed data on prices since the implementation of Medicare on July 1, 1966. As far as prices are concerned, the first phase of the Medicare era may be said to have ended with the implementation of price controls under the Economic Stabilization Program on August 15, 1971. Our concern is with the approximately five years preceding and five years following the implementation of the major provisions of the federal Medicare program and the institution and spread of the federal-state Medicaid program: the former program for the aged, and the latter for a variety of indigent groups in the population, including in particular dependent children and the aged. As Rice and Horowitz have pointed out, during the five years preceding the introduction of these programs the general rise in price levels slowed substantially; this slowing ended rather abruptly in 1966, and was followed by a resumption of the rise at a more rapid pace (171). Needless to say, price indices have continued to rise through this entire period; and what we have described is not a reduction in price followed by a rise, but a deceleration in the rate of increase in prices, followed by an acceleration.

Medical care prices have conformed to the trend, except that the deceleration before 1966 was smaller than the deceleration for all goods and services, and the acceleration began a few months later and was much larger. The largest increases occurred in hospital prices. Table 33 shows the annual percentage increase in the charge for a semiprivate room. Not shown in the Table are "operating room charges" and the charge for "x-ray, diagnostic series, upper G.I.," which have been part of the medical care price index only since 1964; these prices also increased, but at a lower rate. During the five years ending June 1971, daily service charges increased by 95.5 percent, operating room charges by 77.1 percent, and the representative x-ray procedure by 34.7 percent (187, p. 19).

Since these items are all priced separately, there was no index of hospital prices as a whole until January 1972, when seven ancillary services were added to the items priced, and a composite

TABLE 33. Annual Percentage Increases in Specified Prices,[a] Selected Periods, U.S.A., 1960 to 1972[b]

Items Priced	1960–1965	1965–1970	1966	1967	1968	1969	1970	1971	1972
Consumer Price Index									
All items less medical care	1.2	4.1	3.0	2.4	4.1	5.4	5.8	4.1	3.3
All services less medical care	1.8	5.4	3.4	3.7	4.9	6.8	8.3	5.3	3.8
Medical Care Services	3.1	7.3	5.4	8.7	7.3	8.1	7.1	7.3	3.7
Semiprivate room	5.8	13.9	10.0	19.8	13.6	13.4	12.9	12.2	6.6
General physician, office visits	2.9	7.0	6.2	7.9	5.8	7.1	8.2	7.2	2.6
Tonsillectomy and adenoidectomy	2.5	5.2	4.3	5.4	4.9	5.1	6.2	6.9	3.8
Obstetrical care	2.3	6.5	4.5	7.5	5.2	7.9	7.3	5.9	3.7
Pediatric care, office visits	—	7.4	7.8	8.1	4.9	9.1	7.3	7.6	3.2
Dentists' fees	2.4	5.3	3.3	5.0	5.5	7.0	5.8	6.4	4.2

Source: Reference 181, Table 4.

[a] 1967 = 100, for each item.

[b] Medicare went into effect July 1, 1966. Phase I of the Economic Stabilization program was effective on August 15, 1972 and Phase II on November 15, 1972.

index of all 10 hospital services became available (181, p. 4). However, it is possible to derive alternative time series for hospital prices by using information on expenses per patient-day, with or without adjustment for the mix of inpatient days and outpatient visits. For example, Klarman et al. have reported five time series for hospital prices, of which only one series is the daily service charge of the consumer price index (176, pp. 17–19 and Table 13, p. 44). Price increases since the institution of Medicare are of the same order of magnitude, relative to each other, irrespective of which index is used, except that, during the first year of Medicare, there was an increase in the hospital daily service charge that was proportionately much larger than the increase in average expenses per patient day (187, p. 20). This is in line with reports that Medicare brought about a change in the manner in which the different components of hospital care were priced, so that charges corresponded more closely to costs (171, 188). This, however, does not explain the high rates of increase shown for the years 1968 through 1971 in Table 33. Part of this increase is, of course, accounted for by the higher rate of inflation in the prices of all items and of all services, exclusive of medical care; this trend is also documented in Table 33. The rest represents a real increase in price brought about by an increase in factor inputs and a disproportionate increase in their prices.

When data for nonprofit hospitals during 1967–71 are compared to data for 1961–65, one finds the annual increase in plant assets per census to be 1.6 times as rapid, the increase in personnel per 100 census to be 2.4 times as rapid, and the increase in average annual earnings per employee to be 2.2 times as rapid (190, Table 5, p. 9). However, not all of the difference in employee earnings can be attributed to third party payments. Other coincident events include the amendment of the Fair Labor Standards Act, in February 1967, to include hospital workers. As a result, 4.5 percent of nonsupervisory hospital workers received a salary increase (175, p. 3). Even more important has been the spread of collective bargaining for both professional and other workers in the hospital, with a more rapid rise in wages in recent years than in the past. However, it could be argued that the ability to pay higher wages is itself, in part, the consequence of a rising demand for medical care generated by third party payments (170, pp. 52–73).

Another consequence of third party payments has been an improvement in the financial position of hospitals, as shown by Feldstein and Waldman (188) and, more recently, by Davis (189) and by Pettengill (190). The degree of improvement can be seen in Table 34, which gives information for two calendar years—the one which ended 18 months before the implementation of Medicare on July 1, 1966, and the one which began 18 months after that date. For all nongovernmental, short-term hospitals there was, during this period, almost a doubling in net income as a percent of revenue (the net income ratio), while net income per patient day increased by 158 percent. Davis examined the specificity of the relationship between these changes and Medicare coverage, using a multiple regression analysis in which the average net income ratios for each state for 1967–1969 were regressed on a number of state attributes, which included figures for personal income, number of hospital beds, and number of physicians (189). When these and other variables were held constant, there was a significant positive relationship between the ratio of Medicare admissions to all admissions, the ratio of net income to total revenue,

TABLE 34. Specified Net Income and Revenue Data, Community Nongovernmental, Short-term Hospitals, U.S.A., 1964 and 1967

Hospital Category and Year	Net Income as percent of Revenue	Net Income per Patient-day	Revenue per Patient-day
All Hospitals [a]			
1964	2.06	0.89	43.40
1967	4.05	2.30	56.98
Percent increase	97	158	31
Non-profit Hospitals			
1964	1.87	0.81	43.23
1967	3.71	2.12	57.08
Percent increase	98	162	32
For-profit Hospitals			
1964	4.27	1.94	45.55
1967	8.38	4.68	55.80
Percent increase	96	141	23

Source: Reference 189, Tables 1, 5, 7, 8 and 11, pages 12, 15, 28 and 31.

[a] All community nongovernmental, short-term hospitals registered by the American Hospital Association.

and the ratio of net income to plant assets. Davis concludes that "a ten point increase in the proportion of Medicare patients (for example, from 20 percent to 30 percent), other things equal, increases the net ratio by about 1.7 points (for example, from 4.5 to 6.2)" (189, p. 39). The effect of the method of payment is indicated by an inverse relationship between the net income ratio and Blue Cross or Blue Shield enrollment, but no relationship of the net income ratio to membership in plans other than Blue Cross or Blue Shield. It is plausible to suggest that the method of reimbursing according to costs, which is used by Blue Cross, has some effect on reducing excess revenue. Unfortunately, the effect on costs cannot be inferred from the findings.

We may conclude that the advent of Medicare and Medicaid, by sharply increasing the scale of third party payments, has resulted in an increase in the costs of hospital care and a somewhat larger increase in price, leaving hospitals with a larger margin of net revenue. However, the increment of net revenue is a very small component in the increase in prices. Between 1964 and 1967 there was a 45 percent increase in expenses reported by nongovernmental, community short-term hospitals. The additional net revenue attributable to Medicare would, at best, add only 4 percentage points to this figure.

As the reader will recall, one object of our theoretical formulation was to predict the pricing behavior of hospitals with different characteristics. Unfortunately, little attention seems to have been given to documenting variations in pricing behavior, perhaps because the response of Medicare and Medicaid was so pervasive. According to Rice and Horowitz, a special study by the Bureau of Labor Statistics "clearly showed that the growth in hospital daily service charges during 1966 was a universal phenomenon. In 17 of 22 cities covered, all the hospitals reported rate increases for semi-private rooms. . . . During the preceding year . . . . there were only three cities in which all hospitals had reported increases in these rates" (171, p. 20). Nevertheless, the matter of differential response has received some attention which, for obvious reasons, has been focused on the distinction between nonprofit and for-profit hospitals.

Using mainly the annual reports of the American Hospital Association, Pettengill has assembled data for nongovernmental community hospitals during the decade 1961–1971, which can be divided roughly into the five years before and the five years after the implementation of Medicare and Medicaid. The information is summarized in Table 35. Data on use of service, cash flow, and capital assets all show that for-profit hospitals were, and continue to be, a very small segment of the hospital establishment. Comparison of utilization data, prior to Medicare, for nonprofit and for-profit hospitals shows that the latter had a somewhat lower occupancy ratio and a shorter average length of stay, and provided considerably fewer outpatient services relative to inpatient care. With respect to the amounts of labor and capital used to provide services, for-profit hospitals employed fewer persons per patient, paid somewhat lower wages per employee, and had a much smaller capital investment per patient. Perhaps for these reasons, for-profit hospitals had lower expenses per patient day; but since revenue per patient day was almost equal to that in nonprofit hospitals, income per patient day was distinctly higher in the for-profit hospitals. The clearly superior rate of return on investment enjoyed by for-profit hospitals is also shown by the data on the ratios of income to revenue and of income to plant assets. The advent of Medicare and Medicaid tended to accelerate already evident upward trends in use of service, factor inputs, expenses, revenue, income, and rates of return for both categories of hospitals, so that, in the main, their comparative positions have remained essentially unchanged. It is only in detail that one finds possible differences in response. For example, as shown in the last two columns of Table 35, for-profit hospitals were somewhat more successful in achieving relative increases in occupancy and in admissions, while at the same time checking the increase in outpatient services that is so striking a feature of nonprofit hospitals. By contrast, nonprofit hospitals had somewhat larger increases in plant assets, and in income per patient-day, although increases in rates of return were somewhat larger in the for-profit hospitals.

It is difficult to interpret the differences between the two categories of hospitals, either at the outset or in response to the institution of Medicare and Medicaid. To begin with, there may well be defects in the accuracy of the data, which are already biased by the lower response rate of the for-profit hospitals, especially small ones. Moreover, the for-profit hospitals differ from their nonprofit

TABLE 35. Specified Data for Nongovernmental Community Hospitals, by Type of Hospital, U.S.A., Specified Periods

Nature of Data	Non-Profit		For-Profit		1967–71 as percent of 1961–67	
	1961–1965	1967–1971	1961–1965	1967–1971	Non-Profit	For-Profit
Admissions (millions) [a]	18.4	20.4	1.4	1.9	110.9	135.7
Average length of stay (days) [a]	7.6	8.2	6.1	6.8	107.9	111.5
Patient days (millions) [a]	137.2	168.9	10.6	13.3	123.1	125.5
Occupancy ratio (%) [a]	77.3	79.9	67.5	72.8	103.3	107.9
Outpatient visits (millions) [a]	43.9	85.3	3.5 [b]	4.3	194.3	122.9
Total revenue (millions)	5,663	12,738	438	975	224.9	222.6
Total expense (millions)	5,551	12,353	414	901	222.5	217.6
Net income (millions)	112	384	24	74	342.9	308.3
Plant assets (millions)	7,688	12,702	270	411	165.2	152.2
Income ÷ revenue	1.98	3.02	5.48	8.88	152.5	162.0
Income ÷ plant assets	1.46	3.02	7.61	18.07	206.8	237.5
Personnel/100 census	245	285	212	247	116.3	116.5
Earnings/ employee	3,706	5,549	3,443	5,130	149.7	149.0
Plant assets/ census	20,457	27,470	9,279	11,270	134.2	121.5
Revenue/patient day	41.27	75.43	41.17	73.28	182.8	178.0
Expense/patient day	40.45	73.15	38.92	67.71	180.8	174.0
Income/patient day	0.82	2.28	2.25	5.57	278.0	247.6

Source: Several tables in Reference 190.
[a] Unweighted mean of five annual values.
[b] For the 4 years 1962–1965.

counterparts by being generally much smaller in size, and more likely to be located in metropolitan areas and in certain geographic regions, particularly in the South and West. It is likely that a substantial share of the difference between the two categories of hospitals can be accounted for because smaller hospitals tend to have fewer labor and capital inputs and lower expenses per patient day, to operate at lower rates of occupancy, and to have shorter average lengths of stay (191). But, as Pettengill demonstrates (190, pp. 11–19), certain differences do persist even when adjustments are made for hospital size: for-profit hospitals have higher expenses and even higher charges, so that their net income is higher per patient day as well as relative to revenue. The information available, which is admittedly incomplete, suggests that this pattern of income and revenue is achieved by renting rather than purchasing equipment, by more rapid depreciation of capital assets, by contracting for services, rather than producing them on the site, by providing somewhat less intensive care, and by avoiding the provision of services that are unprofitable or little in demand. Unfortunately, we do not know how Medicare and Medicaid may have contributed to these modes of operation, if at all. Nor are we given comparisons, before and after Medicare, adjusted for hospital size. While we wait for such information, all that can be said of the data we do have is that they tend to support our hypothesis that the smaller for-profit hospitals would be better able to improve occupancy and, as a result, to run more efficiently and improve income relative to revenues. As to the effect of size, without reference to type of ownership, Feldstein and Waldman report that the introduction of Medicare had little effect on the ratio of net revenue to total revenue in the smallest hospitals, those that range between 6 and 49 beds. These hospitals were generally not qualified to look after Medicare patients and did well financially without this source of revenue. The greatest improvement in the net revenue ratio was experienced by the groups of small and medium sized hospitals with 50–59, 100–199, and 200–299 beds (188). Although this is in keeping with our expectations, we cannot be certain, since no data are given from which we might infer changes in inputs and in price. However, such data should not be difficult to assemble.

We must now turn to the prices for physicians' services before and after the introduction of Medicare and Medicaid. As shown in Table 33, the increase in these prices has been nowhere near as large as the growth in hospital charges, but has been considerable, nonetheless, and is in excess of the increase in the composite price of all services other than medical care.

Huang and Koropecky, like other investigators before them, dwell on the very rapid increase in fees during the post-Medicare period (1966–1969) as compared to the more than 15 preceding years, but they go beyond this to determine how much of the increase is attributable to the effects of insurance coverage and how much is due to other factors (184). They point out that during 1966–1969 there was an average annual increase in reported physicians' fees of 6.3 percent. Of this, an annual increase of 3 percent was associated with Medicare. Of the 3 percent, 1.25 percent was attributable to the effect of Medicare in increasing the percent of expenditures covered by third parties. However, the remaining 1.75 percent was not attributed to the effect of third party coverage, but to other phenomena associated with the institution of Medicare and Medicaid, or to unrelated factors that distinguished the years 1966–1969 from the immediately preceding decade. Huang and Koropecky suggest that the method of payment used in Medicare may have been responsible, in large part, for the increment of 1.75 percent that is unexplained by advances in coverage during 1966–1969. They also report that changes in per capita income and in supply of physicians had no significant effect on changes in physicians' fees between 1952 and 1969. Though the supply of physicians was found to be an important factor in the differences in price among states, as reported by Fuchs and Kramer (150) and by Feldstein (169), it is not a factor of significance in explaining the secular trend of fees at the national level in recent years.

Table 32 shows some of the internal workings of the market for physicians' service during the early post-Medicare period. It is clear that the expansion in third party payments upon the introduction of Medicare and Medicaid was so large that there was, for the first time in recent years, an actual reduction in average net price. This should have been a powerful incentive to demand, but the market response was paradoxical. Rather than increase services, physicians appear to have raised prices and reduced the quantity produced per physician, so that they could earn higher incomes while they worked less (150, pp. 18–19). How these data, and this interpretation, jibe with more direct information on use of service should be of considerable interest. The reader will recall that a survey of persons 65 and older who were recipients of social security benefits showed that during the year preceding Medicare each respondent experienced an average of 6.6 outpatient visits to a physician and 3.14 days of short-term hospital care. During the year following Medicare the corresponding figures were 6.1 visits and 3.92 days (89). If it is assumed that each hospital day includes one visit by the patient's attending physician, one arrives at a total of 10.02 visits following Medicare as compared to 9.74 visits before Medicare, an increase of scarcely 3 percent per capita. It appears that the two sets of data, one based on expenditures and prices, and the other on direct reports of services received, do not quite correspond, but the difference is not so large as to render implausible the assertion that, in response to Medicare and Medicaid, physicians in private practice reduced rather than increased the supply of their services. In any event, it is difficult to say which of the two sets of data is more credible. The data on services received do not include care provided in nursing homes and extended care facilities, they are not adjusted for mix of services, and they suffer from the usual inadequacies of household surveys. The data on expenditures and prices have their own inadequacies. There is no precise physical equivalent to the figure for "quantity" of services that is obtained by deflating expenditure by price. The periods under comparison do not precisely correspond. And, finally, in the aggregate data of Table 32, effects on those eligible for Medicare may have been counteracted, to some extent, by changes among those not eligible.

A more detailed examination of the increase in reported prices associated with the institution of Medicare and Medicaid reveals a number of other peculiarities that call for an explanation (171). The first of these is that the upturn in the rate of increase in fees began about 6 months before the actual implementation of Medicare, and maintained its pace thereafter. Although hospital daily service charges also show a similar early start, the subsequent trend differs markedly, because the major increases in hospital charges correspond precisely with the implementation of Medicare, and the increases were somewhat smaller after implementation. Another peculiarity is that the increase in professional fees was generalized. It affected services that are particularly relevant to the aged but it also included other services. It was seen about equally in the services of physicians who care for the aged as in the services of other physicians, such as as pediatricians and obstetricians, who do not. Even dentists raised their fees, although they joined the upsurge a quarter of a year late and did not go quite as far in quite as short a time. However, over the five years following Medicare, the percentage increase in dental fees was only 16 percent lower than the increase in physicians' fees. Moreover, the increase in fees over this period was about as large for dentures, an item mostly used by the aged, as for fillings and extractions (187, p. 21).

It is difficult to say how all this came about. The early onset of the rise in physicians' fees could be partly explained by a rise in general prices about this time, and partly by the need to establish a higher benchmark of customary and prevailing fees in anticipation of Medicare. The diffuse nature of the increase in professional fees is somewhat more difficult to explain. One must concede, of course, that because of the concurrent introduction of Medicare and Medicaid, the opportunity to demand more service became available not only to the aged but to younger women and to children as well. In addition, one could postulate that because the services of different categories of physicians are to some extent substitutable, demand for the services of one category becomes diffused throughout. For example, as more aged persons seek care from generalists, the generalists are less likely to be able to care for children and women, who then seek the services of pediatricians and obstetricians, respectively. But neither of these explanations applies with sufficient force to the services of dentists, since they were included to a very small extent under third party payments and are negligibly substitutable for the services of physicians. A possible explanation could be that, as medical care needs are met by third party payments, families have resources released for the purchase of medical care services not covered by such payments. This would influence the purchase not only of dental care but of additional services of physicians as well. To some extent such secondary effects could be generated by the producers themselves through a process of referral. In this way, the properties of substitutability and complementarity, perhaps aided by the discovery effect, could lead to a diffusion of consequences that might have been localized and specific.

Almost all of this, of course, is pure speculation, although some of it is subject to empirical testing, for example, through an examination of the age structure of the caseloads of physicians by specialty. There is also an alternative, or additional, explanation: namely, that pricing has a large social component that goes beyond economics, and involves the maintenance of established relationships of status and prestige, including a hierarchy of incomes. If so, a change in any one component of a set of interrelated parts would initiate a signal for a generalized realignment. In this particular instance, dentists would be assumed to want to maintain a certain income position relative to physicians, and to take action, after some lag, to bring this about. This would mean that the temporal and spatial variations in the fees and incomes of dentists might be better explained by variations in the fees and incomes of physicians than by factors endogenous to the market for dental services. This is a proposition subject to empirical testing. If it can be shown to be at least partly true, its economic consequence would be to assure a degree of comparability in the attractiveness of the two professions, medicine and dentistry, to potential recruits. A third perspective on pricing behavior, which appeals to the epidemiologist, is to regard it as a social contagion, much like other group behavior, and to trace its manifestations in time, place, and person. Although this is pure empiricism, untouched by theory, it has the advantage of being a fresh beginning in the search for causal hypotheses. Somewhat in this spirit, we shall now examine the little that we know about the localization of price increases in different segments of the market for physicians' services.

In order to examine the consequences of Medicare in greater detail, the Social Security Administration has arranged with the Bureau of Labor Statistics to enlarge the panel of general physicians who report the fees for home and office visits that are included in the consumer price index, and to undertake additional pricing for certain services that are particularly important to the aged, though not limited to them. These services comprise in-hospital care for two medical conditions (myocardial infarction and cerebral hemorrhage), and three in-hospital surgical procedures (cholecystectomy, prostatectomy, and fractured neck of the femur). The prices for these items, though collected and reported, are not included in the consumer price index. The prices for office visits, home visits, and the in-hospital care of the two medical conditions are reported by the same panel of about 700 general practitioners and internists. In-hospital care by generalists and internists includes "the cost of admission, hospital write-up, examinations, and other services," but excludes diagnostic and laboratory examinations and medication. The prices for in-hospital surgical procedures are reported by a panel of about 1,300 surgeons. The prices for cholecystectomy are those reported by general surgeons only, whereas general surgeons as well as urologists report prices for prostatectomy, and general surgeons, as well as orthopedists, report prices for fracture of the neck of the femur. All these prices include "the usual single preoperative visit and postoperative care, excluding the fee for diagnosis and tests and the anesthetists' fee." Price quotations for both panels "are obtained in 56 areas located in 34 states and the District of Columbia. Of the 27 largest metropolitan areas, 24 are in the sample used to study physicians' fees. The distribution of sampling units provides rather comprehensive coverage for urban areas, but there is no coverage for services rendered in rural areas" (171, p. 25).

Table 36 shows the increase in the most usual fee charged during the five years following Medicare for each item of care that is especially important to the aged. Other items from the consumer index are cited for comparison. It is clear that the rates of increase in all fees are roughly comparable. A more detailed examination of increases in price during each quarter indicated to Rice and Horowitz that, in the period immediately before and after Medicare, the charges for the services important to the aged rose somewhat more slowly than the composite index of all physicians' fees (171). Accordingly, Rice and Horowitz suggest that the prices that were charged to the aged followed, rather than led, the upward movement of all prices. However, because data on the services important to the aged are not available for a sufficiently long period of time prior to Medicare, and because quarterly fluctuations in all fees for all components of the index are large, it is difficult to ac-

TABLE 36. Percentage Increase in Prices During The Five Years Ending June 1971, for Selected Components of The Consumer Price Index, and All Items in The Special Pricing Survey of The Bureau of Labor Statistics

Items	Percent
Components of The Consumer Price Index	
Hospital service charges	
Daily service charges	95.5
Operating-room charges	77.1
X-ray, diagnostic series, upper G.I.	34.7
Physicians' fee	39.7
General physician, office visits	42.7
General physician, house visits	40.5
Herniorrhaphy (adult)	30.6
Tonsillectomy and adenoidectomy	31.1
Obstetrical cases	40.0
Pediatric care, office visits	42.4
Psychiatrist, office visits	30.2
Dentists' fees	33.3
Denture, full upper	32.0
Special Pricing Survey [a]	
In-hospital medical care	
Myocardial infarction	30.1
Cerebral hemorrhage	29.8
In-hospital surgical procedures	
Cholecystectomy	31.5
Prostatectomy	36.6
Fractured neck of femur	46.2

Source: Reference 187, Tables on pages 19, 20, 21 and 23.
[a] Not included in Consumer Price Index.

cept this conclusion with any degree of confidence. In fact, we might claim to see in the same data a totally different phenomenon at work. It would seem as if the price for procedures for which a backlog of need could have accumulated, such as prostatectomy, responded immediately and in a sustained manner, whereas the prices of conditions that are rather infrequent and episodic, such as fracture of the femur, took distinctly longer to rise. But all this borders on the fanciful. The more sober and defensible conclusion is that the prices for the procedures that are especially important to the aged behaved in a manner essentially similar to all other fees and that, consequently, it is not possible to document a distinctive or specific effect of the Medicare program. Once again, whatever individual currents there may have been are lost in the broader tide of advancing prices. There is, however, one aspect of the increase in prices that is worth remembering. Rice and Horowitz point out that similar relative increases mean larger increments in dollars for the more expensive fees (171). For example, at the end of 1966, the most common fees were $5 for an office visit, $10 for a home visit, $75 for in-hospital care of the "regular" case of cerebral hemorrhage, $110 for the "regular" case of myocardial infarction, and $375 for the "regular" case of each of the three surgical procedures. Accordingly, a 43 percent increase in the fee for an office visit would mean a mere two dollars extra, whereas a 46 percent increase in the charge for treating a fractured femur would mean over $160 extra. Needless to say, this is an observation that applies to all fees, and is in no way characteristic of services to the aged as distinct from other services.

The special survey of prices also provides information on the localization of price increases by person and place. The immediate response of physicians to Medicare appears to have been widespread, but far short of the almost universal response of the hospitals. For example, during 1966 only 37 percent of the panel of physicians who were questioned reported an increase in the fee for an office visit, with an average increment of 24 percent for those who did report an increase (171, Table 6, p. 23). During the four years following Medicare 81 percent of the panel reported at least one increase in the office visit fee, and 33 percent reported more than one such increase. The average increase for all physicians who reported a rise was 39 percent (192, p. 5). From the data provided it is not possible to say what percent of the panel of physicians (excluding surgeons) did not increase any fees at all, since the experience for office visits, house visits, myocardial infarction, and cerebral hemorrhage is reported separately. However, it is reasonable to assume that physicians raise their fees for all or most services, rather than raising them selectively. If so, it is remarkable that during an intensely inflationary period such as this, more than 20 out of 100 physicians on the panel can be presumed to have reported no price increases. It would be interesting to know why they did not increase prices.*

* However, Dorothy Rice has cautioned me that, due to turnover in the panel of reporting physicians, this finding should be regarded as questionable.

Unfortunately, only crumbs of information are available, and that information has been inferred from an examination of physicians' propensities to increase prices according to specialty and location. The differences that are identified by this examination are so small, and so lacking in consistency, that only the most tentative hypotheses can be drawn. For example, when the data for each of the five years following Medicare are examined, there emerges an apparent ordering of procedures according to their susceptibility to fee increases, from most frequent to least frequent, as follows: (1) prostatectomy and fracture of the femur; (2) cholecystectomy; (3) myocardial infarction and cerebral hemorrhage; (4) office visits; and (5) house visits. It would seem as if price increases are more likely to involve: (1) surgical services as compared to nonsurgical; (2) in-hospital services as compared to those outside the hospital; and (3) services that are most likely to be provided by specialists, surgical or medical, rather than by general physicians or general surgeons. Home visits occupy a totally unexpected position in this ordering since one would expect that fees would increase to control "abuse" of this service, which is given so reluctantly by physicians. One wonders why these fees did not increase: because the physicians who provide home services are mainly general practitioners or pediatricians, because they are a peculiar lot in other ways, because house calls have a peculiar geographic incidence, or because house calls tend to be for emergent conditions? It is impossible to say. One does note, however, that when physicians do raise their fees for home visits, the average percent increase tends to be the largest of all the services priced. A plausible hypothesis is that so few physicians make home visits that only the few who make them with any frequency report an increase in fees and that the increase is large enough to act as a deterrent.

As to the average percent increase in fees for services other than house visits, this increase appears to be inversely correlated either with the absolute size of the fee, or with the frequency with which fee increases are made, or with both, since these two phenomena are themselves interrelated. As a consequence, neither the average percent increase for physicians who raise their fees, nor the average percent increase for all physicians, including those who do not raise their fees, produces a clear-cut ordering of the services according to whether they are surgical or medical, whether they are provided in the hospital or outside, or whether they are provided only by specialists or by generalists as well. This ordering, as described, applies only to the percent of physicians who raise prices once or more, and only when the data for each of the five years following the institution of Medicare are examined separately (187). The data that combine reported price increases for a number of years give somewhat different results, as shown in Table 37. It appears that the items listed in the table, which are the services selected as being of particular interest to the aged, are not ordered in the hypothesized manner when one uses as the criterion for ordering the percent of physicians who report raising their prices once or more times during 48 months. However, the propensity to make more than one increase during these 4 years orders the services in a manner that is almost identical to that already described, and which is shown in the third column of Table 37. One may conclude, tentatively, that in an inflationary period the tendency to make repeated increases is a highly differentiated attribute, whereas the making of only one increase is not. We have suggested that the technical content of the service and the degree of specialization necessary to provide it may be major factors in this differentiation.

Additional information by specialty status is available for the

TABLE 37. Percent of Physicians Who Report Increases in the Fees of Specified Services,[a] U.S.A., Specified Time Periods

| | 48 Months Ending Dec. 1969 | | |
Items Priced	One or More Increases	More Than One Increase	Yearly Average [b]
Prostatectomy	82.7 (1)	50.4 (1)	37.4 (1)
Fracture of neck of femur	77.3 (4)	47.6 (2)	37.1 (2)
Cholecystectomy	75.8 (3)	42.0 (3)	31.5 (3)
Myocardial infarction	67.0 (6)	33.6 (5)	29.4 (4)
Cerebral hemorrhage	65.7 (7)	33.7 (4)	28.9 (5)
Office visits	81.1 (2)	33.3 (6)	27.3 (6)
House visits	73.4 (5)	30.2 (7)	22.9 (7)

Source: Reference 192, Table 4, unpaginated, and Reference 187, Table 5, p. 24.

[a] Numbers in parentheses indicate order from most frequent to least frequent.

[b] Arithmetic mean of percent of physicians who report one or more increase in fees during each of 5 years ending June 1971.

four years ending December 1969 (192, Table 5). Unfortunately, while we are given the percentage of physicians who report at least one increase in fees, we are not given the percentage who make more than one increase. Thus we are unable to test our hypothesis of the functionally differentiated nature of repeated increases as compared to single increases. As to the percentage of those who increase their fees at least once, the order, from high to low, excluding house visits, is as follows: (1) generalist, office visits; (2) urologist, prostatectomy, and orthopedist, fracture of the femur; (3) general surgeon, cholecystectomy; (4) internist, office visit; (5) generalist, in-hospital procedures; and (5) internist, in-hospital procedure. We have no hypothesis that explains this progression in a satisfactory manner.

Further data on the pricing behavior of physicians is available by region and by size of community. According to Horowitz there are no consistent regional differences (192). The differences by size of community, though small and not completely consistent, do offer some grounds for speculation. The data, which are summarized in Table 38, are averages for each of five years following Medicare. As a result, they reflect the frequency with which changes are made. Rice and Horowitz report that "very few" physicians raised their fees more than once during 1966 (171, p 23). If this is assumed to hold true for each of the 5 years following Medicare, the product of the percent of physicians who raise fees and the average percent of increase for those who report an increase will approximate the average percent increase in fees of all physicians for each of the items priced.

The items that were priced have been arranged in Table 38 in descending order of the relative frequency with which physicians in all communities combined report a fee increase. We have already described this ordering and offered a rationale in terms of technical complexity of the service and the degree of specialization required to provide it. Now we can examine the possible effect of community size on the propensity to raise prices. When we do so, it becomes apparent that the arrangement in descending order of complexity and specialization holds very well in the two larger size categories, but not in the two smaller.* This may be

* This is not because the larger communities are more heavily represented in the average of all communities. Apparently no weighting according to number of physicians reporting was introduced in computing the averages in the source paper.

TABLE 38. Specified Aspects of Fee Increases by Type of Service and by Community Size, Panel of Physicians and Surgeons in a Sample of Urban Communities, U.S.A., June 1967–June 1971 [a]

Items Priced	All	Community Size			
		Less Than 50,000	50,000–249,000	250,000–1,399,999	1,400,000 or More
Percent of Physicians Reporting Fee Increases					
Prostatectomy	37.4	26.6	40.1	44.0	37.7
Fractured neck of femur	37.1	29.4	43.3	41.4	35.9
Cholecystectomy	31.5	26.6	35.8	32.7	31.8
Myocardial infarction	29.4	26.7	37.8	31.3	26.6
Cerebral hemorrhage	28.9	25.6	37.4	31.9	25.7
Office visits	27.3	26.7	29.3	37.7	23.0
House visits	22.9	22.5	26.3	24.1	21.1
Average Percent Increase in Fees of Physicians Who Raise Fees					
Prostatectomy	16.9	20.6	17.3	13.6	17.6
Fractured neck of femur	20.8	23.0	18.4	14.3	23.4
Cholecystectomy	17.6	17.9	16.5	15.5	19.2
Myocardial infarction	25.7	24.1	21.4	24.4	28.9
Cerebral hemorrhage	25.7	23.7	20.4	26.0	28.8
Office visits	25.5	23.5	22.8	25.3	27.7
House visits	31.5	32.2	27.1	34.8	28.9
Average Percent Fee Increase for All Physicians [b]					
Prostatectomy	6.3	5.5	6.9	6.0	6.6
Fractured neck of femur	7.7	8.8	7.1	5.9	8.4
Cholecystectomy	5.5	4.8	5.9	5.1	6.1
Myocardial infarction	7.6	6.4	8.1	7.6	7.7
Cerebral hemorrhage	7.4	6.1	7.6	8.3	7.4
Office visits	7.0	6.3	6.7	9.5	6.4
House visits	7.2	7.2	7.1	8.4	6.1

Source: Reference 192, Table 7, page 27.

[a] Arithmetic means of data for each of 5 years.

[b] Product of percent of physicians who report increase and average percent increase.

because the functional differentiation of physicians is much sharper in the larger communities, where there are more specialists, and likely to be blurred in the smaller communities, where general physicians and surgeons are more likely to perform more difficult procedures. The data also show that the very rough inverse correspondence between the percentage of physicians reporting a price increase for a service and the percent increase per physician tends to hold in communities of all sizes. As to the product of these two variables, the percent increase in the average fee of all physicians, no consistent order is discernible, except that the average price for a cholecystectomy has risen least or next to least in all community groups. Another phenomenon that cuts across communities is the tendency, which we have already described, for relatively few physicians to report having raised their fees for home visits, but for those few to report relatively large increments. The percentage of physicians who raise fees is smallest for home visits in all categories of communities, whereas the percent of increase reported is the largest in 3 categories and next to largest in one.

In addition to the regularities that cut across all categories of community size, there are tendencies related to size of community that cut across the items priced. These tendencies were identified by ranking the four categories of communities from high to low (1 to 4) according to their position in each row of Table 38. These rankings were appraised, by visual inspection, for order and for consistency. In addition, average ranks and average percentage values were constructed, pooling the data for all the priced items, but without differential weighting by item. These averages are shown in Table 39. It appears that, with respect to the propensity of physicians to raise prices, communities were ordered in a reasonably consistent manner, from highest to lowest, in the following sequence of sizes: (1) 50,000–249,999, (2) 250,000–1,399,999, (3) 1,400,000 or more, and (4) less than 50,000. The last 2 categories were very close together. As to the percent increase in fees for physicians who reported a raise, the communities do not seem to be ordered in a consistent manner, even though the average rankings do show a rough inverse relationship between the propensity of doctors to raise prices and the relative size of the increment in price. In spite of this phenomenon, the ranking of

TABLE 39. Unweighted Average Ranks [a] and Percentages, for Specified Aspects of Fee Increases for All Priced Items, by Community Size, Panel of Physicians and Surgeons in a Sample of Urban Communities, U.S.A., June 1967–June 1971

	Community Size			
	Less Than 50,000	50,000– 249,999	250,000– 1,399,999	1,400,000 or More
Percent of physicians reporting fee increases				
Average rank	3.6	1.3	1.7	3.4
Average percent	26.3	35.7	34.7	27.4
Percent increase in fees of physicians who raise fees				
Average rank	2.4	3.4	2.7	1.4
Average percent	23.6	20.3	27.0	24.9
Percent fee increase for all physicians				
Average rank	3.6	1.9	2.3	2.3
Average percent	6.2	7.1	7.3	7.0

Source: Data in Table 38.
[a] Ranks are 1 for highest and 4 for lowest.

communities by average increase in fees for all doctors, replicates the order for the percent who did increase fees. However, the ranking is not so consistent in detail and the average differences are blurred. The one exception is that communities of size 50,000–249,999 continue to rank highest, mainly because of the great frequency with which physicians in communities of this size raised their prices.

Needless to say, these tendencies, across items and across categories of community size, are easier to describe than to explain, but it is worth making an effort to do the latter. It is reasonable to assume that few physicians in communities of any size are ready to provide home care. The few who do have raised their prices to deter the demand created by the inclusion of home visits under Medicare and Medicaid, which provide benefits for the aged and the young respectively, the two groups most likely to demand visits in the home. The unusually low percent increase in the price of cholecystectomies is less easy to explain unless one attributes it to a combination of characteristics, including the relatively large supply of general surgeons, the nonurgent nature of the operation in many instances, and the relatively large base fee charged for it. A number of factors acting in concert may also explain why prices do not rise so often or so much in the smallest urban communities. General prices may be lower and the costs of practice smaller. Personal disposable income may be lower. More care may be provided by general practitioners or less specialized surgeons. The social ties binding physician and patient may be closer and the restraints on raising prices correspondingly stronger. But none of this would explain why prices increase most often in the category of communities next to the smallest. Accordingly, one is reduced to postulating a relative shortage of physicians in communities of this size. There may also be some interaction between specialty status and community size. As we have mentioned before, the cumulative data for the 4 years following Medicare show that general physicians were more likely than internists to raise fees at least once during this period, and that this was true for all the services priced: office visits, home visits, and in-hospital care for myocardial infarction or cerebral hemorrhage. If these findings are accepted at face value, one would expect a greater tendency to raise prices for these services in the smallest communities, where general practitioners are more likely to be dominant. In fact, the percent of physicians who raised prices once or more times during four years was lowest in these communities (192, Table 5). This suggests that the general practitioners in the larger communities were responsible for the greater average tendency of general practitioners to raise prices. It would seem that there is a progression in the tendency to raise prices at least once, which is as follows, from least to most likely: small-town general practitioners, internists, larger-town general practitioners. It is not clear why this should be so, unless one assumes that general practitioners in the larger towns catered to lower-income persons and were relatively under-paid prior to the advent of Medicare and Medicaid.

To summarize, it is difficult to escape the conclusion that the large increase in third party payments brought about by the institution of Medicare and Medicaid has been responsible for an increase in prices in recent years. However, we cannot unequivocally assert that we understand precisely how this happens, or that these programs have been the only important influence at work. The effect of Medicare and Medicaid on hospital prices is to be seen mainly in the daily service charge, although the prices of other hospital services have also increased rapidly. The increase in daily charges may be partly an artifact of a change in accounting practice, but it is largely real. The specificity of the relationship between the price increase and Medicare is attested to, in part, by a precise coincidence between the implementation of Medicare and the most rapid increase in hospital prices. It is further supported by the positive association between the proportion of hospital admissions paid by Medicare and the net revenue ratios of hospitals, as reported by Davis on the basis of ecological correlations, using states as the units of analysis (189). It appears that the for-profit hospitals experienced smaller relative and absolute increases in price but achieved higher absolute and relative increases in the ratio of net income to revenue. This is in keeping with our expectations, if it is assumed that for-profit hospitals tended to run at inefficiently low rates of occupancy prior to Medicare, and experienced a smaller degree of technological enrichment following its implementation. The relatively more favorable net income ratios observed in small to medium sized hospitals following Medicare is also in keeping with this interpretation.

The increase in physicians' fees that is associated with Medicare and Medicaid has been less marked, and it is less specifically linked with Medicare. The acceleration in the rate of increase began about 6 months prior to the implementation of Medicare, and there was no perceptible change in this rate coincident with the implementation of the program. Moreover, the effects have been diffuse, involving dentists and physicians to an almost equal degree. Among physicians, those specialists who do not cater to the aged have increased their prices as much as those who do; and the fees for services that are particularly important to the aged have been increased about as much as those for other services. There are also suggestions, however veiled, that the propensity to increase prices can be ordered in a hierarchy of services differentiated by complexity and specialization and in a hierarchy of communities differentiated by size; and that there may be an interaction between the two. For example, we have construed the data to mean that services that are more complex and are provided by highly specialized physicians are more likely to have their prices raised frequently; that price increases are more frequent in communities of intermediate size than in those that are very small or very large; and that general practitioners in the larger towns were more likely to raise their prices than internists in communities of any size, or generalists in the smaller towns. It is idle to pretend that all these relationships are demonstrably present or that we have an explanation for them. We have shown, on the other hand, that explanations are possible within the theoretical framework that we have established. Thus, one can postulate that when payment is made according to customary and prevailing prices it is necessary to establish an early benchmark and equally necessary to apply to everyone the prices that are charged to the aged. Supplementarity and complementarity among services and specialties can diffuse localized changes in price so that the increases spread, in ever-widening circles, to include all physicians and services. If we add to this the social forces that maintain established patterns of stratification, we can more fully explain the mass movement of prices. Similarly, we have shown that there are plausible explanations for the way in which the propensity to raise prices is ordered by type of service, by specialty and by community size. All this gives us some assurance that we are on the right track when, through the intermediary of the mechanisms we have postulated, we tie a variety of price changes to the rather sudden growth in third party payments. There is, however, a great difference between true prediction and post hoc justification. In this instance, we knew the essential outlines of the facts before we constructed our theoretical expectations. Thus, we can be justifiably accused of finding what we knew lay ahead at the end of the road. But this has not been entirely true. Besides, our purpose has not been to test theory, but to present the facts as we know them, to provide a framework that would encompass at least some of what we know, and to point the way to the great amount of exploration that remains to be done.

Possible Effects of the Method of Paying Physicians. Among the areas in urgent need of further exploration is the effect that the method of reimbursement has on the price of services and on other aspects of physician and client behavior. Our present concern is with the narrower question of its effect on price.

The Medicare program stipulates that it will pay only the portion of charges for covered services that it considers "reasonable." A reasonable charge is one that is both "customary" and "prevailing." The customary charges depend on what is charged by individual physicians for the services that they provide. The only condition set by Medicare is that the charge for any service be either the same for all patients or, when the charge is not uniform, that it not be larger than 50 percent of the charges made by the individual physician for that particular service during a specified period. Thus, there is a customary charge for each type of service of each physician. The prevailing charges depend on the distribution of the customary charges of all physicians in a defined geographic area. The customary charge of an individual physician for a specified type of service will be accepted as "prevailing" (and hence "reasonable") if it does not exceed a specified percentage (for example, 75 percent) of the customary charges of all physicians for that type of service during a specified period. It follows that there is one prevailing charge for each type of service in a community, and that this prevailing charge is generated by the aggregate of the decisions of individual physicians as they set their own particular fees. Sometimes there are two prevailing charges for each service rather than only one. This is because Medicare permits prevailing charges to be computed separately for generalists and specialists. A final, most important, provision of the Medicare legislation is that physicians are not required to accept the reasonable charges as full payment. They may do so by accepting "assignment." But they may also refuse to be bound by the limits of the reasonable charge determination, in which case they must collect from the patient; Medicare will reimburse the patient for what would have been the reasonable charge. Since physicians can accept or refuse assignment case by case, they have the opportunity to select how they are to be paid so as to earn the most income.

We have already said that the decision to pay customary and prevailing charges and to have physicians, as a group, set the level of what is customary and what is prevailing, was a positive invitation to physicians to raise fees in anticipation of Medicare and to make further increases thereafter. We have also suggested that when the implementation of the payment system is left in the hands of an agency, such as Blue Shield, that is controlled by physicians and responsive to their wants, policy and regulations will be interpreted in a manner most likely to aid physicians in their quest for higher prices.

Anecdotal support for these contentions has been reported by the staff of the Senate Finance Committee (193, pp. 59–69). Huang and Koropecky offer a more systematic analysis (184). We have already referred to their finding that more than half of the annual rate of increase in the reported fees of physicians between 1966 and 1969, which is temporally associated with the institution of Medicare and Medicaid, cannot be explained by the increase in insurance coverage. It can be presumed that at least part of the unexplained increase is due to the peculiar method of reimbursement which was adopted by Medicare, and which as a consequence became a more frequent feature of other insurance plans as well. A more direct test of the effects of the method of reimbursement, and of its component features, was possible because the several carriers that served Medicare in its early years did not use uniform methods of administering the payment system. To study the effects of the variations, the experience of 35 carriers with state-wide jurisdiction was examined. The advantage of selecting these carriers was that information could be obtained concerning socioeconomic and other variables, data which are readily available for states, but not for subunits of states. The disadvantage was that almost an equal number of carriers, many operating in some of the largest states, were excluded. It is not known to what extent this method of sampling may have biased the findings.

The dependent variable in the analysis was the rate of increase in effective charges to Medicare beneficiaries between 1967 and 1969. These are not simply the charges allowed to be reasonable under Medicare, but an average of allowable and actual charges, weighted to reflect the percent of claims for which it is indicated that the reasonable charge will be accepted as full payment. In this way, the charges under investigation reflect the obligations incurred jointly by the Medicare program and its beneficiaries, under the unproven assumption that the average charge in claims that accept the reasonable charge as full payment will be the same as in claims that do not. The independent variables include the previous year's charges, characteristics of the carrier, including the method of arriving at reasonable charges that prevailed in 1967, and a set of geographic and demographic variables. The method of analysis was nonlinear, ordinary least squares multiple regression, using carriers and states as units of analysis.

As expected, it was found that charges increased less rapidly in jurisdictions in which a fee schedule was generally in force, and when a fee schedule was used by the carrier as a basis for determining the reasonable charges. A fee schedule that specified maximum allowable fees was more effective in this respect than one that used relative value scales. Also as expected, the more frequently the carrier recognized that price increases constituted new levels of what is "customary," the more rapid was the increase in charges. This observation justifies the provision, introduced later, that the fees that are considered "customary" for a given fiscal year should be based on the fees that were current during the previous calendar year. Another safeguard, this time in the legislation itself, was that the fees charged to Medicare beneficiaries should be not in excess of fees for comparable services covered by the carrier under other plans. This precaution was only partially vindicated by the findings. Contrary to expectation, increases in price were most rapid when the base for determining customary and prevailing fees was the carrier's experience with its own non-Medicare enrollees. Increases were less rapid in jurisdictions in which the carrier used only Medicare charges as the base for determining customary and prevailing fees, and least rapid where the carrier's Medicare and non-Medicare experience was combined for this purpose. Thus, the statutory provision that the non-Medicare charges serve as a limit to Medicare charges was vindicated by the observation that the increase in effective charges to Medicare beneficiaries was smaller under the jurisdiction of carriers that determined reasonable charges after pooling charges to Medicare beneficiaries and other insured persons than under the jurisdiction of carriers that used charges to Medicare beneficiaries alone. It is not clear why the effective charges to Medicare beneficiaries did not rise even less where the carriers used only the charges to insured persons other than Medicare beneficiaries as the base for determining the reasonable charge.

The regression equation that was used to look into the effect of using different bases for determining the reasonable charge took into account, among other characteristics, whether the carrier was Blue Shield or not, but unfortunately it did not correct for the possible effects of other differences in the method of arriving at reasonable charges (184, pp. 31–32). The effect of the carrier being Blue Shield, rather than a commercial carrier, was also contrary to what we have hypothesized. In states where Blue Shield was the carrier Medicare charges increased more slowly. This was true even when the use of a fee schedule was held constant in one regression equation and the frequency of updating customary fees held constant in another. It is obviously simple-minded to assume that Blue Shield is only responsive to a constituency of physicians who are anxious to charge what the traffic will bear. While such responsiveness may be present in some situations, it appears not to be generally true, at least within the limits defined by this study.

An important concern in the design of reimbursement procedures is whether specialists are to receive special recognition and, if so, to what extent and in what way. Medicare permits separate computation of customary and prevailing charges for specialists and generalists, but not all carriers did so in 1967. Those that did reported slower increases in average charges than those that did not; but the difference was not statistically significant when several variables were held constant: the use of a fee schedule by the carriers, the average level of charges, the standard deviation of charges, the supply of physicians, and geographic region. Some of these variables had interesting effects themselves, on the rate of increase in Medicare charges. The higher the average charges, the less rapid was the rate of increase; the more variable the charges the greater the rate of increase. Contrary to expectation, Medicare did not bring about a greater uniformity or convergence in charges, either within a state or among states. Regional differences were marked, with the most rapid increases in the West, even when corrections were made for the level of charges. Also unexpected was the finding that a larger supply of physicians tended to accelerate the inflation of charges to a small extent, rather than to retard it. This effect persists in spite of correction for every variable used in the analysis, including the level of charges in the preceding year and their dispersion—variables which might be related to the prevalence of specialists in a state. If the mix of specialists and generalists does not explain the relationship observed, it is difficult to say what does. One should remember, however, that the mere prevalence of physicians does not necessarily denote the presence of reserve capacity. It could be that where physicians are most plentiful, they are less willing or able to see more patients. In any event, the observation that, under Medicare, physicians were able to increase their prices even more rapidly where their number relative to population was largest, supports de Vise's contention that revenue from Medicare and Medicaid has made it easier for physicians to locate in geographic areas that are professionally and socially attractive and thus are already well supplied with physicians (194). In this way, it is argued, these programs have contributed to an increase in the maldistribution of physicians, rather than an alleviation, as had been hoped by some.

To conclude, the study by Huang and Koropecky, although it deals only with a selected number of statewide carriers, does support the expectation that fee schedules introduce a retarding effect on increases in physician's charges, and that fees based on customary charges, without reference to a fee schedule, accelerate price increases, especially when these charges are validated at frequent intervals. The reimbursement system, therefore, is an essential consideration in predicting the effect of benefits on price.

Summary of Findings and Policy Implications

Summary of Findings

By definition, third party payment for medical care brings about a reduction in out-of-pocket payments at the time services are consumed. This constitutes a reduction in net price. However, the total cost of delivering health services increases. To begin with, the institution and administration of third party payments, whether it is done for profit or not, adds a cost which has to be reflected in higher fees, premiums, or taxes, in lower wages, or in some combination of these. Secondly, if it is assumed that insured persons are charged the reported price for all services, or that they are charged the reported price only for covered services and a somewhat lower price for noncovered services, one can show that the uninsured pay about two-thirds of the reported price for all services. Under the assumptions, one can postulate rises in the average prices actually paid by those who use service or on their behalf by third parties. Although we have devoted a fair amount of space to studies that illustrate this phenomenon, we need to recognize that the empirical basis for the assumptions remains in doubt.

The third, and most fundamental, effect of third party payments on prices, is the increase in reported prices, which signifies a concurrent rise in average and net prices as well, since these latter are tied to the former. With respect to reported price, the last several years have shown a steady increase, though at varying rates. During the same period third party payments have also gone up. The central theme of this chapter has been that this concurrence in time is not merely coincidental, but that third party payments have caused the rise in price, at least to a significant degree. To develop this theme, we first described its theoretical basis; then, we described the empirical findings that have a bearing on the theoretical expectation.

In theory, third party payments cause a reduction in net price, and this reduction, relative to the prices of other goods and services, in turn causes a rise in demand. The demand is not only for more services but also for qualitatively different services. The result is that prices go up, partly to moderate the pressure of demand on the limited capacity to produce services, but largely to accomodate the richer content of care in amenities and in technology. This is the basic thrust, but it is considerably modified by the characteristics of the medical market and of the producers that operate within it. Consequently, we had to consider in our theoretical construct, as well as in the analysis and interpretation of the empirical findings, several of these factors: the objectives of hospitals and physicians, the response of supply to demand, the characteristics of the technology, features of the method of reimbursement, and aspects of the social organization of the health professions.

The empirical studies that we have reviewed can be classified into two categories. In the first category are studies that have examined the degree of correspondence in the secular trend of third party payments and medical care prices. In these studies corrections are often made for additional influences, with the trend in the prices for all goods and services being perhaps the most important. The second category comprises cross-sectional comparisons between states. Although such cross-sectional studies have the advantage of holding the level of technology relatively constant, they suffer from the limitations inherent in ecological correlations. Their findings, though interesting, remain inconclusive.

As to the comparisons in trends, it is useful to distinguish the period before the institution of Medicare and Medicaid from the period after. For the former period, Feldstein emphasizes that the rise in the average price of physicians' services, while substantial, is less than would be expected from the concurrent rise in insurance coverage (169). He concludes that physicians may be constrained by ethical and other considerations from charging what the traffic will bear. However, the operation of some external constraints, such as fee schedules, cannot be ruled out. With respect to the same period, Fuchs and Kramer emphasize the lack of precise correspondence between the rise in average prices and the increase in the proportion of expenditures for physicians' services covered by third parties, including government (150). They attribute this discrepancy to the changing character of technology during this time period. In contrast to these investigators, who find that the movement of physicians' fees in the pre-Medicare period does not quite correspond to their theoretical expectations, Huang and Koropecky are quite satisfied that they have accounted for the trend in physicians' reported fees, both before and after Medicare, by using only three variables: the price of all goods and services; third party coverage, including that provided by government programs; and a variable that distinguishes the period before Medicare from the period after (184).

As to the period after Medicare, everyone agrees that during this time the prices of medical care services increased quite out of proportion to the rise in prices generally. A rough estimate is that about half of the annual increase in the fees reported by physicians is accounted for by the inflation in the prices of all goods and services. The remaining half is, in turn, divisible into two roughly equal parts. The first part is accounted for by the increase in third party payments and the associated reduction in net price. The second part represents an increment to which many factors may have contributed. Important among these is the method of reimbursement for customary and prevailing fees as implemented during the first three years following the institution of Medicare (184).

Some Consequences

Assuming these findings to be correct, at least in their major outlines, we can now turn to some of their implications for policy. Perhaps the most important of these stems from the effect of rising prices on insured and uninsured consumers. One would expect the heavier burden to fall on those who have little or no coverage, either through private insurance or through governmental programs. Such persons would have to pay, at least in part, the higher prices that have become prevalent because an increasing number of other people have bought insurance or enjoy public benefits. It is generally assumed that the poorest families are reasonably protected by Medicaid. If so, rising prices are likely to hit hardest those who are just beyond the margin of poverty but are not included in a comprehensive plan through membership in an employee group. Even for persons who have private insurance, the rise in price can nullify part of the financial protection afforded by the insurance. According to Feldstein one third of the increased coverage for the physicians' services that occurred between 1948 and 1966 was "diluted by induced price increases" (169, p. 129). This is at the aggregate level. For the individual person with insurance coverage, the loss of protection can occur in three related ways. First, benefits seldom cover all services, so that with respect to non-covered services, persons with insurance are in the same position as those without. Second, with respect to covered services, to the extent that coverage is not complete, protection is reduced so that the enrollee has to participate in payment. Finally, even when coverage is complete, the insured must directly or indirectly bear the cost of premiums that are constantly revised upward in order to keep pace with prices. The erosion of protection for covered services that is brought about by rising prices, when accompanied by deductibles and copayments, is well illustrated by the experience under Part B of Medicare (195). Between 1967 and 1970, the proportion of covered charges that were not potentially reimbursable by the program remained reasonably constant, changing only from 36 to 35 percent. However, as prices and the use of some services rose, the total charges for each person who used the covered services increased from approximately $144 to approximately $195, and the amount that was not potentially reimbursable increased from $52 to $68, an increment of 31 percent. Because of a small drop in use of service and a lower rate of increase in prices, 1971 was the first year following the institution of Medicare during which there was a small reduction in the covered charges per person who used covered services, and this was accompanied by a corresponding reduction in the amount that was not reimbursable, to $67 from $68 in 1970. This reversal of the upward trend was no doubt due to the fact that prices were frozen from August to November of 1971 as a result of the economic stabilization program.

It is clear from the above that a price rise reinforces the rationing effect of coinsurance and deductible payments. These devices are intended to control the level of service and its social distribution. In this respect, the policy considerations that pertain to prices and to participatory payments coincide. The fundamental issue is whether one wishes to maintain financial barriers, at least to some degree, as a rationing device, or whether the social distribution of services is more efficient when prices are not allowed to rise. As we have pointed out, financial barriers tend to penalize the poor more than the rich, and to depress preventive services and health supervision as opposed to therapeutic services for already established severe illness. Should a system of variable participatory payments be adopted to help counter these tendencies, the rise in prices will enhance the effect of the participatory payments and thus should be taken into account in the design.

The price rise that was fueled by the growth in third party coverage would be expected to have a favorable effect on the supply side, where a shortage of physicians is thought to have existed for some time (178). Unfortunately, the empirical studies that we have reviewed suggest that, at least in the short run, the response to a rapid increase in third party coverage may be contrary to expectations, because physicians may prefer more leisure rather than more income (150, 169). If so, this would exacerbate the shortage of physicians, add to public discontent, and invite further governmental intervention in the operations of the medical care market. Limited supplies would also have the largely unintended, but socially valuable, effect of adjusting use of service more closely to need, because there is less room for expanding services to those who already have almost all the care they need. Another effect of the physicians' unwillingness to expand supply would be that use of service and costs to the program would not increase as much as feared. This is a mixed blessing; as we have emphasized, one purpose of third party payments is to bring about increased use of at least some services by some population groups. Furthermore, it is of little consolation to the public program if its costs are increased to almost the same extent, but by an increase in price rather than by an increase in use. Finally, when use of service is controlled by limiting the services of physicians, serious distortions are likely to be introduced into patterns of care, including unnecessary use of costly substitutes for office care, such as the hospital.

In the long run, a rise in prices and incomes should make the health professions more attractive to aspirants. An assessment of the consequences of this is a task that we cannot undertake. It is obvious, however, that the immediate consequence depends on whether the current capacity to train health workers is larger or smaller than the number of qualified applicants. Since there are now more applicants than openings in medical schools, the number of physicians trained is not likely to be affected soon, although medical schools would have more applicants to choose from. Whether this will improve the quality of the product depends on what criteria medical schools use in selecting students and on what constitutes good care in the eye of the beholder.

Another concern on the supply side is geographic distribution. It had been hoped that a rapid increase in third party coverage under Medicare and Medicaid would attract physicians to less favored locations by making it possible for them to earn a decent living while performing a socially meritorious function. We have not seen an even approximately definitive analysis of what has, in fact, happened. Our impression is that the availability of reimbursement under Medicare and Medicaid has made it more feasible to provide care in under-serviced and economically depressed areas through organized programs such as clinics or neighborhood centers. As to the private practice of medicine, Medicare and Medicaid may have materially increased the incomes of those physicians who have, in the past, serviced the poor at lower fees, without adding significantly to their numbers. Some years ago, Rimlinger and Steele argued that the major deterrent to physicians locating in areas with an already plentiful supply of physicians is the difficulty in earning a satisfactory income (196). The ability to charge higher prices in order to earn a satisfactory inccome, even though fewer services are provided by each physician, would remove this barrier and add to the maldistribution in relation to need. The limited data available to Rimlinger and Steele seemed to support their analysis. It appeared that as the physician-population ratio increased, fewer services were produced by each physician, without reduction in average income, presumably because an increase in price compensated for a reduction in work (196). More recently, de Vise has argued in similar fashion, citing data to support the hypothesis that physicians are drawn to locations that are inherently attractive by reason of climate, social amenities, and professional opportunities, not necessarily in that order. Medicare and Medicaid, the argument goes, by creating new purchasing power in these desirable and already well-doctored areas, have removed a major barrier to the further migration of physicians into them. Thus, one observes a continuing depletion of physicians from certain Midwestern states and the inner portions of certain cities, while the proportion of physicians increases in the suburbs and on both coasts (194).

The data cited in these studies could no doubt be questioned on several counts. It is not our intent to use them as convincing evidence, but merely to raise the question of the relationship between rising prices and the redistribution of physicians. A general rise in prices will apparently not bring about a socially desired redistribution. What is needed is a system that creates differential incentives. In this respect, the method of reimbursement under Medicare has features that would seem to promote the opposite of the desired effects. The attraction of high income areas is increased by: (1) giving the physician an option to levy a fee larger than the "reasonable charge" and to accept or refuse assignment on a case-by-case basis; (2) by the greater ease of collecting deductible and coinsurance payments; and (3) by the separation of high income from low income areas in designating the areas within which prevailing fees are to be determined. The findings of Huang and Koropecky are in keeping with these speculations;

they show that during the early post-Medicare period there was no convergence of physicians' charges to Medicare beneficiaries either within or between the 35 states that were studied. Moreover, the increase in charges was most rapid in the West. Unfortunately, the sample studied by Huang and Koropecky did not include California, the state which, according to de Vise, appears to hold the greatest attraction to physicians (184, 194).

The rise in prices following Medicare may also have made physicians less available for recruitment into group practice, except at higher salaries. Huang and Koropecky have reported that the cost of services at the Group Health Association of Washington, D.C. increased at a more rapid rate during 1966–1971 than might have been expected. They speculate that: "The opportunity costs of young, well-trained doctors have been rising rapidly, partly because of higher fees for service, and partly because of improved productivity (technology). Since group practice is already relatively efficient compared to individual practice, the increase in salaries has resulted in an increase in costs" (184, p. 52).

One must conclude that the rise in prices attendant upon the expansion of third party coverage tends, by and large, to thwart the attainment of social objectives while adding to the financial drain on the porgram. The only possible exceptions are that, in the short run, the distribution of services is more likely to conform to severity of illness and, in the long run, the supply of scarce services may be enhanced. In the meantime, it may be necessary to take steps to moderate the rise in prices or its effects on the consumer.

Some Implications for Action

Moderating Prices. There are two lines of attack on the problem of rising prices: one is to deal with the prices themselves and the other is to mitigate the burden that price escalation places on the consumer. Action taken to moderate the rise in prices can, itself, vary in directness. Most indirect, and most congenial to the free market ideology, is to expand supply—for example by building new hospitals or training more physicians. While this may have a moderating effect on the price per service, it may also increase total expenditures and program costs by stimulating additional use of service (170, pp. 78–79). It is not even certain that prices will be appreciably moderated, since the larger number of physicians could reduce their average hours of work and still maintain their income by raising their prices. The attempt to control prices through the expansion of supply appears to have uncertain and hazardous consequences in a market where producers have such a high degree of control.

A more direct approach is to alter the method of reimbursement. We have already shown that the method of reimbursement adopted by Medicare, especially as implemented in the early years of the program, had several features that encouraged physicians to raise their prices. To counteract these price increases, Medicare introduced procedures designed to act as a break to escalation. A longer time lag was established between a rise in fees and the acceptance of the new fees as customary. Thus, the fees recognized as customary for a given fiscal year were based on the fees actually charged during the previous calendar year. In addition, the cut-off point beyond which customary fees are not recognized as prevailing was reduced to the 75th percentile (197). But all this was mere tinkering. Finally, as part of an assault on inflation generally, direct price controls were introduced. Effective on August 15, 1971, prices were frozen for 90 days. This was Phase I of the Economic Stabilization Program. Phase II began on November 14, 1971, when base prices were established and limits placed on the rate at which these prices would be permitted to increase. "Institutional providers, such as hospitals and nursing homes, were permitted only such price increases as were justified by allowable costs adjusted for productivity gains. The regulations permitted a provider to increase its prices over the base prices and thereby increase its aggregate annual revenue up to 2.5 percent without previous approval. Increases from 2.5 to 6.0 percent in the providers' aggregate annual revenue had to be reported to the Internal Revenue Service with supporting justification and to the appropriate Health Insurance for the Aged (Medicare) intermediary; increases above 6.0 percent required that an exception be granted by the Price Commission, based on review of the recommendations of a state advisory board. Noninstitutional providers, including physicians, were permitted aggregate increases in their prices, based on allowable cost increases, of no more than 2.5 percent a year" (181, p. 102). For Medicare, the allowable charges in effect November 13, 1971, were considered base prices under Phase II (197, p. 11). Phase III of the Economic Stabilization Program began January 11, 1973, with the abolition of mandatory controls except for problem areas, including food and the health care industry. On April 30, 1974, even these last remnants of control were abolished. However, since July 1, 1975, reimbursement of physicians' fees under Medicare has been tied to a national economic index, so that these fees will follow, rather than lead, inflationary trends.

Prior to the introduction of direct price controls on medical care, the conventional judgment would have been that they were not an acceptable remedy either ideologically or politically. The establishment of the controls showed that they could be made acceptable. On the other hand, one needs to remember that virtually all prices were controlled, not just medical care prices, and that the controls were explicitly designed to be temporary. Controls that apply only to medical care prices might still be difficult to sustain over an unlimited period of time. The effectiveness of such controls would, of course, be an issue, in addition to their acceptability. On this score, there are data that show how prices behaved under Phase I and Phase II (181), compared to price movements during the two fiscal years preceding Phase I.

It is clear that during Phase I prices were not fully at a standstill, although inflation was much restrained. During Phase II the annual rate of increase picked up a little but remained considerably lower than before. The annual rate of increase in the charge for a semiprivate room was 41 percent of the annual rate of increase during the fiscal years 1969–1971, the rate of increase for operating room charges was 66 percent, and the rate of increase for physicians' fees was 32 percent. In fact, the increase in physicians' fees under Phase II—2.4 percent per annum—corresponds closely to the 2.5 percent permitted under the law. However, these findings are based on the prices reported in the consumer price index and need to be taken with some skepticism, since it may be possible to manipulate pricing procedures to conceal increases in expenditures for a standard package of services.

Manipulation can be checked by examining the revenue of hospitals and the income of physicians. Data on expenses per hospital day, with and without adjustment for the mix of outpatient and in-patient services, are reported by the American Hospital Association. These indices of hospital prices show that while Phase II was effective in moderating the increase in hospital costs, it was less effective than the price index data seemed to suggest (181, Table 2, p. 12). Net income of self-employed physicians in proprietorships and partnerships is reported yearly by the Internal Revenue Service. The income that is cited includes revenue from self-employed practice only, excluding salary and other sources of income. For this reason, and because income tends to be under-reported, the data are an underestimate of true income. And of course, income depends not only on price but also on the services produced by the physician. Nevertheless, it is interesting to note that during 1967, the first full year after Medicare, the net income of physicians increased at an annual rate of almost 14 percent, whereas during 1971, the year the price freeze was introduced in November, there was a decrease of over 2 percent. If these figures are taken at face value, one must conclude, at least provisionally, that price controls had a dampening effect not only on prices but also on gross revenue to hospitals and on the net income of physicians, with a heavier impact on the latter. It is likely, however, that the effect on the net revenue of physicians has not been as large as it seems. This is because, in recent years, physicians with higher income have tended to incorporate, with the result that the average income of the remaining self-employed physicians is necessarily lower (198, p. 55).

An approach to price containment that is more traditional and, in part, more acceptable to physicians, is to use a different method of reimbursement than one based on customary and prevailing charges. Fee schedules are a reasonable compromise, since they permit fee-for-service practice, but also make it possible to moderate inflation through the negotiation of allowable charges by representatives of the insurance program and the profession. The staff to the Committee on Finance, in reviewing experience under Medicare and Medicaid, has in fact recommended a return to the use of scheduled fees; additional limitations would be set on costs so that, in effect, fees would be reduced as total expenditures increased. This would be accomplished by reducing scheduled fees sufficiently to offset any excess in expenditures over the revenue generated by a monthly premium rate fixed by law (193, pp. 67–69).

Payment by capitation and by salary would represent a greater departure from precedent in the U.S. A description of alternative methods of reimbursement and an evaluation of their several features would open up a large new area of inquiry which we cannot now undertake, unfortunately. We must, therefore, be content with emphasizing the need to design the system of reimbursement with extreme care, if prices are to be controlled and other objectives attained.

Service Benefits or Cash. So far, our discussion of what social action might be taken in response to the inflationary effect of third party payments has dealt with methods to control or contain prices. Another social response is to provide some protection to the consumer against inflation in the interim between changes in premium. Within this rather narrow context, it has been traditional to compare service benefits with cash indemnity benefits, and to express a preference for the former. However, the comparison of service and cash indemnity benefits involves a variety of additional considerations which might be usefully explored at this point, even though this will mean some digression from our more immediate concern with prices (199). We propose to compare the relative merits of the two alternatives first from the vantage point of the consumer, then of the insurance program, and finally, of the provider. In this way we hope to gain some appreciation of the remarkable complexity of the situation and to illustrate an approach to evaluation that we will develop more fully in a subsequent chapter.

Service benefits are specified in terms of the units of service to which a beneficiary is entitled, with or without stipulated limits on quantity. Examples of service units are visits to a physician, days of hospital care, specified procedures, and quantities of ancillary hospital services. Cash indemnity benefits are specified as dollar amounts which are paid to the consumer or, with his permission, to the provider, as payment for covered services. Traditionally, service benefits have been the hallmark of Blue Cross and Blue Shield, whereas cash benefits have been the distinctive characteristic of "commercial" health insurance. Consequently, certain additional attributes have become associated with each of the two approaches, so that the two constellations have almost come to represent two opposite ideologies, each with its own mystique. Plans that are committed to service benefits have emphasized the need for complete or near complete coverage of the specified services, without the fiscal barriers of deductibles or coinsurance, or the unpredictable penalty of additional charges levied at the discretion of the physician beyond the fees the third party will honor. Plans that offer cash indemnity benefits, on the other hand, have made much of the need to incorporate deterrents to "moral hazard" and inducements to responsible behavior in the form of deductibles and coinsurance, or through cash payments that are less than the full charge for care. However, faced with the realities of the market, both sides have been willing to offer policies whose attributes fall between the two extremes, so that the distinctions between the two types have become blurred. Benefits under Medicare are an excellent example of a hybrid form that combines service benefits with limits on the amount of service per episode, deductible and coinsurance payments, and less than complete coverage of the physician's bill for insured services when the physician refuses assignment.

Viewed from the vantage point of the consumer, the distinction between the two forms of insurance rests primarily on the degree of protection each offers. At any given time, this is not a function of the difference between service benefits and cash benefits, but of the degree of coverage. If cash benefits are sufficiently large to meet charges, they can be as fully protective as the corresponding service benefits. However, because of the associated characteristics that we have already described, plans that offer service benefits tend to afford a greater degree of protection. In the interim between adjustments of premium, during a period of rising prices, service benefits are distinctly more advantageous to the consumer, since the insurance plan has undertaken to pay for covered services irrespective of price. Needless to say, this obligation is also a spur to upward revision in premiums, which can be a burden to the extent that the beneficiary pays the premium, but which also maintains protection against unexpected medical care costs in the future. By contrast, cash benefits can be rapidly eroded by inflation without creating pressure on the insurance plan to raise premiums, so that the amount of cash indemnity falls progressively behind the financial obligations likely to be incurred by the consumer in the event of illness. Service benefits are, therefore, an excellent hedge against inflation, although the protection they afford can be considerably diluted by deductibles, coinsurance, and other additional charges.

From the vantage point of the program that underwrites benefits, perhaps the major concern is the maintenance of its own financial solvency and integrity. This creates a paradox, because offering protection against inflation to the consumer necessarily means exposing the plan to that same hazard. And this is a hazard of a distinctive kind, which cannot be controlled through the usual underwriting procedures that help define the risks of contracting illness and using service. When specified cash indemnities are paid for a given service, the plan has only to predict how much service will be used. However, if the insurer undertakes to pay a percentage of the charges incurred, the uncertainty created by rising prices remains a hazard. This hazard is greatest when service benefits are offered, since the plan must predict accurately not only use of services by enrollees, but also the price, which it is obligated to pay.

A succession of further developments may be seen to flow from this situation. The plans that have used cash benefits can, as we have said, eliminate the hazard of inflation to themselves by paying specified cash amounts, effectively transferring the full impact of inflation to the consumer. Another solution, much in evidence in group contracts, is to operate on an essentially cost-plus basis, so that premiums are adjusted to the group's experience in the preceding year. This also transfers the effect of inflation to the consumer, but offers protection against unexpected expenditures between renewals of enrollment. Finally, the cash benefit plan, by paying only a proportion of the charges for care, shares the risk with the consumer.

As we have pointed out, these, or analogous, remedies are also available to plans that provide service benefits, but if they are adopted, they represent a departure from the tradition and ideology characteristic of these plans. The distinctive line of development dictated by the commitment to service benefits is to enter into arrangements with the providers of service with a view to defining the bases for reimbursement and, in that way, achieving some degree of control over prices. Thus, service benefit plans are necessarily more intimately involved with the providers of service and with the way they are organized to provide care. No wonder, then, that service benefits have been a distinctive feature of plans that are sponsored, and largely controlled by, hospitals (Blue Cross) or physicians (Blue Shield). Provider sponsorship has been necessary to make procedures that are, in fact, an infringement on free enterprise, seem acceptable and legitimate. Thus, the insurance plan may have to negotiate and institute fee schedules, and enter into agreements that bar additional charges for covered services. Uniform procedures have been developed to establish the allowable costs of care in institutions. When this has been accomplished, it is still necessary to agree on what is a reasonable margin of revenue over costs, and it may be necessary to negotiate a discounted price in recognition of what amounts to a wholesale purchase of service by the plan on behalf of its enrollees. Such activities, which in effect involve price-fixing and discriminatory advantages to the provider-sponsored plan, have required special legislative dispensation. This dispensation has not, however, prevented a perennial sprinkling of challenges in the courts.

But these challenges are only a minor nuisance compared to the more serious tensions that develop between a plan intent on reducing cost and uncertainty to itself, and professional or institutional providers equally intent on protecting their income and their autonomy. The tension is heightened when, as is not infrequently the case, the plan has to accommodate to the rival claims of providers who demand special treatment in recognition of their superior quality, their greater contributions to medical education, or for other reasons. Thus, the commitment to provide service benefits is often associated with the need to become both involved and embroiled in the affairs of the providers, an eventuality that those who pay cash benefits have been anxious to avoid.

Another disadvantage of service benefits may be seen to flow from the need to have frequent increases in the premium if service benefits are to be maintained in the face of inflation. This is likely to damage the competitive position of the plans unless the purchaser can look beyond the immediate price to the protection that is purchased. When revisions in premium require public hearings prior to approval by the insurance commissioner of a state, as is often the case for provider-sponsored plans, the general discontent is heightened by adverse publicity.

There are, however, considerable advantages to the marriage of provider-sponsorship with service benefits. At the broadest level, the provider-sponsored plans could use the considerable leverage that they have through the mass purchase of services to bring about socially desirable changes in the organization of health services. More realistically, the peculiar relationship with providers allows these plans to play some role in regulating prices and moderating inflation. The plan could also persuade the providers to accept prorated reductions in payments should the obligations incurred by the plan exceed its resources. Thus, if worse should come to worst, the immediate hazard of inflation is passed on to the providers, rather than the consumers. Finally, service benefits usually imply direct payments to the provider, rather than the consumer, a feature that can considerably reduce the number of individual transactions and reduce administrative costs accordingly. But the plans that pay cash benefits accomplish the same end if the patient signs a release that permits the provider to collect directly from the plan, a procedure that providers are likely to demand.

From the vantage point of the provider, cash benefits offer the least interference with autonomy and traditional modes of practice. However, if cash benefits are paid to the patient rather than to the provider, and particularly if the cash indemnity is significantly lower than the provider's bill, it may be difficult to collect from the patient. Thus, the provider loses the assurance of being paid, which is such a comforting feature of service benefits. For that reason providers, individually or collectively, may prefer to put up with the restrictions associated with service benefits provided the fees are reasonably adequate. For the same reason, they appear willing to enter into agreements to accept prorated reductions in charges should circumstances require it, especially since improvements in actuarial and underwriting procedures have rendered such an eventuality rather remote. On the other hand, it is possible for providers to assure collection of fees under cash benefits by requiring the patient to assign such benefits to the provider.

If, in addition, cash benefits are generous, there remains little reason for providers to prefer service benefits over their counterpart in cash.

It follows from this analysis that service benefits and cash benefits can be viewed differently by the several participants in the transaction: the consumers, the providers, and the "third party." It can also be inferred that the comparison is often not between service benefits and cash benefits as ideal types, but between alternatives that combine features of both. Hence, in evaluating the form of benefits in any plan it is necessary to probe beyond the mere identification of whether benefits are in service or in cash. We need to examine the benefits in detail, using criteria such as the ones we have considered above: protection of the consumer against unexpected expenses, the presence of barriers to seeking or receiving needed care, protection of the fiscal integrity of the insuring agency, ease of implementation and administration, acceptability to providers, and so on.

Redistribution

General Considerations

We have seen that the provision of benefits can have a profound effect on the volume of services used, on the differential use of some services in comparison to others, and on price. The provision of benefits can also bring about a redistribution in the command over resources; this redistribution may be intended and desired, or it may be fortuitous and, sometimes, contrary to public policy. Under prepayment, there is always a transfer of resources from the well to the ill. There may be, in addition, transfers among population subgroups characterized by age, sex, social class, and geographic area or jurisdiction of residence. Resources may even be transferred between generations, as when those who use services now place a burden of debt on those in the future. The providers of care are themselves involved in these transfers by being favored to varying degrees by different programs.

The degree and direction of redistribution are determined by who pays and how much he pays, by who receives the benefits and in what quantities, and by who gets paid and how much he is paid. The answer to the question "Who pays and how much?" depends, quite obviously, on the details of financing. To the extent that a program is publicly financed, it must draw on tax revenue. Since different taxes have different effects on redistribution, it is necessary to know precisely what taxes are used and what proportion of revenue is generated by each. This is the first step in the tedious, and sometimes inconclusive, process of tracing the consequences of each tax. Next, it is necessary to know the tax base and the rate structure (200). The base is the object that is taxed; for example, personal or corporate income, payroll, property, the manufacture of some commodities, the sale of most, and the importation of others. The rate defines the manner in which the tax that is imposed and collected relates to the value or the physical quantity of the base. The relationship may be a fixed percentage of the base, in which case the tax is "proportionate." Alternatively, as the value of the base increases, the tax may become an increasing or decreasing percentage of the base, in which case the tax is, respectively, "progressive" or "regressive." Knowledge of the tax base provides the first intimation of who pays the tax. However, this immediate impression may be erroneous, since it is often possible for the person, or category of persons, who ostensibly pay the tax to shift its burden to someone else. The tax on a commodity is shifted forward when the burden is borne, fully or in part, by the consumer. It is shifted backward to the extent that the burden is borne by the producer.

It is, therefore, necessary to fix the incidence of each tax: which is where the burden ultimately falls (200). Unfortunately, the direction of the shift and the amount of the burden that can be shifted depend on so many attributes of so many markets, that the precise incidence of any given tax can remain open to considerable debate and conjecture. For example, the payroll tax, which plays such a large role in financing the social security system that includes Medicare, is ostensibly paid by the employer. However, only part of the burden may fall, in the form of reduced profits, on those who own the enterprise. Some or all of the burden may be passed on to the worker as lower wages, and to the consumer as higher prices. But the distribution of the burden among owners, workers, and consumers varies from firm to firm, and it depends, among other things, on how well organized the workers are; whether the production process is susceptible to the substitution of machinery for labor; whether prices can be raised without reducing demand; and whether it is possible to reduce quality without reducing price (201, p. 162).

Knowing about the base of a tax is the first step towards finding where the tax finally comes to rest. Knowing about its rate structure leads us to a judgment concerning its fairness. Both are germane to a determination of its redistributive effects. The fairness of a tax and the appropriateness of its redistributive effects are judgments that derive not from economists but from social values

(200, p. 54). The "benefit principle" in tax equity demands that the advantages that flow from the use of revenue from a tax (or from taxes collectively) be enjoyed by those who finally pay the tax in a manner that is proportionate to their contribution to the tax. The "ability-to-pay principle," on the other hand, requires that the tax burden be distributed in accordance with income, or some other measure of the ability to pay, so that those with equal ability are required to pay equal taxes (which is "horizontal equity"), and those with greater ability are required to pay more than those with less (which is "vertical equity"). It is clear that in order to achieve vertical equity, the contribution to the tax must be at least proportionate to the ability to pay. A society may, however, decide that it is more fair to require proportionately more as the ability to pay increases. Thus the notion of proportionate, progressive, and regressive taxation applies both to the relationship between the tax rate and its base, and to the relationship between the incidence of the tax burden and the ability to pay. These dual connotations may give rise to some confusion; for example, a proportionate tax on the purchase of food is regressive with respect to ability to pay, since the poor spend a larger proportion of their more limited resources on food. It is also necessary to note that the benefit principle and the ability-to-pay principle are often in direct contradiction. The former tends to gear benefits to effort or achievement, and is "libertarian" in orientation. The latter is a means of distributing benefits in a manner more congruent with need and is, therefore, "egalitarian" in spirit (1, pp. 1–12). It is possible, knowingly or unwittingly, to design taxation so that the poor pay a greater share than is warranted by their income, and to arrange access to benefits so that the poor receive less than is called for by their need, thus combining the worst of both worlds.

It is clear that an understanding of the tax structure that generates revenue for government services in general, and for medical care programs in particular, is essential to any estimation of the redistributive effects of these programs and services, separately as well as collectively. But taxation also impinges on what seems, at first glance, to be the private financing of non-governmental health services. As we shall see in a subsequent section, "voluntary" health insurance in the U.S. is largely financed by contributions made by the employer. Since these are considered to be a cost of doing business, they constitute a tax-exempt deduction from employer income. This exemption amounts to governmental subsidy of insurance coverage in the private sector. The subsidy is further augmented by allowing individuals to deduct from taxable personal income a share of their medical expenditures, including payments for health insurance premiums up to a specified limit. Since a loss in tax revenue from one source must be made up in some way, this indirect subsidy involves the imposition of a compensatory tax burden which may be distributed in a manner different from the distribution of the subsidy. Thus, government intervenes to bring about at least the potential for redistribution in the private financing of health insurance.

The private insurance sector also has the potential for shifting the burden of paying the premiums for benefits. It is generally conceded that the unsubsidized expenditures made by individuals or families are borne by them alone. However, contributions made by employers under collective bargaining, or other private arrangements, can be shifted in the same way as the payroll tax. Deductible and coinsurance payments under private insurance offer another parallel to taxation. It does not stretch the imagination to see the deductible as a flat tax and the coinsurance as a proportionate tax on the use of health services. Thus, deductibles and copayments raise the same issues of horizontal and vertical equity as are raised by taxation. Needless to say, deductibles and copayments are also important because they must figure in the determination of who pays for care and how much is paid.

The answer to the difficult question "Who pays?" is only part of the information necessary to determine the presence and magnitude of distribution. The next object of inquiry is to determine who receives the benefits and how much is received (202). The answer depends on the nature of the benefits, who is eligible to receive them, and how much behavior changes in response to the availability of benefits. The nature of the benefit and the characteristics of the eligible are, to some extent, interdependent. For example, maternity benefits and preventive immunizations are designed to favor young women and children, respectively; nursing home benefits are designed to cater to the aged, in general, and to very old women, in particular. But benefits can also be channeled by more direct specification of eligibility. For example, Medicare is designed for the old, Workmen's Compensation and a great deal of voluntary health insurance is directed at the labor force, and public assistance medical care serves those who are destitute, or close to it. The specification of benefits and of eligibility are elements of program design which explicitly signify the intent of public policy to favor specified groups. But an element of uncertainty, which may result in unforeseen and unintended consequences, enters the picture because of the way persons behave when benefits become available. After all, it is those who seek and use the services who actually realize and enjoy the benefits of medical care programs. In this way, benefits that seem to be equally available to all may actually result in a redistribution in favor of the rich if they use relatively more service than the poor. As we shall see when we describe certain empirical studies, there are additional systemic repercussions to the introduction of a medical care program; these repercussions alter the state of affairs so as to influence not only the distribution of benefits but also the incidence of costs (203, pp. 81–102).

The professional providers of service occupy a distinctive position in the calculus of redistribution. As consumers, they take their place among those who bear the burden and receive the benefits of health programs, although their expenditures for medical care are modified by considerations of profesional courtesy and reciprocity, the implications of which have remained unexplored. For example, assuming that physicians do not ordinarily pay the full charge for the services of a colleague when they are uninsured, but do so when covered by insurance, the incremental value of insurance is lower for them than for non-physicians who pay the same premium. But more important than this is the income that providers derive as producers of services. Since these services are benefits that are assigned to the consumer, they cannot figure yet another time as benefits to the provider. However, to the extent that, as a result of increasing demand, a physician can raise his prices at a more rapid rate than is justified by his costs and by his contribution in taxes, a form of redistribution may be said to have occurred (203, pp. 105–106). Still another kind of redistribution may take place when a medical program, through the selectivity of its benefits, its methods of reimbursement, or other means, favors one category of providers more than another, so that an alteration is made in the proportionate distribution of medical care expenditures among providers.

Empirical Observations

A fair amount of material that has a bearing on redistribution has already been described and discussed in previous sections of this work. We have seen, for example, in what direction and to what extent use of service is altered by the provision of prepaid benefits, by the nature of the benefit package, and by the imposition of deductibles and copayments. It is clear that the provision of benefits under voluntary or statutory prepayment brings about far reaching changes in the incidence of consumption. But so far we have not had corresponding information on the incidence of financial contributions towards the benefits received, which would allow us to compare contributions and returns across categories of persons. It is these comparisons that now claim our attention, and lead us to an examination of three major instrumentalities: Medicare, Medicaid, and voluntary health insurance.

Medicare and Medicaid

For a study of the redistributive effects of Medicare and Medicaid, we turn to the pioneering work of Stuart and Bair at the Michigan Department of Social Services (203). Their study provides data for Michigan and for the United States for each of two fiscal years: 1966/67 and 1967/68. We shall focus our attention on the second of the two years, and consider only the redistributive effects nation-wide. The basic unit involved in redistribution is the household, because it pays the costs and receives the benefits. The definition of a "household" is that used by the Bureau of Labor Statistics in its Survey of Consumer Expenditures for 1960 and 1961: "(1) a group of people usually living together who pooled their income and drew from a common fund for their major items of expense, or (2) a person living alone or in a household with others but who is financially independent, i.e. his income and expenditures were not pooled" (203, pp. 26–27). The authors' object was to trace the balance of exchanges among groupings of households. The groups chosen for this purpose were: (1) households of Medicare eligibles; (2) households of Medicaid recipients; (3) non-recipient households; (4) households of physicians;

(5) households in each of four income groups; and (6) households in each state plus the District of Columbia.

Needless to say, the population of the United States is not neatly packaged for the investigator's convenience. To achieve the partitioning, the authors laboriously assembled information from several sources and pieced it together, using a variety of approximations and assumptions, which no doubt imparted a certain roughness to the final results (203, pp. 67–73). Certain additional features of the classification deserve some comment. It should be noted that the first category includes all who were eligible for benefits under Medicare, defined as all persons 65 or over, whereas the second category only includes those who were reported to have actually received services "free or at reduced cost" under the Medicaid program during each fiscal year. Aged persons who are eligible for Medicare, but also receive services under Medicaid, appear under each of the first two categories, but are counted only once when the two are combined to represent the joint class of "recipients." The category of nonrecipients is a residual one, since it comprises all those who are not identified as either eligible for Medicare or having received benefits under Medicaid. The category of physician households is constructed on the assumption that each household contains only one physician; it includes only active physicians who are not in training, and it is further divided to distinguish the subgroup of households with a physician who has at least some private practice.

The categories of households having been identified and the number in each category estimated, the next task is to estimate how much each category contributes towards the costs of Medicare and Medicaid and how much each receives in benefits under these programs. This can be done under two different sets of assumptions, corresponding to somewhat different purposes and interpretations. The first is to compare only direct benefits and costs. This shows the "gross effects" of each program. The second is to estimate the incremental benefits and costs of each program, taking into account not only direct benefits and costs, but also the additional gains and losses which have resulted from major changes that can be attributed to the institution of Medicare and Medicaid. This second approach reveals the "net effects" of the program. In either approach, the direct benefits are the vendor payments made by each program, and the costs are payments that the households make toward each program through taxes or premiums. In estimating the net effects, additions and substractions are made on both the benefit and cost sides for each of the three categories of households: recipients, nonrecipients, and physicians. The credits and debits are the results of changes brought about by Medicare and Medicaid, including: (1) the discontinuation of medical assistance programs in states that adopted Medicaid; (2) a greater tendency by aged veterans to use community hospitals in preference to Veterans Administration facilities; (3) the increase in medical care prices that is not explained by changes in the remainder of the consumer price index; (4) increased labor costs in the production of physician and hospital services; (5) reduced charity care and fewer bad debts incurred by physicians; (6) changes in the income tax law that effectively increased the tax liability of the aged; and (7) a multiplicity of adjustments in tax payments that are a consequence of the preceding factors. It is clear that each of these changes can figure differently in the credit and debit columns of the accounts of the several categories of households. For example, the end of the pre-Medicaid medical assistance programs is a loss to many Medicaid and some Medicare recipients, but it is a gain, in the form of tax relief, to some groups, particularly nonrecipients. The reduction in charity care and the rise in prices is a loss to the recipient category, although the loss is somewhat mitigated by tax deductions for medical expenses. The same changes are a gain for physician households, though the advantage is somewhat reduced by the increased labor costs of providing care and by higher income tax payments. The higher income tax payments by physicians mean, in turn, that others will pay relatively less in taxes. In this manner, each change sets in motion a new chain of events, until the entire complex machinery has come to rest in a new configuration of benefits and costs for each group of households. It is the difference between this configuration and the pattern that was prevalent prior to Medicare and Medicaid that represents the net impact of these two programs.

Of the many items of information necessary to estimate the gross and net effects of Medicare and Medicaid, the most important are the estimates of direct benefits and costs. Data on benefits, which are equivalent to vendor payments, are obtained from program reports and "include all administrative expenses of the two programs" (203, p. 74). It is assumed that the benefits from the consumption of medical care services remain within the households that consume them. For that reason, hospital benefits under Medicare are allocated to each income class in a manner proportionate to the number of persons aged 65 or over in that class, based on the expectation that patient-days of hospital care are equal across classes. The benefits of Part B of Medicare, which covers the services of physicians, are also considered to be distributed equally by income class, after allowing for the percent of aged persons in each class who elect to participate in Part B through premium payments, and for the 50 percent of the aged in the lowest income class for whom Part B coverage is assumed to be purchased by Medicaid (203, pp. 108–109).

Medicaid benefits are also assumed to be equal for all recipient households irrespective of income. Under this assumption, all that is necessary is to estimate the number of recipient households in each income class and in each state. This is done by first assuming that the potentially eligible households from which Medicaid recipients are drawn are: "(1) all families and unattached individuals earning less that $3,000 per year; (2) all families of four or more members earning between $3,000 and $5,000 per year; and (3) all families of six or more members earning between $5,000 and $7,500 per year" (203, p. 219). Given the reported number of Medicaid recipients, and assumptions about the household size of the recipients (203, pp. 70–72), it is possible to estimate what proportion of all potentially eligible households actually received Medicaid benefits during a given year. Assuming this proportion to be equal for each of the three categories of potentially eligible households, the recipient households are distributed among the three income classes (203, p. 116). The distribution of Medicaid recipients by state is accomplished using a similar procedure, except that the differing eligibility requirements of the states are taken into account in distributing recipient households among the three categories of potentially eligible households (203, p. 219).

The estimation and allocation of direct costs is more difficult, because program funds come from many sources, through routes that are made devious by "shifting." The portion of Medicare that pays primarily for hospital care is financed by the social security tax that is levied on the payrolls of employers, the wages and salaries of employees, and the earnings of the self-employed. A specified percentage of each of these, up to a limit, is earmarked for Medicare. The component of Medicare that pays for the services of physicians, as well as some other services, is financed in equal parts by the federal general fund and by premium payments made by those who are insured. Both parts of Medicare receive contributions from Medicaid funds, because the states are required to pay the deductible and coinsurance that are incurred under Part A of Medicare by their indigent aged, and are also allowed to enroll them in Part B by paying the premium on their behalf. Medicaid funds are themselves derived from a combination of federal and state funds. The federal contribution is designed to subsidize more heavily states that are less able to care for their own poor. Based on their per-capita income, states derive anywhere from 50 to 83 percent of Medicaid expenditures from the federal general fund. The states finance their own share of Medicaid expenditures in a great variety of ways. For the purposes of their study, Stuart and Bair assume that the contribution of local units of government comes from property taxes and the rest of the expenditure from each state's general fund. The overlap between Medicare and Medicaid, which comes about because Medicaid funds are used to finance benefits for the indigent aged under Medicare, is handled by including these expenditures under Medicare as well as under Medicaid when the two programs are considered separately. When the two programs are combined, the Medicaid contribution to Medicare is counted only once.

The manner of financing each program having been determined, the next step is to allocate to each group of households its contribution to the financing of each program. Premium payments by self-supporting households are considered to be borne by themselves alone. Since all remaining program funds come from taxes, it is necessary to determine: (1) which specific taxes are involved; (2) what is the incidence of each tax; (3) how much each group of households used in the analysis contributes towards each tax, and (4) how much each tax contributes to program funds. As we have already determined, the relevant taxes are the federal social security tax, the local property tax, and the taxes that garner the general funds of the federal and state governments. The major components of the general funds are taxes: on wages and salaries; on dividends; on corporate earnings; on estates and gifts; on retail sales; and on specific commodities and services such as alcohol, tobacco, automobiles, motor fuel, utilities, telephone and telegraph services, and on group and other life insurance. Accurate information is available on the amount of each of these taxes and others collected by each level of government. The problem is to determine the incidence of each tax and, taking incidence into account, how much of each tax is contributed by each category of households (203, pp. 205–221).

Needless to say, there is no complete agreement on the incidence of the taxes in question. Stuart and Bair used "only the most commonly accepted hypotheses relating to tax incidence within a short-run partial equilibrium framework . . ." (203, p. 206). Their major assumptions are : (1) the employer's contribution to the social security tax is shifted, so that it is borne in equal amounts by the worker, as lower wages, and by the consumer as a rise in prices; (2) personal income and property taxes fall on those who pay them; (3) gift and estate taxes are paid entirely by households with an annual income over $15,000; (4) taxes on corporate profits are borne equally by consumers and stockholders; and (5) general sales taxes and taxes on specific commodities and services are borne by the consumers of the commodities and services in question (203, pp. 206–207). Another kind of tax shift occurs because states are able to pass on some of the burden of their taxes to other states. To correct for this, it is assumed that the burden of state corporate income taxes and state severance taxes is distributed among all the states: one half of the burden being allocated on the basis of dividend income, and the other half on the basis of retail sales, reported by each state. The burdens of all other state and local taxes are assumed to remain within each state (203, pp. 254–259).

Given information on the total revenue from each tax and an assumption concerning its incidence, we can now estimate the contribution of each category of households to the tax. This means that the fraction of tax revenue that is specified by the assumed incidence is to be further partitioned among the several categories of households. This is done by assuming that the tax revenue in question is collected in proportion to the distribution, among the categories of households, of a "tax allocation base," which is the thing taxed or some proxy for it. For example, half of the corporate income tax is distributed in proportion to total consumption and the other half in proportion to dividend earnings attributable to each category of households. The excise on cars is attributed in proportion to the purchase of cars, the excise on alcoholic beverages in proportion to personal income, and the tobacco excise in proportion to population.

In order to arrive at these allocations it is necessary to have information concerning the relevant attributes of primary population modules; from this information the same attributes may be inferred for the categories of households used in the study. The basic modules are groups of households that are characterized by the age of the head of the household (below 65, or 65 and over), family size and composition, income class, and state of residence. A survey conducted by the Bureau of Labor Statistics gives data for 1960–61 on expenditures for specified goods and services for households categorized in this manner, except that residence is classified by four regions rather than by state. The classification of households by state is available on a current basis, but without data on consumption.

A combination of these two sets of data—consumption expenditures and household characteristics—can yield the information needed to characterize the categories of households used in the study by Stuart and Bair, and to allocate the tax burden accordingly. However, this requires assumptions and approximations that, added to the ones we have already described, further compromise the accuracy of the findings. These assumptions are as follows: (1) The relative positions of the several population modules with respect to consumption has not changed between 1960–61 and the two years of the study, fiscal 1967 and 1968. This means that only a correction for price is necessary. (2) The levels and patterns of consumption, by a population module within a state are those of the region within which a state is located; this, no doubt, has the effect of reducing variability among the states; but it is not known to what extent. (3) The consumption patterns of Medicare households are the same as those in households headed by a person 65 and over, as reported in the survey of consumer expenditures. (4) The consumption of Medicaid recipients in each state is the same as that of all households of the same type and income in the region. Finally, (5) households of physicians are assumed to have the same consumption patterns as those of all households with an annual income of $15,000 and over in the 1960–61 survey.

Having derived the attributes of the categories of households used in this study, we can now determine the contributions of each category to each tax in the manner already described. Briefly, this requires: (1) an assumption concerning the incidence of each tax, and (2) the choice of a household attribute (the tax allocation base) in proportion to which each tax is distributed among the categories of households. All that remains is to convert the estimates of the contributions of each category to the several taxes into a corresponding statement about their contributions to program costs. For this purpose, it is assumed that "each family or group of families contributes to program costs in proportion to its payment towards each contributing tax," and that "program expenditures from general funds are financed from each contributory tax in direct proportion to the relative importance of that tax to total general funds" (203, p. 35). In other words, the proportionate contribution of a group of households to a given program is the product of two fractions: the fraction of each tax that is contributed by that group and the fraction of program funds that is contributed by that tax. In this tortuous manner, subject to all the inaccuracies in the primary data as well as those introduced by the many assumptions necessary to adapt the data to their needs, Stuart and Bair arrived at an estimate of the transfers among groups of households.

The direction and magnitude of transfers can be expressed in a variety of ways (203, pp. 36–38). Stuart and Bair use three measures of redistribution: the benefit-to-burden ratio, the net dollar grant, and the net dollar grant per household. The benefit-to-burden ratio is, obviously, the ratio of the benefits received by each category to the program costs borne by that category. The net grant is the algebraic value of benefits minus costs. When the benefit-to-burden ratio is 1.0, the net grant is zero. When the benefit-to-burden ratio for a given category is above 1.0, that category has a net grant gain. On the contrary, there is a net loss when the benefit-to-burden ratio is below 1.0. The benefit-to-burden ratios for two categories can be directly compared as an indication of the relative advantages they enjoy under a given program. For example, households in a category with a benefit-to-burden ratio of 2.5 receive a rate of return from the program twice as high as that received by households in a category with a benefit-to-burden ratio of 1.25 (203, pp. 37–38).

We are, at last, ready to take a look at the findings. We shall examine, first, gross and net transfers among households of recipients, nonrecipients, and physicians; then, gross transfers among households in four income classes; and, finally, gross transfers among the states, with attention to household income. Gross transfers result from the total costs and benefits of Medicare and Medicaid, whereas net transfers restrict themselves to the additional benefits and costs of these programs and take into account the secondary effects of these programs on the medical care system. Table 40 shows gross and net transfers among households of recipients, nonrecipients, and physicians. It is clear that both Medicaid and Medicare involve considerable transfers of funds to households who, respectively, receive the benefits of the former and are eligible for the benefits of the latter. As to gross transfers in fiscal 1967/68, each household that received Medicaid services obtained, on the average, the equivalent of $896 in excess of its own contribution to Medicaid. Each household that was entitled

TABLE 40. Benefit/Cost Ratios and Net Grants per Household under Medicare and Medicaid for Households of Recipients, Nonrecipients and Physicians, U.S.A., Fiscal Year 1967/68

Categories of Households	Gross Transfers		Net Transfers	
	Benefit/ Cost Ratio	Net Benefit Grant per Household [a]	Benefit/ Cost Ratio	Net Benefit Grant per Household [a]
Medicaid recipients	34.78	$896.30	3.16	$ 637.61
Medicare eligibles	3.23	244.21	1.82	175.51
Total "recipients" [b]	4.99	401.67	2.16	287.29
Nonrecipients	0.00	−160.16	0.44	−114.56
Physicians in private practice	0.00	−405.30	3.97	3,923.20

Source: Reference 203, Table 5D, page 78 and Table 5H, page 104.
[a] Benefits minus costs per household.
[b] Medicaid recipients plus Medicare eligibles.

290 Benefits in Medical Care Programs

to benefits under Medicare received an average of $244 in excess of its contribution to that program. The rate of return per dollar contributed was $3.23 for each household eligible for Medicare, and an impressive $34.78 for each household that received Medicaid. The benefits-to-costs ratio and the net benefit grant per household are larger for Medicaid than for Medicare partly because Medicare beneficiaries make direct current contributions in the form of premiums, they probably bear a larger current tax burden because of their higher average income, and they include eligibles who have not received service during a given year. The net transfers are somewhat more modest because they only include benefits *additional* to those formerly available, mainly under public assistance programs, to households who subsequently became beneficiaries of Medicare and Medicaid; and because they include adjustments to the impact of Medicare and Medicaid, chief among which is the rise in medical care prices. Nevertheless, Medicare and Medicaid represent a considerable improvement in the ability of the aged and the sick poor to command health care. Naturally, the advantage enjoyed by these segments of the population is at the expense of the nonrecipients who must foot the bill. In 1967/68, nonrecipient households contributed an average of $160 towards the costs of Medicare and Medicaid, of which $115 was a new burden attributable directly and indirectly to the institution of these programs. This transfer of funds from nonrecipients to recipients during any given year is, of course, a universal feature of all prepaid programs, so that what we learn from these findings is the magnitude of the transfers rather than their direction, the latter being predictable on a priori grounds. We should note, however, that the transfers we have described are essentially contemporaneous. This is an important limitation to the analysis since, especially in the Medicare program, beneficiaries have contributed over a lifetime to receive benefits during a relatively short period of eligibility.

There is a subset of nonrecipients who are the object of much curious attention. This subset is the households of physicians. Because of their relatively high income, these households are heavily taxed to finance benefits to others under Medicare and Medicaid. Each physician household contributes a yearly sum of $405, which is 2.5 times the average contributed by all nonrecipient households. But, in spite of this, the net effect of Medicare and Medicaid has been to add almost $4,000 to the income of the average physician household. For each dollar contributed towards the costs of Medicare and Medicaid, each physician household enjoys a return of $3.97, which is more than twice as high as the return per dollar garnered by those eligible for Medicare, and 25 percent higher than the return even for recipients of Medicaid. This increment to the net income of physicians does not include the yield from additional services provided by the physician. The increment is mainly that portion of additional income which is unexplained by the larger number of visits provided by each physician and by the inflation in general prices during the post-Medicare period. About a third of this increment is attributable to improved collections, because of less charity care or for other reasons, and the remainder is due to the unexplained rise in medical care prices. One could question the accuracy of these estimates. In particular, it is not clear whether the count of visits included the greater amount of hospital care provided by physicians. One can also argue that an improvement in collections is not a gift to the physician, since this is payment for work done. But even under these provisos, it is difficult to escape the conclusion that physicians may have been the chief beneficiaries of Medicare and Medicaid. If so, one can symphathize with the rather bitter conclusion of Stuart and Bair that "it is difficult to defend a policy which provides, at public expense, the greatest gains to one of the highest paid professions in the nation" (203, p. 106).

The key findings concerning gross transfers by income class are presented in Table 41. The transfers shown are the resultant of two opposing tendencies: one regressive, and the other progressive. The distribution of costs is regressive in the sense that costs, as percent of disposable income per household, become smaller as income increases. On the other hand, benefits as a percent of disposable income per household decreases even more rapidly with income. The result is an essentially progressive distribution of benefits, net of costs. This means that households in the higher income classes receive less than they contribute, whereas households in the lower income classes receive more than they pay to the program. The dividing line for Medicare, as well as Medicaid, is within the income class $5,000–9,999. Medicare and Medicaid,

TABLE 41.   Specified Measures of the Redistribution of Gross Benefits and Costs of Medicare and Medicaid by Income Class and Region, U.S.A., Fiscal 1967/68

Disposable Income Class of Households (dollars)	Medicare and Medicaid	Medicare	Medicaid		
			Total	North East Region	South Region
Benefits Minus Costs per Household (in Dollars)					
0– 2,999	368.64	173.37	195.27	504.41	51.80
3,000– 4,999	107.44	69.02	38.42	68.73	8.97
5,000– 9,999	− 59.23	− 35.67	− 23.56	− 31.78	− 17.18
10,000–14,999	−160.31	− 83.30	− 77.01	−109.88	− 50.35
15,000 and over	−363.45	−152.31	−211.14	−314.96	−153.83
Benefits as Percent of Household Disposable Income Minus Costs as Percent of Household Disposable Income [a]					
0– 2,999	23.5	11.1	12.4	30.1	3.2
3,000– 4,999	2.5	1.5	0.8	2.0	0.2
5,000– 9,999	− 0.7	− 0.4	− 0.3	− 0.3	− 0.2
10,000–14,999	− 1.2	− 0.7	− 0.6	− 0.8	− 0.4
15,000 and over	− 1.2	− 0.5	− 0.7	− 1.1	− 0.5

Source: Reference 203, Tables 6B, 6E, and 6H, pp. 111, 118 and 123 and Tables 6F, 6I, and 6J, pp. 119 and 124.

[a] Computed from data in the source tables.

taken together, add an average of almost $369 each year to the disposable income of each household below the poverty line ($3,000), representing a net increment of 23.5 percent of income. In contrast, the average household with an annual disposable income of $15,000 or over suffers a loss of $363, which is, however, only 1.2 percent of income. The rate of return for each dollar contributed (not shown in the table) is $9.63 for households in the lowest income class, but only 12 cents for households in the highest income class (203, Table 6L, p. 128).

A comparison of Medicare and Medicaid shows that Medicaid is more steeply redistributive than is Medicare. However, because much larger sums of money are involved in Medicare, this program has the greatest impact on income redistribution. Medicare has the additional peculiarity of ceasing to "tax" progressively beyond a yearly income of $15,000. Although a household with an income between $10,000 and $14,999 suffers a net loss of $83.30 per year, compared to $152.31 for each household in the highest income group, these sums are 0.7 percent of the disposable income of the first group, and only 0.5 percent of the disposable income of the second group. Stuart and Bair conclude that one effect of Medicare is to have "widened the gap between the upper and middle income classes" (203, p. 115). A further consideration, which has already been mentioned and is particularly applicable to Medicare, is that all the data cited deal with transfers during one year only. Medicare recipients make contributions over a lifetime of employment in return for benefits during a relatively short period of eligibility. If it transpires that Medicare beneficiaries in the higher income classes live longer and use more and costlier services after age 65, then the total balance of lifetime contributions and benefits might reveal a change in the magnitude, and perhaps even the direction, of redistribution.

Medicaid differs from Medicare in being a joint enterprise of the federal government and the states. The states determine how much money they will put up, and how stringent the levels of financial eligibility are to be. The federal government, in an attempt to transfer funds from the wealthier to the poorer states, augments the state contribution by 50 to 83 percent in a manner inversely related to the per capita income of the state. The result is considerable variability in the characteristics and consequences of Medicaid by state and geographic region. Table 41 shows the redistributive effects of Medicaid, by income class, for the two regions that are most sharply in contrast. In both regions there is a transfer of funds from the rich to the poor, but in the North East region the wealthiest households contribute twice as much, and the poorest households receive almost ten times as much, as their counterparts in the South region.

Stuart and Bair also studied the transfer of funds among states and regions with special attention to the extent to which Medicaid has accomplished redistribution in favor of the poorer states (Reference 203, pp. 142–154 and References 204 and 205). Two rather conservative tests of distributive equity are proposed: that program costs be distributed in proportion to the per-household disposable income of the states, and that benefits be distributed in proportion to the distribution of households that have a disposable income below $3,000 (205). Using these criteria, it is possible to compute for each state the degree to which costs, benefits, and the net grant (which is benefits minus costs) deviate from the standard of equity. When the 51 jurisdictions—the 50 states plus the District of Columbia—are arrayed in order of diminishing per-household disposable income, Nebraska is at the median of the array, with 25 jurisdictions above and 25 below. Table 42 shows that the wealthier states spend more than called for by the standard, but receive as benefits an even larger excess over the standard. The net result is that the wealthier states receive a larger flow of net benefits. Another way of assessing the same array of data is to count the states in which the net grant exceeds the standard. Table 42 shows that, irrespective of whether one uses as the

TABLE 42. Measures of Deviation of the States from a Specified Standard of Equity for the Distribution of Medicaid Costs and Benefits, U.S.A., Fiscal 1967/68 [a]

Measures of Deviation from Standard	States above Median Income [b]	States below Median Income
Costs minus standard costs	$343,818,000	−$334,843,000
Benefits minus standard benefits	$973,412,000	−$962,900,000
Net grant minus standard net grant	$629,594,000	−$628,057,000
Number of states in which net grant exceeds standard	14	3
Number of states in which net grant per household exceeds standard	13	2
Number of states in which net grant per poor household exceeds standard	12	1

Source: Reference 205, Table 2, pages 174–175.

[a] The standard of equity is that costs be proportionate to per-household disposable income of the state and benefits be proportionate to the number of poor families, defined as those with per-household disposable income below $3,000 per annum. The array includes all states plus the District of Columbia, with Nebraska occupying the median position. The net grant is defined as Benefits minus Costs. The net grant per poor household is computed assuming the entire net grant is allocated to this category.

[b] The per-household disposable income of the median jurisdiction.

criterion the net grant, the net grant per household, or the net grant per poor household, the favored states are heavily concentrated above the median income, with very few below.

Several phenomena underlie these findings. The first is that, in 1968, 14 states had not initiated Medicaid programs. Of these, 8 were below the median in per-household income and 6 were above it. The balance of payments was very adverse to these states, since they received no benefits from Medicaid but continued to support it through the contributions of their residents to the federal general fund. Stuart and Bair estimate that "In fiscal 1967, the 23 states without Title XIX plans contributed an average of more than $10 million each toward the program costs of the remaining 27 states. During fiscal 1968 the average state cost for non-participation reached $25 million" (203, p. 147). A second underlying factor is that, of the states that did participate, those that were wealthier tended to make larger state appropriations for Medicaid and to get bigger federal grants, even though the federal matching ratio was lower for them. Furthermore, these relatively larger combined funds were spent on a relatively smaller number of poor families. In 1968, taking the Medicaid states alone, there was a rank correlation of 0.1183 between per-household state income and net grant per household, showing a weak positive relationship. However, under the assumption that the net grant for a state was entirely allocated to households with an annual disposable income below $3,000, there was a rank correlation coefficient of 0.6255 between per-household disposable income for the state and the net grant per poor household. This relationship is shown in graphic form in Figure 10. It is clear that as a state becomes wealthier, the benefits that it can make available to its poor become considerably larger. Finally, there were in 1968, and still are, a few states, notably Massachusetts, New York and California, that had programs so disproportionately generous as to distort markedly the entire distribution of costs and benefits. It is no exaggeration to say that the dollar gains of these states were so great that they were "enough to guarantee a net redistribution of income away from virtually all of the less affluent states" and that "perhaps the most accurate discription of the program's regional impact is to say that California and New York gained at the expense of all four major regions" (203, p. 174). The conclusion is

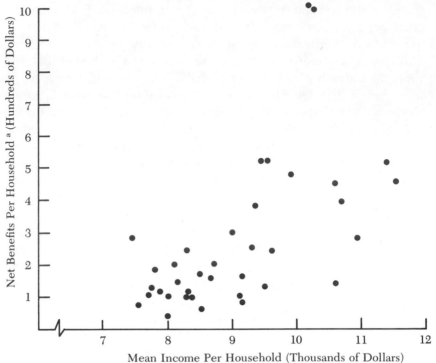

FIGURE 10. States by net Medicaid benefits per household [a] and by mean state income per household (States with Medicaid programs, fiscal year 1968)

Source: Reference 204, Table 5, pp. 28–29. Reproduced by permission from *Medical Care Chart Book,* School of Public Health, The University of Michigan.

[a] Federal Medicaid benefit expenditures per household with income under $3,000 minus Medicaid-related tax burden per household with income under $3,000 that is attributed to that income class.

that "as a redistributive mechanism, Medicaid must be judged a failure. The program was designed to reduce inequities in the distribution of welfare payments among states. Instead it has widened an existing gap in assistance levels. . . . At the same time the Medicaid program has in many cases redistributed real income from the poor to the wealthy states. In so doing, it has violated even the weakest standards of horizontal and vertical equity" (205, p. 176).

In contrast to Medicaid, there is no explicit or implicit intent to use Medicare to redistribute income among the states. Nevertheless, considerable transfers do occur, ranging, in fiscal 1967/68, from a benefit of $50.36 per household in Florida, to a loss of $66.22 per household in Alaska. Such transfers bore no consistent relationship to per-household income. Both wealthy and poor states can be found among those that subsidize others as well among those that receive subsidy. The contribution of the states to Medicare seem to be best described as being proportional to per capita income, an attribute that explains about three-quarters of the variability in state contributions. Benefits, on the other hand, seem to be largely dependent on the number of elderly persons in each state, but this factor explains only 60% of the variation in benefits among the states. There is indirect evidence to suggest that differences in price and use of service may account for some of the remaining variation in the money value of benefits. Thus, Medicare appears to transfer funds from the wealthier states to those that have relatively larger numbers of eligible recipients.

To sum up, both Medicare and Medicaid transfer considerable funds from non-recipients to recipients during any year. They are also responsible for the redistribution of income from the well-to-do to the poor. Medicaid is more steeply redistributive with respect to income classes, but Medicare has the greater redistributive effect because it has a larger budget. Medicare has the effect of transferring funds from the wealthier states to the states that have a proportionately larger number of aged persons. Medicaid, on the other hand, has failed to equalize state differences in medical care expenditures on behalf of the poor and has, contrary to its intent, transferred funds from the poorer to the wealthier states. When the major secondary effects of Medicare and Medicaid are taken into account, one arrives at the remarkable conclusion that of all the categories of households considered, the households of physicians have reaped the greatest additional benefits, followed by those who receive public assistance, with the elderly coming last.

Voluntary Health Insurance

As we have already said, the transfer of funds from those who do not receive care during any given year to those who do is a necessary feature of risk sharing. Consequently, some transfer must take place in any form of health insurance, whether voluntary or governmental. It is expected that, over a longer period of time, all those who are insured will experience their "fair share," as it were, of illness and its attendant expenditures. If premiums are assumed to be proportionate to this fair share, there would be no transfer of funds among those who are insured during this longer, but undefined, period. However, even over fairly long periods of time, transfers could occur if certain categories of insured persons were consistently more likely to be ill, to use more services, or to use costlier services, without having paid proportionate premiums. As we shall see, this matter of transfers under voluntary insurance has been a subject of serious social concern. But, strangely enough, one finds very little empirical documentation of the magnitude and direction of transfers under voluntary health insurance. There is much material on the use of service and expenditures by various categories of insured and uninsured consumers with different demographic and socioeconomic attributes. We have reviewed some of this literature in a previous chapter. What we do not seem to have is commensurate information concerning premiums and disbursements under insurance, so that the two can be compared for different categories of insured persons.

Under voluntary insurance, transfers occur when premiums do not correspond to benefits for designated categories of persons, during any specified period of time. Another, less obvious, source of transfer is through public subsidy of insurance premiums. This occurs in two ways: First, employer contributions towards health insurance premiums for their employees are considered to be a legitimate business expense which is not subject to either the corporate or personal income tax. Second, personal payments for health insurance are also deductible from taxable income, up to a limit. Feldstein and Allison have estimated the aggregate loss to the Federal treasury from the total exemption of premium payments to have been $1.63 billion in 1969, and from the partial exemption of personal premium payments to have been somewhere from $339 to $389 million during 1968. Thus, the Federal government subsidizes the purchase of voluntary health insurance to the tune of almost $2 billion a year (206). Feldstein and Allison have examined the distribution of each of the two components of the subsidy according to family income, under a certain set of assumptions.

Their estimation of how the employer contribution, and the tax loss associated with it, is distributed, begins with information on: (1) the average employer contribution per employer, and (2) the distribution of employees, by earnings, for each of 32 major industries that employ, all together, 48 million persons, excluding married women. It was assumed, by Feldstein and Allison, that married women "typically" obtain benefits under their husbands' rather than their own insurance plans. Consequently, they were excluded from the number of employees in each industry. This was done by reducing the number of women employed in each industry by 65 percent, which is assumed to be the proportion of working women who are married (206, pp. A3–A5). There is no information about variation in the employers' contribution according to the earnings of the employee within each industry. As a result, the investigators had to be content with the assumption that within any one industry all employees, irrespective of earnings, receive the same contribution from the employer towards the health insurance premium. But the earnings distribution of workers varies by industry, and this distribution is known. It is possible, therefore, to aggregate the 32 industries and arrive at a distribution of employer contributions by earnings class, assuming that the contribution does not vary by earnings *within* each industry. Next, the distribution of employees by earnings is converted to a distribution of employees by family income, using national data concerning (1) the relationship between the earnings of married men and the earnings of their wives, and (2) the unearned income of each husband-wife combination (206, p. A6). Given an estimate of family income, it was possible to compute marginal income tax rates by income class using Pechman's estimates of the average effective tax rates (206, p. 6). Finally, if it is assumed that in the absence of employer contributions, the same amount would have gone to the employee in wages and, thus, be subject to the income tax and to the social security tax on wages below $8,000 (in 1969), it is possible to compute the loss to the Federal treasury in taxes. This loss, in effect, is equivalent to a subsidy to the employees. Interpreted and estimated in this manner, the total subsidy for 1969 was found to be $1,629,364. As shown by curve A in

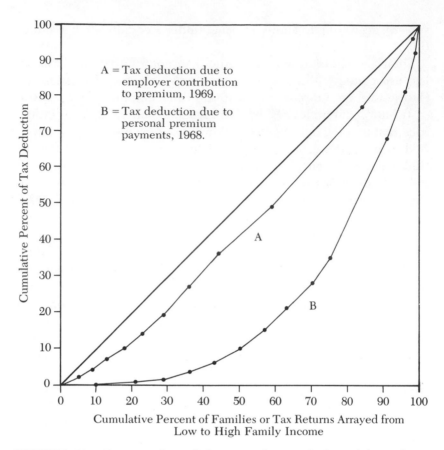

FIGURE 11. Percent of tax deductions that result from (A) employer contributions to insurance premiums and (B) personal premium payments, that are realized by each percent of taxpaying units, arranged in ascending order of family income.

Source: Reference 206, Tables 3 and 6, pp. 8 and 13.

Figure 11, the distribution of this subsidy by family income was distinctly more favorable to the rich. This is partly because employer contributions per family increased progressively with family income, and partly because the tax reduction on a given contribution also increases with family income. For example, a family with a yearly income below $1,000 received an employer contribution of $96 and a tax reduction of $12, whereas a family with an income of $25,000 or more received a contribution of $162 and a tax reduction of $59.

As to the reduction on personal income tax payments, it was possible in 1968 to deduct 50 percent of a health insurance premium up a maximum deduction of $150. Data on deductions claimed by families in each income class are available from the Internal Revenue Service. Using two alternative methods of computing the marginal tax rates, Feldstein and Allison estimated the total tax reduction attributed to deductions for premium payments to be either $339 million or $389 million. The distribution of these sums by income class was even more heavily biased in favor of the rich than was the distribution of the larger total reduction attributed to employer contributions. As shown in Figure 11, the 50 percent of families in the lower income range realized about 40 percent of the total tax reduction attributable to the contribution of employers to health insurance premiums, but only 10 percent of the tax reduction attributable to personal payments for health insurance premiums. It must be remembered, however, that the regressivity of the tax reduction due to employer contributions may have been underestimated as a result of the assumption that all employees in an industry receive equal employer contributions.

Further subsidies to personal health services in the private sector occur through income tax deductions on a variety of medical expenses, including medical and dental care as well as drugs and appliances, provided that the former exceed 3 percent and the latter 1 percent of adjusted gross income (207). However, we have not seen an analysis of the redistributive effects, if any, of these exemptions. More indirectly, personal health services in the private sector are also subsidized by direct government support and by tax exemptions accorded to a variety of activities in the health field, including research, professional education, and the delivery of care through nonprofit institutions. While the redistributive effects of such activities do not usually figure in assessments of "welfare policy" as it is more narrowly defined, they can, nevertheless, be large and socially significant (202).

Policy and Action Implications

As one might expect, the primary policy issues that are relevant to the redistributive effects of program benefits are related to social concepts of equity and to the role of public and private enterprise in implementing these concepts. Implicated in this is the ability of the private sector to solve the problem of financing health care for groups who suffer from the twin handicaps of high risk and low means. As we shall see, the very survival of private financing may hinge on how this problem is handled. The redistributive effect is also linked to another fundamental issue: allocative efficiency.

This issue arises because the groups that receive what is, in effect, a subsidy are encouraged to use more services. The cost of a specified increment in use of services is relatively fixed, but the benefits from that added use depend on the level of prior use, which determines the magnitude of unmet need in the user. But unmet need does not have a fixed measure, being perceived differently by those who use the additional services and by others in the society. This means that by changing the amount and distribution of the subsidy one can change the average benefit derived from a unit of expenditure, and that the valuation placed on that benefit is itself variable depending on whose interests and wants are being taken into account (3, pp. 37–42).

As we have already pointed out, there are two conflicting principles within the concept of tax equity. One is that the tax should be distributed according to the benefits received from its use, and the other is that the tax should somehow be related to ability to pay, irrespective of the social distribution of the benefit (200, pp. 54–55). It is now widely accepted that government may use the tax system to redistribute access to certain services of collective concern, including health care. But two contrary arguments are also heard from time to time. One is that, in programs separately funded for particular purposes (for example the social security system and, by extension, Medicare), the benefits should be proportionate to the contributions made by or on behalf of the beneficiaries (201, pp. 27–37). The other argument does not question the appropriateness of redistribution but rather the means for achieving it; it holds that it is more efficient to alter the distribution of income than the distribution of the ability to purchase specific services. In this argument, a financial subsidy that improves a family's ability to purchase health care would be preferable to a system of benefits that would, in effect, direct people to receive health services when other goods and services might be of higher priority to them.

Contrary to these points of view, one could argue that once society has accepted a generalized commitment to redistribution, there is no reason, *in principle*, why "social insurance" programs should be exempt from this obligation. One could also argue that no choice need be made between financial subsidies that improve purchasing power in general, and health care benefits that improve the ability to purchase a specific set of services. Why health care services deserve special attention has already been discussed in our introductory statement on social objectives. What remains, then, is to agree on the direction and magnitude of redistribution, and to make sure, by monitoring the operations of the system, that socially validated objectives are being achieved, and that no unintended and unwanted redistributions have taken place. As an example of the failure to achieve an explicit redistributive objective we have cited the redirection of funds from the poorer to the wealthier states during the early years of Medicaid. As possible examples of either unintended or undesirable consequences, we have cited the large subsidy to the households of physicians under Medicare/Medicaid, and the use of tax exemptions that result in greater subsidization of the purchase of private health insurance by families with higher incomes than families with lower incomes.

Contrary to the general agreement that redistribution is legitimate under tax-supported programs, there is much disagreement concerning the social validity and practical feasibility of using private insurance to bring about redistribution. The consequences of redistributive policy to allocative efficiency, and the action implications of these consequences, are also matters for current debate. We shall consider these matters under the two headings of: (1) "Community and Experience Rating," and (2) "Variable Subsidy Insurance."

Community and Experience Rating

In the field of private health insurance, "equity" acquires a narrower meaning than the one we have given it in our discussions so far. It relates merely to the "benefit principle," and signifies the strict proportionality of benefits to contributions. In effect, it rules out redistribution as inappropriate and undesirable. This is, in part, an ideological position, congenial to a free enterprise system. In part it is a practical necessity in a competitive market (208). Competitive necessity dictates that the price at which insurance is sold to a specific category of persons should reflect the probability and magnitude of the loss that is predicted for that category, the "credibility" of that loss (which means the likelihood of error in predicting it), and the additional costs of acquiring and administering the insurance business of the category. If the price is lower than is dictated by these factors then the insurance agency will take a loss; if the price is higher than is dictated, a competitor may be able to underbid the original insurer, depending on what considerations go into determining the profit margins that are possible and acceptable to the competitors.

For these reasons, part ideological but mainly pragmatic, equity theory has governed the practice of private insurance since its early days (208, p. 153). In this tradition, special or preferential rates have been used in employers' liability insurance since at least 1896, if not earlier. With the advent of workmen's compensation, the application of these special rates to industries with lower records of loss was called "experience rating" or "merit rating," because it adjusted the price of insurance to the occurrence of compensable injuries, and it rewarded employers who had a better record of safety (209, p. 39). Since then, the meaning of experience rating has been extended to embrace the pricing of health insurance, especially in underwriting large groups of employees, the very size of which confers credibility on the prediction of loss as well as considerable economies in acquisition and administration.

Under any system of rate setting it is necessary to begin with some estimate of the losses that might be incurred, based on a knowledge of the characteristics of the insured and the relationship between these characteristics and the frequency of loss. For example, given age, sex, employment status, and family size it is possible to make predictions about the incidence of illness, the corresponding use of service, and expenditures under a prevailing set of prices. The peculiarity of experience rating is that it makes these estimates for subgroups of clients, either because they are large collective purchasers (such as an employee group), or because they share a set of characteristics that makes them similar in their susceptibility to loss. Furthermore, the estimates of risk are modified in accordance with the actual experience of the losses incurred by each category and, perhaps, the costs of administering the policy as well. The resulting adjustment in premiums may be prospective, retrospective, or a combination of both (208, pp. 162–164).

In prospective rating, immediate past experience is used as a guide to introduce an upward or downward adjustment in the premium for the following year. This means that the insuring agency exposes itself to the possibility of incurring a loss that can be corrected only if the insured group remains a client for still another year, which in turn exposes the insurer to the possibility of another miscalculation. Because prospective rating has those limitations, retrospective rating is more congenial to the insurer, and is the more usual practice. In retrospective rating, the insurer sets a higher rate than is actually needed, but at the end of the contract period the insurer shares with the insured group the surplus over the losses and other expenses generated by the group. This procedure means that the policyholders have advanced considerable funds to the insurer, the use of which is enjoyed by the latter but denied to the former; a combination of prospective and retrospective rating may be used to reduce the size of these advances. Carried to its ultimate extreme, retrospective rating becomes, in effect, a cost-plus operation in which a large group of insured persons contracts with the insurer to have its claims processed at a specified price, with the insurer carrying no risk and maintaining no reserves insofar as the business of that group is concerned.

The advantages of experience rating are that it satisfies a restricted notion of equity, maintains and encourages competition among insurers, and rewards groups that have a low experience of loss, allegedly encouraging both health maintenance and restraint in the use of insurance. There are also disadvantages. The pegging of premiums so closely to the loss experience of each employee group could discourage the hiring of workers who are more likely to become ill (210, p. 8). In a more general sense, the analogy to merit rating in workmen's compensation may have become overly strained when it is applied to health insurance as a whole. The employer has control over the work environment, but there is very little that can be done to reduce the general incidence of illness or the behavior of individuals seeking care. Besides, it is not clear that restraint in the use of health services is a commendable social objective in all situations. One purpose of health insurance is to encourage health care when it is appropriate. But the most fundamental problem created by experience rating is that individuals and groups with a high expectation of illness and low income must be required to pay high premiums, which they cannot afford. Thus, the lowering of premiums for young, relatively healthy, employed groups is accomplished at the expense, so to speak, of the much higher premiums that are required of other groups, either because they are more likely to become ill, or because they must purchase insurance at retail as smaller groups or as individuals, or for both reasons. In fact, carried to its ultimate extreme, experience rating would negate the concept of risk sharing by parceling the insured into subgroups of precisely equivalent risk and exacting the corresponding premium from each. Thus, insurance would become merely a mechanism for budgeting one's health care obligations in the short term as well as in the long. Fortunately, this reduction to absurdity is not likely to be fully realized, partly because the need for credibility in the estimate of loss limits the minimum size of each category of the insured, but, mainly, because collective purchasers are socially structured into irreducible market units. Nevertheless, the tendency of experience rating is to press constantly in the direction of that absurdity that "equity" and competitiveness both seem to favor.

Experience rating has contributed to the emergence of a residual population of hard-to-insure people, and this population, in turn, has been a major concern of social policy (43). A central preoccupation in the formulation of social policy, in the past as well as now, has been whether the voluntary system can solve this problem unaided, whether government must help private insurance and in what way, or whether government must take on the function of health insurance and, if so, to what extent (211–213). "Community rating" could be one solution within the private sector. Under community rating all the clients of an insurer are lumped together for the purpose of estimating losses as well as paying administrative expenses. This means that everyone with equal coverage pays the same premium, irrespective of *known* differences in their likelihood of illness and their liability of incurring medical care expenditures, of whatever magnitude. In this way, the risk of illness and of medical care expenditures is fully shared, so that many more people can afford to purchase reasonably protective insurance, with a relatively small increase in average price.

It is clear that community rating, in the form described, involves a large variety of transfers, not only in the short term, but also, more consistently, over a longer period of time. Thus, resources are transferred from the more healthy, including the young, to the less healthy, including the aged. Given equivalent health status, transfers are made from those who are less likely to use services to those who are more likely to use them, and from those who pay low prices for care to those who pay high prices, whether because of geographic differences in prevailing prices, the type of provider used, or the mix of services received. Transfers also occur from larger groups, for whom the costs of acquisition and administration are lower, to smaller groups and individuals for whom such costs are higher. Unless adjustments are made for family size and composition, there are also transfers from small, stable families of adults and adolescents to actively breeding, larger families with many small children.

Needless to say, such transfers are not entirely eliminated under experience rating as it is practiced. However, the intent as well as the consequence of experience rating is to reduce transfers to the minimum possible, whereas community rating *knowingly* permits, and even encourages, transfers. The primary intent of community rating is to facilitate access to care by disseminating insurance coverage. The nature and social significance of the other transfers that attend the achievement of this primary objective are often unexamined and ignored. In general, it is assumed that the transfers are equitable, in the sense that they impose a higher burden on those more able to pay. As we have already pointed out, information on this point is remarkable by its absence. But we know enough to say that the transfers are not always equitable. They are often inequitable because persons with higher income pay the community-rated premium but are more likely to use the services, and particularly to use services that cost more. For example, Shain has reported that under Blue Cross and Blue Shield in Michigan, prior to a recent modification in rate-setting, "the plan under community rating had been heavily subsidizing the relatively high-paid, strongly unionized employees of some of the largest corporations in the state, whose premiums were paid entirely by their employers, at the expense of lower-paid groups in smaller companies. Furthermore, residents of rural and small-town areas of the state, where hospital costs (and generally, hospital bed supply) were lower, were contributing to the expenses of residents in the major industrial cities" (214, p. 1696). Under such circumstances community rating becomes harder to justify, but this is not, by far, the major problem it faces.

In their early days, Blue Cross and Blue Shield marched under the banner of community rating. As a result, they were subject to the depredations of the "commercial" insurers who were able to lure away larger, low-loss employee groups by offering equivalent protection at lower premiums. To survive, the Blues had to modify community rating, often to the point of virtual abandonment. Thus, community rating as we have described it is an ideal type with few representatives in real life. In practice, community rating is often modified to account for group size; family size and composition of enrolled groups; geographic area of residence; eligibility for Medicare and Medicaid; retirement; termination of employment; individual enrollment; and so on (210, Appendix A, pp. 3–4). Even the legislation authorizing aid to "health maintenance organizations," which requires community rating of all the enrollees of each such organization, permits modification of premiums by family size, group size, geographic area, and eligibility for Medicare and Medicaid (215). Whatever remnants of community rating there are in Blue Cross-Blue Shield, or in the prototypical "health maintenance organizations" that are now extant, are possible because of support by powerful union-management funds (as in Michigan), and because of the lowered costs stemming from tax exempt status, from preferential prices agreed to by hospitals, and, under group practice, from reductions in hospital use and other claimed, but mainly unproven, economies of large scale organization.

It is generally agreed that, in a competitive system, community and experience rating cannot coexist without modification of the former almost to the point of extinction. However, under a mandated health insurance program that uses private insurers to underwrite and market a specified minimum package of benefits, community rating of this basic package could be required by law. There are those who support this course of action, mainly in order to achieve equal access at equal cost. The oppenents point out that this provision would be difficult to implement and would most likely lead to covert and socially undesirable means of competition. These might include selective selling only to more favorable risks, transfer of costs from the health insurance component to other forms of insurance sold as a package, and the offer of other considerations such as financial loans to support businesses that buy insurance from the lender (210, pp. 4–6). The opponents of community rating propose as their solution to the problem of access the establishment of a subsidized fund, with or without government contributions, that could help a private insurer to underwrite small, high-risk groups, as well as individuals, at a reasonable price, without excessive risk to the insurer (210, pp. 6–12). There is, of course, a third body of opinion that finds no place for private underwriting in a national system. In a national program, it would be feasible to have true community rating on a regional or national scale, as is the practice under Medicare now.

Variable Subsidy Insurance

In this chapter we have been concerned with the relationship between the distribution of costs and the distribution of services, both under private insurance and under government programs. A disparity between the two distributions means that a transfer of resources has taken place, often undetected and sometimes unintended. One purpose of social policy is to expose these transfers, and then either to eliminate them, or, if they are socially desirable, to permit and encourage them. Thus, transfers become an explicit and planned feature of social policy rather than fortuitous and concealed events. If transfers are not only to be permitted but also to be purposive instruments of social policy, an egalitarian orientation demands that costs be distributed in a manner that is positively related to ability to pay. The precise nature of the relationship between the burden of cost and the ability to pay, whether progressive or merely proportionate, and, if progressive, to what degree, is a matter for social decision. But this decision cannot be divorced from an equal concern with the distribution of services, because it is the balance of services against the burden of costs that determines the direction and magnitude of redistribution. If services are proportionate to the burden of costs, there is no redistribution. The consequence is that redistributive social policy must separate the distribution of services from the distribution of costs.

If this separation is made, what rule governs the distribution of services or of the benefits that attach to these services? In our introductory chapter we offered a variety of choices. One was that services should be distributed according to valuation placed on them by consumers. Another choice was to distribute services according to a hierarchy of needs as defined by health professionals in general, and physicians in particular. Still another alternative was to distribute services according to the payoff in health potential, which was defined as an increment of health measured over a life-time. Presumably, the hierarchy of payoffs corresponds to the professional ordering of need, but this is not a foregone conclusion. The professional estimates, whether of service needs or of payoffs, may be different from the short time preferences of consumers, although we have argued that the degree of correspondence would be very high if the consumer were able to take an informed and long term view of the consequences of his decisions concerning health care. In any event, society, through the legitimate process of government, must decide what distribution of services is desirable, and whether this distribution is to be achieved by taking action or refraining from doing so.

In the absence of insurance, and under a given distribution of incomes, the relative value that consumers assign to goods and services is revealed by their purchasing behavior. Without insurance, the rich appear to be more ready than the poor to seek care; they receive more care, and they receive care for less serious illness. Under equivalent health insurance, the poor may be expected to increase their consumption of health services to a proportionately greater degree than the rich, but the rich also increase their consumption, so that a gap remains between them and the poor. If it is assumed that, in the absence of insurance, the rich have already met all or most of their significant health needs (according to their own valuation or the valuation of others), whereas the poor have not, the increment of use under insurance is clearly of much less value to the rich than to the poor. Pushing one step further, we could assert that if uniform insurance coverage is provided for everyone, and if the coverage is so complete that it assures the receipt of a socially desirable level of care for the poor, the consequence would be the receipt of redundant care by the rich. There are those who do not accept this construction of events. First, they believe that even the rich have a long way to go before the care they receive may be properly called redundant. Second, they would propose a certain redundancy of access to care for everyone, with use of service subsequently adjusted to need or payoff through professional decisions supported by organizational safeguards. There are others who find direct organizational controls on the use of service distasteful, or who doubt that these controls will be efficacious or will remain responsive to consumer preferences. They propose instead a system of financial disincentives that are graduated to income, so that the rich and the poor have more comparable access to care, relative to their needs, as well as comparable protection against the burden of costs, relative to their ability to pay. By altering the design of the system of disincentives, one can, presumably, attain any desired distribution of costs and benefits relative to income.

One such proposal has been put forward by Martin Feldstein under the name of "major risk insurance" (216). Under this proposal a deductible equivalent to 10 percent of family income would be a feature of a national health scheme. The deductible would also be the limit on out-of-pocket payments. Alternatively, there might be a deductible of 5 percent of family income with a 50 percent copayment on charges beyond the deductible, until the sum of the deductible and copayments equals 10 percent of income, beyond which all further charges would be paid in full by the insurer. In order to help consumers pay the deductible and copayment amounts, when these become large during any given year, Feldstein proposes loans, guaranteed by the government, which would spread the burden over a longer period of time. For families below the poverty level, there could be a yearly grant equal to their expected health spending. This amount, provided the family puts it to the intended use, would reduce the maximum out-of-pocket expenditure that would be borne directly by the family during any year to about 3 percent of income. All the percentages cited are merely illustrative. The key feature of the incentive-disincentive system is that the maximum payment that is demanded of any family during any year should be large as a proportion of the average expected yearly medical care expenditures for that type of family, but that the maximum payment should be small in relation to family income. This means that the family, while having full protection against anything exceeding 10 percent of income, would, most of the time, be paying its own medical bills. According to Feldstein, this would result in more careful purchasing of care, a lower rate of inflation, lower administrative costs, and a smaller tax burden, all without the imposition of unacceptable regulation on the medical care system, or serious financial hardship to the consumer. Needless to say, the key element in this design could be negated by the purchase of private supplementary insurance against the deductible and coinsurance payments expected of each family. Feldstein argues that this is not likely to occur, because the cost of such insurance would be high relative to the possible returns from it. It is a moot point whether this is sufficient or whether, in a national system, the purchase of such supplementary insurance should be banned.

More recently, Pauly has provided a detailed analysis of some of the theoretical bases for this approach to health insurance design (3). Under the rubric of "variable subsidy insurance" he has also offered some specific, illustrative, incentive-disincentive schemes (109, pp. 43–48). The features shared by these proposals are: (1) a deductible; (2) a relatively high coinsurance rate for a specified range of expenditures beyond the deductible; (3) a second, much lower, coinsurance rate for a range of expenditures beyond the first one; and (4) a maximum out of pocket payment. All four features are adjusted to family income, because the object of the design is to discourage the receipt of less necessary care by the rich and to encourage necessary care for serious illness by poor and rich alike. As family income increases, the deductibles become larger, the two intervals within which the two coinsurance rates successively apply become longer, and the maximum out-of-pocket payment becomes greater. The payments are progressive relative to imcome up to a point, beyond which they become proportionate. For example, under one proposal, a family with an income of $2,000 would pay a deductible of $50, followed by a copayment of 35 percent for aggregate charges between $51–199, followed by a copayment of 7.5 percent for aggregate charges between $200–999, with full coverage beyond that. The maximum out-of-pocket payment would amount to $163, which would represent 8.1 percent of income. For a family with an income of $8,000, the deductible would be $480, followed by a 50 percent copayment for aggregate charges between $601–1,999, followed by a copayment of 15 percent for aggregate charges between $1,999–4,999, with full coverage thereafter. The maximum out-of-pocket payment would be $1,400 per year, which would be 17.5 percent of annual income. These relationships between aggregate annual charges and out-of-pocket payments for the two income classes are shown graphically by the interrupted lines in Figure 12.

Figure 12 also shows, for comparison, the relationships that flow from Feldstein's proposal for a deductible equal to 5 percent of income, plus a copayment of 50 percent of additional charges, up to a limit of 10 percent of income in out-of-pocket payments. It is clear that the Feldstein proposal, in which the maximum out-of-pocket payments required are the same proportion of income (for example, 10 percent) in all income classes, is more regressive than Pauly's proposal, in which, as income rises, the maximum out-of-pocket payments become an increasingly larger proportion of income, up to a point (in this example, an annual income of $8,000) beyond which increases in out-of-pocket payments are proportionate to rises in income.

The design characteristics cited above, and the maximum out-of-pocket payments that they generate, do not provide sufficient information to permit a judgment concerning redistribution. It is necessary also to know the consumption of services and the corresponding charges in each income group, as well as how the schemes are to be financed in order to meet the costs that exceed out-of-pocket payments. Thus, assessment of the probable redistributive impact of an insurance scheme requires: (1) further specification of its features, beyond those given above; (2) a set of analytic tools; and (3) a set of value criteria.

Feldstein et al. have described a method that permits the simulation and assessment of the redistributive effects of a properly specified insurance proposal. The general approach underlying their method is already familiar to us from our discussion of the redistributive effects of Medicare and Medicaid. What is new about their proposal is that it does not examine the actual effects of an

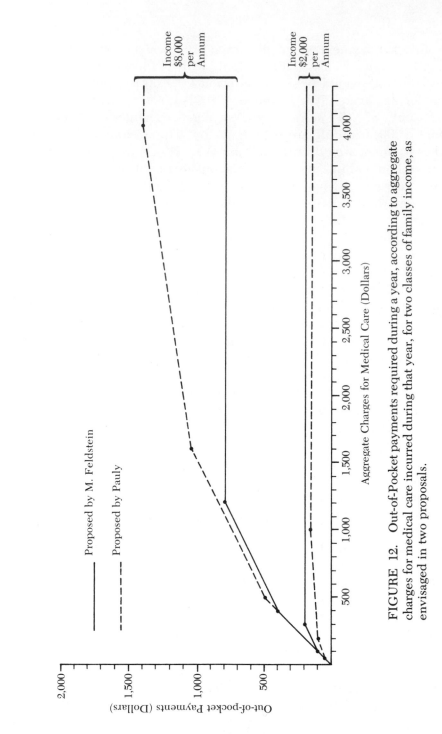

FIGURE 12. Out-of-Pocket payments required during a year, according to aggregate charges for medical care incurred during that year, for two classes of family income, as envisaged in two proposals.

Source: Reference 109, Tables I and II, pp. 45 and 46.

existing program but attempts to predict the probable consequences of alternative insurance schemes prior to implementation.
It also offers criteria of redistributive equity that are additional to
those used by Stuart in his assessment of Medicaid (204).

The first requirement of the simulation is to specify the design
of the insurance scheme including the method of financing. For
example, Feldstein et al. examine the probable effects of a "standard plan" with the following characteristics:

Deductible:
Basic: $50 per adult and $25 per child.
Income-related: $50 per $1,000 of family income in excess of
                   $3,000 to a maximum of $450 at an income of
                   $12,000.

Coinsurance:
Basic: 8 percent of charges.
Income-related: 4 percent per $1,000 of family income, to a
                   maximum of 56 percent at $12,000.
Maximum: Coinsurance is payable by the family on all
                   charges between the deductible and a total
                   of $14,000. There are no copayments on ag-
                   gregate charges beyond that.

Premium:
Basic: $50 per family.
Income-related: 1 percent of income between $3,000 and
                   $12,000.
Maximum: $140 per family.

Additional financing:
Payroll tax: 1 percent on wages and salary earnings on self-
                   employment income, to a maximum of
                   $9,000.
Income tax: The remainder; in this instance a 7.1 percent
                   increase in revenue from each tax bracket.

A critical feature of any design, of course, is the nature of benefits.
In this instance, Feldstein et al. do not go beyond the specification that the benefits be "comprehensive." It is possible to proceed with this minimal degree of specification only because the
method has certain features that will soon become evident.

Given some specification of the insurance scheme, such as the
one above, it is next necessary to determine the charges incurred

and the distribution of their burden by income class. This requires, first, information on the distribution of expenditures to uninsured families with a specified income and family composition. Second, it requires an estimate of how the deductible and coinsurance features of any particular insurance proposal would influence that distribution. The distribution of expenditures for the reference population of uninsured persons was derived from data concerning charges incurred by employees, spouses, and dependent children under the "high option" policy for federal employees. This policy provides "very comprehensive" coverage with low deductible and coinsurance rates. "This implies that the basic expenditure distribution is not distorted by differences among families in insurance coverage or by levels of insurance coverage that discourage expenditures. . . . Both of these have been problems in previous use of survey data to derive [a] *potential* expenditure distribution" (217, p. 5). Given the charges incurred under this plan, and its deductible and coinsurance features, the underlying distribution of the charges that would have occurred in the absence of insurance was derived under the assumption that insurance has no effect on the price of services, and that the price elasticity of demand is constant at either 0, -0.33, or -0.67. Thus, there are three different estimates of expenditures in the absence of insurance. These estimates of expenditures for employees, spouses, and dependent children were used to construct, numerically, the estimates of expenditures, in the absence of insurance, for families of various size and composition. The implicit assumption is that the expenditures of individuals remain constant irrespective of what type of hypothetical family the individual is in. Family income also does not figure in these estimates, either because the price elasticity is assumed to be constant across incomes, or because the families covered by the federal employees' program are assumed to comprise a reasonably representative cross section of families.

For each type of family, characterized by size and composition, these manipulations yield three hypothetical frequency distributions by expenditures, assuming each of three price elasticities and no insurance. These are the basic data from which are derived the estimates of the effects of any insurance proposal. To accomplish this, a large number of random drawings are made, as in a lottery, from each distribution for each family type. Each of these is converted to the equivalent expenditure under insurance using the corresponding assumption concerning price elasticity, and given the deductible and coinsurance features of the proposed plan. Having derived the expenditure under the proposed plan, and given the deductible and coinsurance features of the plan, it is also possible to compute what is the out-of-pocket payment for each drawing, the frequency distribution of such payments and their average. The difference between average expenditures and average out-of-pocket payments is the actuarial value of payments by the insurance plan, which is the average family benefit, for any specified type of family.

These procedures yield, for each family type, three distributions (corresponding to the three assumptions concerning price elasticity) for each of: (1) aggregate charges incurred, (2) out-of-pocket expenditures, and (3) reimbursements by the insurance plan. In order to apply these nine distributions to the population for which insurance is being designed, it is necessary to know the make-up of that population with respect to family size and composition. Feldstein et al. derived this information for the U.S. from the "data file" of the 1967 Survey of Economic Opportunity (217, p. 11). In this way, they obtained estimates of the distribution of benefits and out-of-pocket expenditures. In order to estimate the redistributive effect of the insurance plan, it is necessary to allocate not only benefits and out-of-pocket expenditures, but also all other costs of the plan by income class. As we have already pointed out, Feldstein et al. have not considered income as a factor in the incidence of benefits and out-of-pocket expenditures, except to the extent that income may have been correlated to family type. Both benefits and out-of-pocket expenditures are considered to attach to the families that experience them. The incidence of other costs depends on the method of financing the plan and on the assumptions made concerning the degree and direction in which these costs may be shifted. For example, in simulating the effects of the particular insurance proposal described above, Feldstein et al. assumed that premiums are borne by the families that pay them; the employer's contribution to the payroll tax is shifted forward to be borne in proportion to family income; and the personal income tax is not shifted, so that its incidence is based on the average tax rate for each income class (217, pp. 9–10).

The data which are generated by the procedure described

above, and which are used to evaluate any specified insurance proposal, are: (1) gross benefits, (2) out-of-pocket payments, (3) costs, (4) average total payments, (5) net benefits, (6) the net benefits expressed in terms of uniformly distributed dollars, (7) the marginal gross tax rate, (8) the marginal net tax rate and (9) the maximum out-of-pocket expense. The gross benefits are the actuarial value of the payment by the insurer, derived in the manner already described, from estimates of total charges and out-of-pocket expenses incurred. The costs are the premiums plus the burden of taxes, after adjustment for any shifting that is assumed to have taken place. The average total payment per family is the sum of costs and out-of-pocket payments. This is the measure of the financial burden on each family, or on the average family in each class. The net benefit is the gross benefit minus cost (the latter being premiums plus taxes). The "uniformly distributed dollar" is proposed as a way of expressing numerically the notion that the same net or gross benefit may be valued differently when received by families of different income class. It is proposed that this be done by deriving a weight which is a negative exponential function of income, so that:

$$\text{Weight} = \text{Income}^{-\alpha}$$

Feldstein et al. examined the distributions of gross and net benefits using 5 values of α: 0, 0.5, 1.0, 1.5, and 2.0. An exponent of 0 means that family income does not modify the dollar value of benefits. An exponent of -1.0 means that a given dollar amount in benefits becomes half as valuable as income doubles; an exponent of -2.0 means that the benefit becomes 4 times less valuable as income doubles. The marginal gross tax rate is a measure of the rate at which costs (premiums plus taxes) increase as income goes up. The marginal net tax rate is a measure of the rate at which net benefits go down as income goes up (217, p. 15). Whether there is a maximum out-of-pocket payment and, if so, how much it is, depends on the design of the insurance policy. It is not often that families will pay the maximum, but it is reasonable to assume that the maximum liability is an important consideration in the purchase of insurance. Hence, Feldstein et al. propose that the maximum out-of-pocket expense should increase with income, but that at no income should it be so high as to encourage the purchase of additional insurance. Needless to say, the purchase of such insurance would invalidate the analysis described above and neutralize the social objectives implicit in the design of variable-subsidy insurance.

Feldstein et al. give data that reveal the consequences of the insurance proposal that they cite, under the assumptions already specified. For a family of given size and composition, as income goes up, out-of-pocket payments and other costs also go up. On the other hand, gross benefits and net benefits go down. Beyond a family income of $8–9,000 the net benefit becomes a progressively larger negative value, which means that these families pay more in premiums and taxes than they receive in benefits. Over most of the income range (namely, from $3,000–$14,999, inclusive), the average total payment (which is out-of-pocket payments plus premiums plus taxes) remains about 6 to 7 percent of income, and the maximum out-of-pocket payment about 7 percent of income. But this constant proportionality breaks down at the two extremes of the income range, to the detriment of the poor and the relative advantage of the wealthy. The average gross benefit, which is the actuarial value of insurance, is $288 for all families with two adults and two children. But the mean net benefit is −$38, which means that these families pay somewhat more in taxes and premiums than they expect to get. We are not told whether this is due to horizontal transfers among families of different size or due to differences in their income structure. In any event, the degree of progressivity, by income, of gross and net benefits is considered to be substantial. When the net benefits are weighted so that the value of the dollar is doubled when income is reduced by half ($\alpha = 1.0$), the average net benefit has a value of $89; this goes up to $256 when the exponent is taken to be 2.0.

Feldstein et al. add a brief but instructive section on the consequences of discrete changes in the design of the insurance package (217, pp. 29–31). Regressive consequences, which favor the well-to-do relative to the poor, flow from increases in the deductible, the coinsurance rate, and the premium. An increase in the income-related component of the coinsurance rate has somewhat progressive consequences, whereas an increase in the income related component of the deductible helps the two lowest and two highest income classes while making those in between slightly worse off (217, p. 29). "It should be stressed that distributional effects of each of these changes reflects not only the change itself but the induced change in the income taxes that provide the 'residual' finance for the plan" (217, p. 31). We thus have a tool, subject to the limitations introduced by the assumptions that have been described, to test the fiscal consequences of alternative insurance proposals. The administrative and political feasibility of such alternative proposals is, of course, another matter altogether.

PART THREE

Benefits and Program Objectives

A major theme in this book has been the evaluation of the consequences of benefit design, with reference to a variety of objectives. We began by introducing the two social objectives that seem to have motivated the development of organized financing for personal health services. The more traditional, and perhaps the more powerful, objective has been protection against unpredictable medical care expenditures. The second objective, more ambitious and increasingly more insistent, has been the adjustment of use of service to a measure of need that involves some social valuation of the health benefits to be derived from the services. These objectives are obviously related. The threat of unforeseen and unbudgeted expenditures can effectively serve as a barrier to care, just as the actual incurring of such expenditures can mean financial ruin. But, in spite of this not so subtle linking of the two objectives, it remains true that existing social programs and instrumentalities, as well as more general social policy orientations, may be differentiated by whether they put emphasis on one objective or the other.

Further consideration of the second objective, of assuring access proportionate to need, reveals that not all needs are of equal merit, so that, given limited resources, some needs have a greater claim to social attention than others. It is a short step from this insight to the postulation of a third objective, which is the attainment of allocative efficiency. This objective gains further force and relevance from the theoretically expected, and empirically observed, capacity of prepayment to distort use of service in favor of the persons and services covered by it. The tendency to use covered services as substitutes for other services focuses attention on a fourth objective: efficiency in production. This is a matter of concern because the preferential use of a substitute may be wastefully costly or less effective. Fifth, and finally, the transfers involved in the incidence of the costs and benefits of medical care programs highlight the social objective of equity and the different ways equity can be interpreted.

These five objectives—financial protection, access proportionate to need, efficiency of allocation, efficiency of production, and equity—have been the touchstones we have used to test benefit design in medical care programs. In this part we propose to treat these and some additional objectives in somewhat greater detail. For this purpose, we shall use a classification of objectives that we have called "orientational" (1, pp. 38–39). The distinctive feature of this classification is that it relates objectives to the groups whose interests they primarily serve and who, therefore, attach the greatest weight to these objectives as they engage in complex interactions to influence the formulation of social policy. In this way, we get an impression of the competing forces engaged in the political arena. Incidentally, we are also able to test the utility of the classification as a means for ordering and rendering more comprehensible a rather diverse and complicated set of elements.

Client-Oriented Objectives

It seems reasonable to assume that what clients look for in purchasing insurance, and in assessing the merits of alternative health plans, is the degree of protection against the expense of care, the stability and continuity of that protection, and the value received for the money spent to obtain protection.

Degree of Protection

Possibly the most elemental expectation that the consumer has of health insurance is that it protect him against unexpected expenditures. But it is likely that people differ in their aversion to risk-taking and in the price they are willing to pay for a given degree of protection (218). Psychological or personality factors no doubt have a part in influencing this propensity. The social situation of the consumer, in its broadest sense, is also a factor. It is generally assumed, for example, that the wealthy are more willing to assume risk, provided all other things are equal (218, p. 254).* But they seldom are. The rich are more likely to be healthy, to have a lower expectation of illness, to pay higher prices for medical care, to have higher social aspirations to maintain, and, should truly catastrophic illness strike, have a longer and perhaps more anguished fall down to the depths before they reach the level where welfare medical care may be expected to come to their aid.

The hazards faced by persons in different social situations are obviously very different, so that it is difficult to speak of risk aversion without first considering the component elements of the risk

---

* Feldstein refers to the basic work by Pratt (219) and by Arrow (220) relative to the relationship between income and risk aversion, and points out that the correlation of risk aversion with income need not always be positive.

itself. In so far as unexpected medical expenditures are concerned, the first element is the probability, actual or perceived, of the occurrence of illness in varying degrees of severity, the severity being assessed in terms of threat to life or physiological function. The second element in determining risk could very well be the corresponding probabilities when care is received in specified degrees of completeness. The hypothesis is that what motivates persons to receive care, and to seek the means of assuring care, is at least partly the perception of the difference that care makes in the probability of death or physiological dysfunction. But the valuation placed on death or physiological dysfunction is itself, in part, psychologically and socially determined. The valuation might be expected to differ depending on the extent to which physiological dysfunction interfers with one's usual work and with the discharge of this and other obligations: marital, parental or more general. Even the aversion to death is not a constant, but is graded in relation to the psychological and social threat that it poses to oneself and to others.

If we have reasoned correctly the third element in our formulation of risk is the conversion of the first and second elements into the corresponding probabilities of the threats that we are socially and psychologically conditioned to perceive. The risk of not receiving care can then be expressed as the risk of foregoing the benefits of receiving care, the benefits having been valued by taking into account physiological, psychological, and social factors. In a most fundamental sense, insurance is sought as protection against the consequences of absent or deficient care. In a more derivative sense, insurance is sought against the consequences of having to pay for appropriate care. The fourth element in risk, therefore, is the money value of care. Here again, the social situation of the consumer intrudes, since it influences the ability to pay the price of care out of current income or other assets, either with or without reductions in the current standard of living or in future social aspirations. Eligibility for welfare can be considered as part of ability to pay. But it also has a price. Part of the price is that resources must be depleted and social aspirations abandoned before eligibility is granted. Another part is the devaluation the recipient suffers in his own eyes as well as the eyes of others, given the dominant values of our culture.

A fifth element in the evaluation of risk is its degree of uncertainty; the confidence with which the risk can be predicted for any individual or family. Both very common and very rare events can be predicted with higher degrees of certainty than events which have an equal probability of occurring or not (33, p. 15). Individuals differ with respect to their tolerance of uncertainty; social factors are also likely to be relevant, because the consequences of having guessed wrongly obviously vary with one's social situation.

In the preceding exposition we have used risk as a rather undifferentiated concept that includes the probability of occurrence of a particular peril (in this instance, disease episodes of specified severity), the probability of occurrence of a loss (in this instance, the consequences of not receiving appropriate care, or the charges incurred when such care is received) and, finally, the uncertainty involved in predicting the probability of occurrence of the peril or the loss.* To put it simply, we have reasoned that a person faced with buying insurance asks himself how likely it is for him or for a member of his family to become ill; how severe the illness is likely to be; what the consequences would be if he could not afford care; what the consequences would be if he had to pay bills of varying orders of magnitude; and, finally, how likely he is to guess wrong concerning any of these probabilities, and what the consequences of a wrong guess would be. We have also suggested that each one of these elements in the calculus of decision-making is influenced by the social situation of the consumer. While all this appears, on the face of it, eminently reasonable, at least as a basis for empirical expectation, we must also remember that the decision whether to buy health insurance and what kind of health insurance to buy is often not a matter for individual choice, but a necessary concomitant of employment. One accepts whatever health insurance goes with the job. However, some health insurance is bought individually, some employers do offer a choice of plans with varying degrees of protection at differing or comparable premiums, and, in some cases, it is conceivable that health insurance and other fringe benefits are a factor in the choice among employers.

* According to Dickerson, "peril" is an event which may produce "loss," and "risk" means "uncertainty as to loss" (33, pp. 108, 15). However, it appears to us that he also uses "risk" in a more undifferentiated sense, as we have done.

Empirical evidence of the behavior of consumers choosing health insurance comes from a series of studies that have attempted to explain how auto workers chose between Blue Cross-Blue Shield and a prepaid group practice plan that offered more benefits for the same premium (221–225). An early finding was that workers who selected the prepaid plan were more likely to be older, to be married, to have children, and to have higher incomes. Two related notions were briefly alluded to in explaining these findings. One was that these subscribers had a "greater expectation of need for health services" (221, p. 25), and the other that "an objective position of economic vulnerability is a primary basis for the choice of prepaid group practice" (221, p. 44). The notion of vulnerability was differentiated and expanded to comprise three elements: "physiological susceptibility, social responsibility and lack of social support," which were taken to correspond to "aging, child rearing and anomie" (222, p. 84). This further elaboration was offered as a post hoc explanation of the observation that when people were queried about the importance of specified benefits in a health insurance plan, the "demand" (or desire) for such benefits seemed stronger amongst older persons, married persons with children under 18, persons who were widowed, separated or divorced (especially if they had children under 18), and persons who rated their incomes as above average for the area.

From these rather tentative formulations, one could infer that vulnerability is associated with an expressed desire for more benefits under insurance, even at greater cost, and with a tendency to actually enroll in a prepaid plan that offers a broader range of benefits, even when the competing plan is more familiar and offers the advantages of free choice. However, it soon became apparent that the notion of vulnerability might have broader ramifications. A striking finding of the initial study in this series was that 32 percent of the workers who had chosen Blue Cross-Blue Shield did not remember that the choice of another plan had been offered at the same time (221). Analysis of the data showed that the variables that had been subsumed under the rubric of "vulnerability" were positively associated with remembering that a choice had been offered. Accordingly, it was hypothesized that an additional way in which vulnerability influences behavior is by creating greater interest in, and awareness of, information concerning health insurance plans, and that this greater interest produced the differences in recall observed in the study (223). If one accepts this formulation, it is interesting to note that differences in income had the largest effect on recall, that recall increased with income and that the largest difference observed was between respondents in the lowest income class (under $4,000) and those in the next highest class ($4,000–$5,999). Thereafter, recall continued to improve with income, but at a much lower rate. Although there were no data concerning families with much higher incomes, the relationship observed suggested to the authors that perceived vulnerability is highest in the middle range of income and lower at both extremes. Presumably, very poor families have very little to lose (or have a lower price to pay for welfare medical care), whereas the very rich have the resources to take care of their losses. While this formulation is both plausible and theoretically attractive, the reader should remember that it involves an extrapolation from data which are themselves at one remove from demand, since they relate to a consumer's remembering a choice rather than to the nature of the choice itself.

It is possible to pursue the notion of vulnerability along two lines. One is its relationship to information and the other its relationship to choice. Richie pursued the former route by postulating that vulnerability leads to an awareness of information concerning features of alternative health care plans, either by sensitizing persons to the information that comes their way, or by motivating them to actually seek the information. The acquisition of information, by whatever means, leads in turn to the choice of the health care plan that best meets a person's needs (224).

The notion of vulnerability itself is considered to have three components, which are "perceived physiological susceptibility," "social responsibility for others," and "lack of social support," as postulated by Bashshur and Metzner (222). Alternatively, these three elements might be seen as three types of vulnerability. In order to test this formulation, Richie used data from another of the studies of health plan choice made by Metzner and Bashshur, this time in Cleveland (224). Respondents who had chosen either Blue Cross-Blue Shield or a competing prepaid group practice plan had been asked by the original investigators what they knew about each of 14 features of these and other health insurance plans. The criterion of knowledge used by Richie was simply whether the respondent had given any information, irrespective of its accuracy, or answered "don't know." In the process of analysis the 14 items of information had to be clustered and ordered in a Guttman scale so as to arrive at three levels of not-knowing: "high," "moderate," and "low." These three categories were the dependent variable. As to the independent variable, which was "vulnerability," respondents who said they were concerned or worried about something that might go wrong with their health were considered to exhibit "perceived physiological susceptibility"; those who had children below 18, whether they themselves were married or not, were considered to have "social responsibility"; and those who were single, widowed, divorced, or separated, irrespective of whether they had children, were considered to have a "lack of social support." As expected, persons who were considered to have responsibility for others, in this instance dependent children, were found to have lower levels of not-knowing. However, contrary to the investigator's hypothesis, "lack of social support" was related to higher levels of not-knowing; in other words, respondents who were married exhibited lower levels of not-knowing. Richie speculates that the factor of "responsibility for others" concealed the effect of "lack of social support." In fact, respondents who were both married and had dependent children were most likely to have information about health plans, irrespective of the accuracy of that information. Finally, "perceived physiological susceptibility," as defined, was found to be unrelated to the level of not-knowing. Thus, the notion of vulnerability, as formulated and tested by Richie, was only partially supported by the findings.

When a variety of other factors, which might independently influence exposure to information, were taken into account, the relationships between not knowing and the several elements of vulnerability became even less general and distinct. The relationship to income is particularly interesting in view of the expected nonlinear relationship postulated by Bashshur and Metzner, as described earlier (223). In the data used by Richie, the measure of income was the respondent's report that income was "more than adequate," "adequate," or "less than adequate" to meet basic family needs, including paying bills and buying things the family needed. Among persons who had elected the prepaid group practice plan, the level of not-knowing decreased as the perceived adequacy of income increased; but among respondents who had elected the Blue Cross-Blue Shield plan there was no clear relationship between the two variables. Although Richie had not considered perceived income adequacy as a component of vulnerability, the findings of the study suggest that the notion of vulnerability remains no more than a possibly viable concept in explaining the level of information as that level was defined by Richie.

There has been no further explicit testing of the relationship between vulnerability and either the actual demand for insurance or the choice among alternative plans. However, one finds in other studies evidence of the relationship between the purchase of insurance and some of the variables which Bashshur and Metzner construe to signify vulnerability. For example, Moustafa et al. have reported on how employees of a university chose among 6 plans, either initially or when they had the opportunity to switch from one plan to any of the others (226). About three-quarters of the new employees chose one of three plans with comprehensive benefits. Those who changed plans were more likely to join the prepaid group practice plan than to leave it. Although the employees' detailed knowledge of benefits was defective, choice was judged to depend upon a realistic estimate of cost and breadth of coverage. Persons who chose comprehensive plans usually did so to obtain broader coverage; those who chose the basic plans did so because of lower premiums. The demographic characteristics were not as important in determining choice as were plan characteristics. Nevertheless, middle-aged married persons, many of whom had children, tended to choose the comprehensive plans, whereas younger single people tended to choose plans that offered fewer benefits at correspondingly lower cost.

In another study from California, which we have described earlier, Roemer et al. found that the clients of two "representative" prepaid group practice plans, when compared to those enrolled in similarly "representative" commercial and provider-sponsored plans, were more likely to be old, to have suffered chronic as well as acute illness during the previous year, to pay attention to symptoms and to be of lower class, as judged by education and occupation (52, pp. 14–17). The authors conclude that, although the differences are not large, prepaid group practice tends to attract people who are at highest risk, and commercial plans tend to sell to people of lowest risk, even when only group insurance is considered, as was the case in this study. Needless to say, this differential propensity is a matter of great concern to insurers; the reader, no doubt, has recognized the affinities between the notion of vulnerability and the more familiar phenomenon of "adverse selection," which is the universally recognized tendency for persons who expect to use the benefits of insurance to be more likely to buy it, and to buy more of it. Another component of vulnerability, namely, the perceived susceptibility of illness, has also recieved considerable theoretical and empirical attention as a detriment of use of service (though not of demand for insurance), first by Hochbaum (227) and later by Rosenstock, Kegles, Haefner, and others (228).

So much for differences in consumers' perceptions of their need for protection against the unpredictable costs of care. Let us now turn to an assessment of benefit design relative to the perceived need for protection. Here the key features are: (1) the range of benefits (services and commodities) included; (2) the quantities of these benefits, expressed as charges or physical units; (3) the nature and amounts of participatory payments, such as deductibles and coinsurance; (4) susceptibility to unpredictable out-of-pocket payments, due to inflation in prices or to optional acceptance of "assignment" by the physician; and (5) the presence or absence of maximum limits either to the liability of the insurer or to the liability of the insured. Several of these features have already received attention in other relevant contexts. Deductibles and co-payments have been discussed in detail in Chapter 2, on use of service. Protection against inflation has been discussed in Chapter 4, on price, where, among other things, we spoke of the protective effect of service benefits, compared to cash. We have also considered the range and quantity of benefits as determinants of use of service and as factors in the substitution of some services for others. The money value of the benefits received, as compared to the incidence of costs, was a key element in plotting the redistributive effect of insurance. What remains to be done is to synthesize these various elements into some way of measuring the protective efficacy of alternative benefit designs, both in absolute terms and relative to the consumer's ability to pay.

The problem of rating health insurance plans with respect to their protective efficacy has puzzled and frustrated medical care experts almost as much as consumers. The confusion has been enhanced by the bewildering, and seemingly irrational, variety of policies. One simple, but useful, approach to the problem has been to merely list the "good" and "bad" features of a policy in order to gain an overall impression of its likely efficacy. In this tradition is the almost notorious *Shopper's Guide,* published by Herbert Denenberg in his capacity as insurance commissioner in Pennsylvania (229). One can infer from the *Guide* that even before the buyer examines the provisions of the policy, he should be cautioned by the way it is sold and by the identity of the seller. Group plans are likely to be more protective than plans bought individually, and individual plans bought from Blue Cross and Blue Shield, or some other reputable organization, are likely to be more protective than policies bought from a commercial concern that gets a great deal of its business by mail orders or through hard-sell solicitation in the press, radio, or television. The financial stability of the insurer is also important; Denenberg advises that no firm be patronized unless it has earned one of the two highest ratings in *Best's Insurance Reports.*

A more detailed examination of a policy will reveal several critical features. One is the number of different services and commodities covered. Another feature is the limits placed on benefits, with particular attention to whether there are waiting periods before benefits become operative, whether so-called "pre-existing" conditions are excluded, and whether maternity benefits and coverage for infants from birth is included. If the policy does not offer service benefits, it is important to check the going prices and assure oneself that the cash benefit covers a large percentage of the charges for each service. Even then, problems may arise if care is required in a larger city where prices may be higher. Denenberg also offers a primer of the more misleading terms in the insurance jargon that may lead the customer to believe that he has the protection which he does not, in fact, have.

In the Denenberg tradition is a *Consumer's Guide to Health Insurance* published by the Comprehensive Health Planning Agency of Massachusetts (230). One of its useful features is a dummy table which the buyer can use to visually display the benefits, exclusions, and other limitations in his health insurance policies, so that he can determine his situation at a glance (230, pp. 16–17). The New York State Department of Health takes a somewhat different tack (231). It proposes that the protective efficacy of an insurance policy can be rated by the extent to which it can meet the aggregate charges of typical, frequently encountered disease episodes. Since different types of families are subject to different perils, the typical disease, or set of diseases, that is selected would be adjusted to family type. Pending the development of a more comprehensive system, the following test conditions are proposed: (1) for a single person, appendectomy; (2) for a married female without dependents, maternity care; (3) for a married male without dependents, myocardial infarction; and (4) for a married couple with two children under 18, cholecystectomy. The index of protection for each of these situations is the fraction of expected expenditures for the entire episode of care that is expected to be met by insurance under the provisions of any given policy. It is proposed that this numerical index be converted to a set of letter ratings, such as A +, A, A −, B +, and so on, based on an expert judgment of how high expectations of coverage should be. This entire approach, while not fully developed by the author, has hidden in it a set of important conceptual advances that we shall presently return to. But first, we should briefly describe the most ambitious attempt we know of to rate health insurance plans. We refer to "HPGS," the Health Plan Grading System, developed under the direction of Breslow by his coworkers at the Los Angeles and Berkeley campuses of the University of California (232).

The development of the Health Plan Grading System began with the identification of critical features of health insurance plans. The features were classified under 5 headings: (1) organizational and administrative arrangements established to carry out the plan; (2) extent of coverage, for example, whether family members are included; (3) scope of benefits; (4) administrative provisions to assure quality of medical care provided under the plan; and (5) the amount of money which members of the plan spend for health services, in addition to the health insurance premium. The full list of features is reproduced in Appendix B; it was assembled from several sources of information and the opinions of many experts, representing the academic community, the organized purchasers, and the insurers. The key features of a plan having been identified, the next step was to assign an order of importance to each, so that an aggregate index of adequacy could be constructed. This was done by requesting the opinions of persons who represented "various phases of interest in the medical care field." Taking these opinions into account, the investigators have developed a system of scoring that assigns a numerical value to each feature of the plan, with an overall maximum value of 1,000 points. The rating system clearly represents normative consensus and defines client protection more broadly than we have done so far. At the heart of the rating system is the assessment of protection against unpredicted expenditures, which embraces categories 2, 3, and 5, and accounts for 600 points out of the total score of 1,000. As shown in Appendix B, pages 398–99, item III, "scope of benefits," comprises 15 services which differ in weight from 40 points for hospital room and board to 5 points for the provision of ambulance service. These weights represent the points earned by an insurance plan that pays for the service in full. For each benefit there are five lower steps representing progressively less complete payment; at each of these steps a plan earns correspondingly fewer credit points. The maximum possible score for "scope of benefits," when all services are paid in full, is 300, which is almost one third of the total score for all features.

The proposed system was tested on 10 California plans. The premiums charged by these plans and the scores they earned were highly correlated, which suggests that one gets what one pays for. But this correlation did not always hold, which indicates that the scoring system could detect a poor buy. The rank order of the ten plans by scope of benefits corresponded rather closely to the overall rank order. In part, this indicates the large weight given to this feature, but it also indicates the necessary intercorrelation between scope of benefits and out-of-pocket payments, and between the latter and extent of coverage. The investigators responsible for the system do not comment on this lack of independence of some components of the scoring scheme. They do recognize, however, that several parts of the scheme, and in particular the quality assurance component, require much further refinement. Nevertheless, taken as whole, the Health Plan Grading System is impressive in the breadth of its concern for the consumer and in the care with which it was constructed. It can be accepted as a good representation of the norms among the community of scholars and administrators who are knowledgeable in health insurance. But the conceptual framework that underlies these norms is not made explicit, and is itself subject to challenge. One must consider, therefore, whether it is possible to develop a more explicit and precise measure of the protective efficacy of health insurance plans.

There are two extremes in the specification of benefits. At one extreme the benefits are specified simply in terms of how the insurer and insured will share in paying the expenses of care, with no limit on the scope of services included. At the other extreme, each category of services is listed and the amount of each service for which the insurer will pay is specified in physical quantities, in dollars, or in both. The first type of specification is rarely, if ever, encountered in real life, since very few plans cover all or almost all of the medical care services that are likely to be needed. We have, however, encountered such a specification in the work of Pauly (109) and of M. Feldstein (216). The importance of this formulation is that its protective efficacy can be assessed by a reasonably simple method. This method was developed by Feldstein et al. to test the redistributive effects of alternative health insurance proposals, and has been described in Chapter 5 (217).

Given a plan that places no constraints on the range of services covered, the assessment of protective efficacy begins with the construction of a hypothetical universe that specifies, for families of given size and composition who do not have insurance, the frequency distribution of annual expenditures for medical care. As the reader will recall, this hypothetical universe was extrapolated from actual expenditures by subscribers, spouses, and children under the most generous policy offered to federal employees. Given this hypothetical universe of expenses, and a family of given size and composition one can, by repeated sampling from the universe, construct a probability distribution of expenses, assuming no insurance. For each entry in this distribution one can specify the shares paid by the insurer and by the insured, given the characteristics of the policy. It follows that one can also compute the average out-of-pocket payment, as well as the likelihood of paying any specified sum or more. These are the measures of protection, without reference to the ability to pay or to the likelihood that insurance will increase use of service and, therefore, alter the degree of protection offered by the plan. Feldstein et al. account for the effect of insurance on use of service by assuming a range of price elasticities of demand and adjusting the distribution of expenditures accordingly. They do not, as we understand it, consider the effect of income on these elasticities. They also do not take into account inflation in medical care prices. It would seem, however, that a correction for the latter could be rather easily introduced. The method devised by Feldstein et al. also seem to be applicable, though much less precisely, when all we know about the universe of expenses is the mean for each family type, provided we are willing to assume that expenses by family type conform to a Poisson distribution, or to some other defensible shape. It appears, therefore, that this method is a conceptually valid means of judging the protective efficacy of a health insurance plan when the benefits are stated exclusively in money terms, without reference to the services covered or excluded. Unfortunately, an extension of this approach to the more usual plan, which excludes certain services and covers others in variable amounts, poses certain difficulties.

To begin with, the probable occurrence of the need for different services, or the actual use of services, varies considerably from person to person. This probability differs according to the characteristics of the person or population insured. For example, the aged are not likely to use maternity services or orthodontia, though they are likely to need dentures and nursing home care. Thus, the matching of benefits to needs is a critical issue. A corollary to the variable nature of need and use of service is that, in certain population subgroups, the need for certain services is so highly probable as to be predictable and budgetable, while other services are highly unpredictable. The probability of occurrence is closely related to the amount of service that is likely to be needed. Both together contribute to the magnitude of the hazard, but they do not determine it entirely. There is another property that might be called the "degree of indivisibility" or the "lumpiness" of the risk associated with each category of services. This property is itself an amalgam of the severity of the illness episodes and the aggregation of services needed for different episodes of care. The concept of lumpiness can be illustrated by contrasting the one or two office visits necessary for preventive care, or for the management of each of a succession of minor illnesses, with hospitalization for a more serious illness. The contrast is much like that between several slaps on the face and a hammer blow to the head. The cost of the hospitalization may not exceed the total cost of repeated care for minor conditions during a year, but the financial impact is larger for at least two reasons: expenditures are concentrated within a short period of time and the patient has less choice in adjusting the amount of care to his financial ability. This leads us to consider another attribute of the risk, namely the necessity or cruciality of the service, or the bundle of services, that correspond to that risk; by this we mean the consequences to the client if care is not received. Obviously, one has discretion in the use of some services but not in the use of others. The degree of discretion depends on two related factors: the severity of the illness and the therapeutic efficacy of the service. One can ignore efficacious services for minor illnesses, as well as nonefficacious services for serious illnesses. This means that one cannot evaluate the cruciality of the service benefits of a plan without at the same time knowing about illness, unless it is shown that, when all disease episodes are considered together, certain cetegories of service continue to differ in average cruciality from others. The final difficulty in assessing the relative protective efficacy of providing one configuration of service-defined benefits versus another is the extent to which services are interrelated by being mutually complementary and substitutable. Moreover, as we have shown, different benefit designs can elicit and reinforce different patterns and degrees of complementarity and substitution. Services must be seen as a tissue of interrelated parts. At best, types of service may be separated into clusters or fields. For example, it may be true that much (though not all) dental care or "vision care" is functionally separable from other care. If so, it is reasonable to separately consider protection for each of these clusters of care. But most health care involves such an interdependence among component services that it is not realistic to consider each service separately in the assessment of the benefit package. If this is true when protective efficacy is being assessed, it is even more true when broader issues of social utility are evaluated.

A recognition of some of the characteristics of services as they relate to protection against risk is implicit in some of the attempts we have described to rate health insurance plans. For example, Shapiro's proposal that plans be tested for their ability to meet the expenses of caring for important and frequent health problems (such as maternity, myocardial infarction, appendectomy, and cholecystectomy), appears to be based on some awareness of the properties that we call cruciality, lumpiness, and interdependence among services (231). The HPGS scheme developed by Breslow and his aasociates ignores the interdependence of services, but does recognize, without making the rationale explicit, that services differ in importance (232). Under Breslow's scheme, if we assume that maternity services, dental services, psychiatric services, and preventive services belong to separable clusters, then the remaining services are arranged as follows, according to the credit points assigned to plans that provide full payment: hospital room and board, 40; surgical care, 35; hospital services, 30; doctor's hospital calls, 25; hospital diagnostic x-ray and laboratory services, 20; outpatient diagnostic and laboratory services, 20; doctor's office calls, 20; doctor's home calls, 15, anesthetist, 15; prescribed medicines (office or home), 10; and ambulance, 5. By comparison, preventive services are rated 20, and maternity care, psychiatric care, and dental care each receive 15 points, when they are paid in full. Since the reasons for these ratings are not given, the reader is as competent as the author to speculate about what considerations of predictability, magnitude, lumpiness, and cruciality may have gone into the weights proposed.

The weights that are attached to the several benefits in the HPGS rating scheme represent the normative consensus of a group of experts. It is also possible to derive norms in a more empirical manner, from observed behavior under specified assumptions. For example, it could be argued that the use of various services, and the expenditures made for them, are roughly equivalent to their utility and to the importance of including them in a health insurance plan. One might also argue that the average of charges incurred for any service per claim is a measure of the lumpiness of that service. Some combination of these two attributes: total expenditures for each service and average size of claim for each service, might yield a measure of the importance of each service as a component of a benefit package. Another way to measure the perceived importance of a service could be the frequency with which the service appears as a benefit of health insurance plans. This approach was taken by Loebs in developing a measure of state effort under the Medicaid program (233, pp. 94–114). Loebs' measure, an "index of comprehensiveness" of medical benefits, has two components: an "index of coverage" and an "index of scope." The index of coverage is designed to show the extent to which the costs of medical care are met by any Medicaid plan; a value of one is assigned to the average expenditure per eligible person in the state with the highest such expenditure. A decimal fraction represents the average expenditure per eligible person in other states, after corrections are made for price differences among the states. The value of the expenditure per eligible person is itself the product of two terms: the proportion of eligible persons who receive any covered services and the payments on behalf of those persons. Hence, the index of coverage shows the effects of varying and unspecified combinations of access to care and of the amount of care received once access has been achieved.

The index of scope was designed to show how many different services were included as benefits in each state's Medicaid program, taking into account the importance of the services. In 1970, there were 30 optional services under Medicaid, in addition to the 5 mandatory services. The importance of each optional service was considered to be represented by the percent of states that provided that service. The sum of these percentages for each state (one percentage for each service covered) represented the scope of the benefits provided by that state. Since no state provided all the optional benefits, the state with the largest score was taken to have a value of 1 and the scores in all other states were expressed as decimal fractions of this value. The benefits and their relative weights, arranged in order of diminishing value, are shown in Table 43. This ordering, it must be noted, does not take account of differences in the quantities of services covered by each benefit, although it seems plausible that these differences would be related to the notion of importance. The quantity of service for all services combined is, of course, a component of Loebs' index of coverage. Presumably, an analogous score for coverage could have been computed for each service, had the information been available. The index of "comprehensiveness," as computed by Loebs,

TABLE 43. Mandatory Medicaid Benefits and Optional Benefits, Arranged in Diminishing Frequency of Inclusion in State Medicaid Programs, As of January 1, 1970

Benefit	Proportion of States that Provide the Benefit
MANDATORY	
Inpatient hospital services: general hospital	1.00
Outpatient hospital services	1.00
Laboratory and radiology services outside of hospital	1.00
Skilled nursing home services: general	1.00
Physicians' services	1.00
OPTIONAL	
Home health care	0.96
Prosthetic devices other than eyeglasses, dentures and hearing aids	0.93
Transportation: ambulance—emergency	0.90
Services of podiatrists	0.90
Physical therapy	0.88
Prescribed drugs	0.85
Family planning services	0.81
Speech therapy	0.75
Emergency hospital services	0.73
Occupational therapy	0.71
Services of optometrists	0.71
Inpatient hospital services: institutions for mental disease	0.69
Clinic services other than hospital	0.67
Dental services	0.67
Prosthetic devices: eyeglasses	0.65
Early and periodic screening and diagnosis for persons under 21	0.58
Prosthetic devices: dentures	0.58
Inpatient hospital services: institutions for care of tuberculosis	0.56
Transportation: other than ambulance—emergency	0.52
Services of chiropractors	0.46
Prosthetic devices: hearing aids	0.46
Private duty nursing	0.44
Audiology	0.44
Skilled nursing home services: institutions for mental disease	0.40

(continued on next page)

Table 43 (*continued*)

Benefit	Proportion of States that Provide the Benefit
Other diagnostic, screening and preventive services	0.40
Skilled nursing home services: institutions for care of tuberculosis	0.25
Care and services in Christian Science Sanitarium	0.25
Services of licensed practitioners other than podiatrists, chiropractors and optometrists	0.21
Personal care in patients' home	0.15
Services of Christian Science nurse	0.04

Source: Reference 233, Table A4-1, page 298. Originally from U.S. Department of Health, Education and Welfare, Assistance Payments Administration and Medical Services Administration, *Characteristics of State Medical Assistance Programs Under Title XIX of the Social Security Act.* Public Assistance Series, November 49: 1970 Edition; As of January, 1970.

was merely the sum of the two decimal fractions representing coverage and scope. Accordingly, it could theoretically range from 2 to 0. In fact, the scores of comprehensiveness varied from 1.791 for Wisconsin to 0.573 for Louisiana. The components of these scores can be examined to distinguish states that cover fewer services in greater depth from those that cover many more services but cover them less thoroughly.

The construction of methods of measurement such as those proposed by Breslow et al. and by Loebs, no matter how plausibly and ingeniously it is done, leaves many questions unanswered. For example, we do not know what rationale was used by Breslow et al. to arrive at the weighted values they proposed. For the Loebs index, similarly, there is no proof that the importance of benefits is directly proportionate to the frequency with which they are included in state Medicaid programs, or that the scores of coverage and scope should be equally weighted in arriving at a measure of comprehensiveness. While these scales may have some useful properties, they tend to measure indirectly properties that may be subject to a more direct and precise measurement.

The method proposed by Feldstein et al. to study the redistributive effects of alternative health insurance proposals might be extended to provide a direct measure of the degree of protection when the benefits are specified in terms of the services that are included and the quantities of these services that will be provided (217). Let us assume a health plan that covers a very broad range of available services and which pays physicians by salary, so that the clinically most appropriate mix of services is selected, but with due regard for cost. From the experience of this plan it should be possible to obtain the yearly consumption of specified services by individuals and families with given characteristics. The characteristics should include age and sex, at least, since illness and care differ so markedly according to these attributes. After the consumption of services in this plan has been calculated for the clients in each category, and the quantity of services has been specified in physical units as well as dollar amounts, it should be an easy matter to test the extent to which any other plan or insurance policy meets this standard. The standard itself is specified in a manner that takes account of the interrelationships among services, so that the functional integrity of the medical care process is safeguarded. A plan that provides, for any given category of clients, more of any given service than is almost ever needed, while it provides much less than is frequently needed of another service that is a supplement or complement of the first, could be downgraded using some reasonable conventions. The one major aspect of services that escapes assessment under this proposal is cruciality. This is a difficult problem, since the cruciality of a given service is largely a matter of clinical judgment, which must be applied on a case by case basis. It is not inconceivable, however, that a representative sample of services could be rated as to cruciality, at least for the sake of research. If this were done, we would be well on our way to solving the problem of rating the protective efficacy of health insurance proposals. However, the cruciality of services could not be definitively assessed unless there were also a quantifiable measure of the impact on health status of not receiving specified kinds and quantities of care in defined clinical situations. The assessment of insurance is linked to the assessment of the health outcomes that result from receiving or not receiving care, and the latter assessment is itself a subject of active current concern (234 and 1, pp. 136–164).

In the proposal that we have sketched, the standard universe of care was derived from a plan with hypothetical characteristics. Certain prepaid group practice plans may approach this ideal or, to the extent that they place limits on some services, they could provide a clue to the relative perceived importance or cruciality of services. A more purely normative approach to the derivation of the standard universe of care is suggested by the original work of Lee and Jones (235), which has recently been replicated and extended by Falk, Schonfeld, and their associates (236). We have reviewed this work in detail in another publication and a different context: that of deriving estimates of requirements for services and resources (1, pp. 572–622). It seems to us, however, that the information developed by these studies is applicable here also. The key aspect of this work is that expert physicians are asked to estimate the services necessary for "good" care for each of a series of disease and health states. Using these estimates, and given data on the incidence and prevalence of disease states, one can arrive at an estimate of normative service requirements for any specified population (237). No distinctions of cruciality are made, fortunately or unfortunately; in keeping with established medical norms, all the elements of "good" medical care are taken to be equally necessary. A major limitation, for our purposes, is that service requirements are generally stated only as averages for the typical patient. Hence, one does not have the probability distributions, showing the probable needs of different patients, that are a required feature of our standard universe of care. However, the data generated by Falk, Schonfeld et al. do include at least some frequency distributions. From mean values it might be possible to extrapolate the probability distributions of illness, of the quantities of services, or both assuming a Poisson or other plausible shape. However, the precise suitability of the data for our present purpose cannot be determined until they are published in more complete form.

Among the more precise measures of protection (or of its absence) are the probabilities of incurring specified out-of-pocket expenses and the average out-of-pocket expense incurred. If the insurance plan places a limit on the liability of the insured, it is important to know how large this maximun liability is and how frequently it will be reached (216). These three factors are absolute measures of risk. It is also important to assess risk in relation to the ability of the family or the household (depending on how one defines the economically interdependent basic unit) to pay for the costs of care. The usual measure of ability to pay is disposable income, possibly with adjustments for family size and composition. When benefits or out-of-pocket expenses are expressed as a proportion of disposable income, a doubling of income renders benefits, as well as out-of-pocket expenses, relatively half as large. Implicit in this calculation is a hypothesis as to how benefits and risks are viewed as income changes. As Feldstein et al. have pointed out in their study of redistribution, one could postulate some other relationship between costs and ability to pay, such as a quadrupling of the "value" of the same dollar amount of benefits or out-of-pocket expenses as income is halved (217). Another set of considerations arise if one posits that some measure of wealth other than current income is a more appropriate referent in evaluating the relative impact of out-of-pocket expenses. It could be argued that all liquid assets should be available to pay for medical care. One may go further and insist that all the surplus of income, plus all assets beyond those needed to maintain a minimally adequate standard of living, with some minimum reserves, should be available to pay for medical care and should constitute the measure of ability to pay. The reader will recognize this extreme position as the one taken by our public assistance system (238). A somewhat more generous approach would permit a higher standard of living, a larger quantity of reserves that would be immune from the depredations of medical expenditures, and a slower rate of depletion of the remaining assets (239). But these considerations have taken us into an area that more properly belongs under the heading of eligibility for public assistance, a subject we hope to consider in greater detail at some future date.

Stability and Continuity of Protection

The most generous of benefit packages avails the client little if his protection is swept out from under him by the financial collapse of his insurer. Accordingly, the Denenberg *Shopper's Guide* (229) advises the consumer to consult *Best's Insurance Reports* at his local library to determine the rating of the company that proposes to protect him and to select only from among companies that are designated "most substantial" or "very substantial," bypassing those that are merely "substantial" or "considerable"!

But the stability and continuity of the client's protection is more frequently threatened by the terms of the policy itself than by the insurer's instability. Under an outpouring of insurance double-talk, the policy may have taken away with one hand what it may seem to be giving with the other. In this regard, Mayerson has warned that "most health insurance policies are, in form, 1-year contracts, and the absence of a cancellation clause merely guarantees protection for 1 year. Unless this right is specifically stated in the policy, nothing requires the insurer to renew an individual health policy" (240, p. 30). At the anniversary date, the insurer may refuse to renew for any reason, including the fact that the client has been ill and, therefore, needs insurance! If greater candor is desired, this implicit option is made explicit by designating the policy "renewable at the option of the company." But the client's position could be even more precarious if the language of the policy specifies that it is "cancelable"; this means the insurer has the right to cancel at any time, usually on five day's written notice. Needless to say, cancellation occurs just as the client has incurred or is about to incur large medical expenses, so that he is stripped of protection when he needs it most. Fortunately, market competition and state laws have reduced the prevalence of cancelable policies, and the trend has been towards agreements that give the insured a greater degree of protection (240, p. 32).

Various degrees of protection against cancellation, ranging from negligible to appreciable, are offered by policies that are designated "conditionally renewable." If we understand our sources, the distinguishing characteristic of these policies seems to be that they specify the conditions under which a policy may be canceled, and in the absence of which there is a "renewal guarantee." Provided these conditions exclude deterioration in the health of the individual, the client has reasonable assurance of continued protection. The restrictions on cancellation often include the provision that the insurer cannot cancel or refuse to renew an individual's policy, although an entire *class* of policies may be terminated, so that if an individual loses protection it will be in the company of others of his ilk. In a fog of semantic confusion, Dickerson designates such policies "collectively renewable,"

while Mayerson considers them typical of the "conditionally renewable" category (33, pp. 112–113 and 240, pp. 31–32). Still another category of policies, called "guaranteed renewable," specifies
a period of time (for example 5 years, till age 50, or till age 65) during which the policy cannot be terminated for any cause. However, in this type, and in all the other types mentioned so far, the
insurer has the right to change the premium rate for any class of
policy holders. According to Mayerson, "the term noncancelable
is reserved by industry usage and NAIC rule, to policies that guarantee not only the right to renew, but also the right to renew at a
specific premium. For obvious reasons, few if any such policies
include hospital or medical care coverage" (240, p. 32). Thus, the
best that one can usually hope for under voluntary health insurance is a policy that is guaranteed renewable, but with possible
changes in premiums, until age 65, when Medicare should take
over.

It is clear that a precarious state of eligibility is a major factor in
rendering protection equally precarious. Eligibility can be terminated by the insurer when the client becomes too great a liability. The client is also exposed to loss of eligibility because of
unemployment, retirement, or disability (210, Appendix B, pp. 1–7).
Death of the wage-earner also exposes the family to a loss of coverage under group insurance. Finally, a child outgrows, so to speak,
the coverage he enjoys as a member of his family when he ceases
to be a "dependent"; should he suffer from some serious illness,
the purchase of individual insurance could be very difficult. A
major feature of insurance coverage, therefore, is how long the insured and his family are protected under the original policy in situations that could lead to the termination of insurance; whether
insurance can be extended, for how long, and under what terms;
and, finally, whether insurance can be converted so that it can be
carried on an individual basis, and the conditions under which
this is possible. Unfortunately, conversion of coverage from a
group to an individual policy is almost always associated with less
protection at higher cost, because those who choose to continue
coverage are suspected to be at higher risk than those who do not,
in addition to being, on the whole, at higher risk than those who
remain with the original group (241).

Precariousness of protection through instability of eligibility is also a major problem in welfare medical care. Here, eligibility depends partly on the economic status of the client and partly on the occurrence of medical expenditures. Since both of these are likely to fluctuate, there is a group of families who remain for long periods in a twilight zone of possible, but questionable, eligibility (242). Needless to say, this poses no small barrier to rational behavior, both by the individual and by the program.

Value For Money Spent

It is reasonable to assume that clients are concerned about what they receive in benefits as compared to what they pay in premiums. The broader, social aspects of this comparison have been considered under the heading of redistribution and in the notions of equity related to it. A narrower, though by no means unimportant, issue is how much of the premium dollar is "lost" to the client due to the profit margin retained by the insurer, and through the costs of merchandizing and administering the program. The most important distinction, in this regard, is the very low return on individually purchased insurance as compared to insurance available under group contracts. Individual policies, when purchased from insurance companies, are so costly to merchandize and administer that, on the average, they return in benefits little more than 50 cents of the premium dollar—a record of poor performance that has remained constant during the last decade (243, p. 37). Smaller, though appreciable, differences in the returns in benefits relative to premium result from the type of benefits covered by a policy. For example, hospital expenses occur less frequently and in larger bundles than physicians' services, and they involve a relatively smaller number of producers. Hence, the cost of administering insurance that covers hospital expenses is smaller than the cost of administering payments to physicians, especially when the latter is for services outside the hospital. Accordingly, Blue Cross loses less in administrative costs than Blue Shield, and "major medical insurance is regarded as the most costly type of coverage to administer" (243, p. 32). One should remember, however, that high administrative costs are not a necessary feature of comprehensive benefits, unless the benefits are provided in piecemeal fashion through an unorganized, fee-for-service system (245).

Important differences in the return in benefits relative to premium arise from whether insurance is bought individually or in a group, from the nature of the benefits covered, from the nature of the medical care system through which the benefits are provided and paid for, as well as other features of benefit design that may increase administrative costs by requiring verification, recording, and so on. All these factors are correlated with the auspices under which insurance is sold. In addition, insurance companies pay federal and state taxes from which Blue Cross-Blue Shield and other nonprofit plans are exempt. Accordingly, one observes that different categories of insurers make different returns to the consumer, as shown in Table 44. We have already referred to the greater returns under Blue Cross as compared to Blue Shield. The Blues as a whole offer greater returns than the insurance companies, but only because the latter write a great deal of individual insurance. Most advantageous of all to the consumer are the independent plans under employer-employee-union auspices. However, there are only very small differences between these independent plans, group policies under commercial insurance, and Blue Cross and Blue Shield combined. In 1972, claims expense as

TABLE 44. Claims Expense, Operating Expense and Net Underwriting Gain Expressed as Percent of Premium Income, Private Health Insurance Organizations, U.S.A., 1972

Type of Health Insurance	Claims Expense [a]	Operating Expense [a]	Net Underwriting Gain [a]
Blue Cross-Blue Shield	90.6	6.9	2.5
Blue Cross	92.0	5.2	2.8
Blue Shield	87.2	11.3	1.5
Insurance companies	83.6	21.4	−5.0
Group policies	93.3	13.4	−6.7
Individual policies	52.6	47.0	0.4
Independent plans	92.2	7.5	0.3
Community	91.9	6.5	1.6
Employer-employee-union	93.9	7.6	−1.5
Private group clinic	78.5	15.9	5.6
Dental service corporation	86.7	10.2	3.1

Source: Reference 243, Table 13, page 32.
[a] As percent of premium income.

a percent of premium income for these three categories of plans was 93.9, 93.3 and 90.6 percent, respectively. Commercial group plans were able to offer a favorable rate of return even though their operating expenses, on the average, were about twice as high as for the other two categories. In making this return, they incurred an underwriting loss of 6.7 percent of premium income. These losses have occurred every year since 1962, and have tended to increase, from 3.5 percent of premium income in 1962 to 8.9 percent in 1970, with a small decline during the following two years. According to Reed and Carr, losses such as these are made up, in part, from the investment of reserves. But in 1967, when the loss equaled 6.7 percent of premium income, it appeared that these investments were not sufficient to cover the loss, so that "sizable subsidization of group health care coverage by the wage-loss and life insurance business seems indicated" (244, p. 19).

This is the only authentication known to us of the widely held belief that group health insurance is often used as a loss leader to achieve the sale of a larger package of coverage by insurance companies. To the extent that the losses are made up by revenue from other insurance sold to the same group, no transfers are involved. To the extent that this is not true, there are redistributions of undermined degree and direction. Such transfers, as well as differences in other sales procedures, administrative practices, and profit margins, account for the different returns to consumers from comparable policies written by different insurance companies. Since information about these differences is difficult to come by, perhaps the unkindest cut that Denenberg dealt the insurance industry was to publish, in his *Shopper's Guide*, a list of 25 large companies, giving the "loss ratio" for each (229, p. 17). The loss ratio is "the percentage of premiums which a company pays back to its policyholders in benefits." For "hospital, medical, surgical policies, other than noncancellable and collectively renewable" that were bought individually, the rate of return (indicated by the loss ratio) for the 25 insurance companies ranged from 29.8 percent of premium, which is deplorable, to 76.3 percent, which is not too bad. By comparison, the rate of return for 6 Blue Cross or Blue Shield plans in Pennsylvania ranged from 98.8 to 133.6 percent. In all the Blue Cross and Blue Shield plans, purchasers of individual insurance received more in benefits than the sum of their claims plus operating costs. This means that there are transfers from group policies to individual policies under some degree of "community rating."

Finally, in considering value received for money spent, consumers should be concerned about the quality of the goods and services they buy under insurance. To the extent that insurance results in the consumption, for one reason or another, of inferior, unnecessary, and possibly harmful services, the client has received low value for the insurance dollar (218, 246). While consumers are very likely to put a high value on quality in the abstract (247), they are equally likely not to be aware of differences in the technical quality of care they consume, unless it is almost scandalously bad (248, p. 79). This suggests that appropriateness and quality of care are likely to be taken as a near-constant by the general public. However, consumer organizations, such as labor unions, that are involved in the wholesale purchase of insurance, are becoming more sophisticated in this regard, so that the demand for a quality product will be increasingly insistent (249, 250).

Organization-Oriented Objectives

All who participate in the delivery of health services, whether directly through the provision of care or indirectly through financing it, seem to find it socially necessary to give obeisance to client-oriented objectives. They insist that they serve the interests of the client, if not out of altruism at least for reasons of enlightened self-interest. To varying degrees, this may be true, since a sound program is a necessary safeguard to the client. There are, however, other objectives that are of more immediate concern to any organization that pays for health care, whether through insurance or some other arrangement, and whether public or private. These can be described as organization-oriented objectives, even though the organization is, to some extent, mindful of the interests of the client, and the clients, collectively, are mindful of the legitimate interests of the organization.

It takes no originality to perceive that the organization is concerned primarily, and most immediately, with its own survival, integrity, and growth. For public agencies, this requires a sensitive adaptation to their political environments, a subject we shall allude to under another heading. Both public and private agencies must also maintain fiscal integrity; the agency must remain solvent and, where appropriate, make a profit. Fiscal integrity requires that the liabilities be highly predictable and that their magnitude be controlled to some extent. Of the two requirements, predictability is the more important, since, theoretically, anything that can be predicted can be insured against, provided the appropriate premium is charged. However, very expensive health plans are difficult to sell, whether in the political arena or in the market.

Hence, a great deal of attention goes to keeping costs low as well as predictable. Both of these are necessary in order to maintain a competitive advantage over other plans in the marketplace. We find, then, a set of interrelated objectives which we perceive as primarily, though not uniquely, the concern of the plan. These can be briefly designated: solvency; profitability, predictability and control of liabilities; saleability; and competitive advantage. Among these objectives, the need to predict and control the financial liability of the plan occupies an obviously central position. From this need are derived many features of health insurance that seem to work contrary to the clients' equally crucial need for predictable protection. For what is meat to the insurer may be poison to the insured.

This discrepancy in interests arises from something fundamental to insurance, namely, the properties of an "insurable hazard." To paraphrase McIntyre, "conventional insurance theory" has demanded that certain conditions be met before insurance may be offered (209, p. 21). First, the thing insured against must be precisely defined (with respect to identity, time of occurrence, duration, place, etc.) so that there can be no appreciable difference of opinion concerning what it is, or how it is to be measured. Secondly, what is insured against must be something that the client does not want to happen, but which may occur due to circumstances beyond his personal control. In this way, the insurer is protected against willful acts by which the client increases the liability of the insurer. Thirdly, the occurrence of what is insured against for one person must be reasonably independent of its occurrence for others, so that it is unlikely to occur simultaneously among large numbers of insured persons, leading to "incalculable catastrophic loss." Fourthly, the thing insured against must be fairly rare, so that its occurrence is highly unpredictable for any individual during any given period of time, but not so rare that its occurrence cannot be made highly predictable to the insurer when a reasonably large number of insured persons are taken as a group. The thing insured against must be unpredictable to the individual because losses that are very likely to occur can be handled by budgeting; but it must be predictable in groups of insured persons because, otherwise, the insurer is in danger of incurring large losses.

The key concept that gathers all these stipulations into one meaningful whole is that an insurable hazard must be a precisely defined, relatively rare event, as close to being truly random as possible, so that it can be actuarially predicted by applying the laws of probability. This is the basic theoretical requirement. An additional, more pragmatic, stipulation is that the thing insured against must represent a significant loss to the client and the cost of insuring against it must be reasonable. It is difficult to sell insurance unless its cost, in absolute terms as well as relative to the magnitude of the loss, makes sense to the consumer.

The requirements that we have described obviously raise serious questions about the insurability of medical care expenses. In many instances, the thing insured against cannot be precisely defined because of imperfections in medical knowledge and because of great variability in the methods and costs of treatment. Mental illness is an excellent example of this uncertainty. Occurrences of illness are not independent; some illnesses do occur in epidemic or even pandemic forms. Perhaps even more important, although illness is largely involuntary and undesirable, the consumption of health services is voluntary, desirable and, worst of all, influenced by having insurance. Finally, many medical care expenses are small and recurrent, so that handling them through insurance is relatively costly and inefficient, unless the delivery system is reorganized. It is no wonder then that the insurance companies had to be "half-dragged, half-lured" into the field of health insurance, which they entered in significant numbers only after Blue Cross and Blue Shield had made a go of it (251). But, having entered the field of medical care, the commercial insurers used a variety of devices to make what was insured against conform to the requirements of an insurable hazard and, to the extent that this was not possible, to protect themselves against the consequences.

The devices used by the insurers are easy to enumerate and describe. They are more difficult to classify in conceptually meaningful fashion because of the interrelationships that permit any given device to serve a variety of purposes. We shall try to describe these devices in an orderly fashion and say enough to give the reader a feel for the subject, but no more, since there are a number of standard texts in which these features of health insurance are exhaustively (and exhaustingly) described (33, 252). We perceive the insurance agency taking action to control its liabilities by first defining the thing insured against as precisely as possible. Secondly, precautions are taken to reduce the non-randomness and bias introduced primarily by volitional acts of clients in the purchase of insurance, in the occurrence of the peril, and in the use of service after insurance is purchased. Finally, there are a set of devices used by insurers that can be perceived as controls over any residual degree of unpredictability as well as over high costs in general. In all this, attention is focused on protecting the insurer. The consequences to the insured, usually in the form of reduced protection, receive scant attention, if any.

The thing insured against may be defined by a series of successive specifications: first, of the "peril" that causes the loss; second, of the loss itself; and third, of the benefit that the insurer undertakes to provide relative to the loss incurred by the insured. Certain perils are so ambiguous that they are either excluded or are covered only subject to formidable restrictions. Mental illness is a good example in the field of health insurance. In the more traditional field of accident insurance there is much difficulty in defining an accident and determining whether a distinction should be made, or indeed can be made, between an accidental injury and an injury by accidental means. For the former, all that needs to be established is that there has been an unusual and unexpected injury as the result of some activity or event. But for the latter, it is necessary to exclude any nonaccidental factors either in the injury or the event that caused it. If this second approach is adopted, the concern of the insurer is to exclude preexisting or subsequent nonaccidental factors (such as illness or disability) related to the injury, as well as any injuries that were either intended by the insured or that he should have anticipated. It would seem that sufficiently searching examination would reveal something nonaccidental in almost every accident, or in its consequences, so that the insurer need rarely pay! Equally bemusing sophistries are encountered in the definition of "disability" and the losses that it produces, an important aspect of insurance, but one we shall not pursue.

The losses in health insurance are expenditures for medical care, and the benefits are the contributions made by the insurer towards meeting these losses. It is not always easy to define the loss and, therefore, the benefit pertaining to it. Consider, for example, how a hospital can be distinguished from a nursing home or, more difficult still, a "skilled" nursing home from any other; how certain kinds of dentistry are to be distinguished from oral surgery; what constitutes a surgical operation; whether two or more surgical procedures are stages of one operation or constitute several separate operations; and under what circumstances, for purposes of insurance, a second hospital admission is considered a continuation of a preceding one rather than a new episode. These and similar matters are of considerable importance to the traditional insurance approach, and they must be carefully specified in the insurance policy (235, pp. 468–473). Needless to say, the quantity of the benefit must also be carefully specified. If they can be specified in dollar amounts, so much the better for the insurer, since uncertain changes in price need not enter the actuarial calculus.

A second set of constraints introduced into the field of health insurance are intended to assure that those who are insured are similar to the hypothetical reference population used in computing premiums. One way in which a difference might arise is that those who expect to use the benefits of insurance are more likely to buy it. In insurance language this is called "adverse selection" or "antiselection" because, unless it is recognized and corrected for, it introduces errors in prediction that mean loss to the insurer. But, from a broader social perspective, this behavior, far from being "adverse," is both rational and laudable. It is unfortunate, therefore, that it should carry such a pejorative label. But whether we call it "adverse selection" or merely "noncongruence," it is most likely to be present when insurance is purchased on an individual basis, it is progressively less likely to pose a problem when insurance is bought by groups of increasingly larger size, and it is totally absent when there is universal coverage—unless distinctions among population subgroups continue to be maintained.

As a result of efforts by insurers to control adverse selection, the purchase of insurance by individuals is most encumbered by restrictions. The purpose of the restrictions is to control those characteristics of the beneficiary that increase the likelihood of being ill or the propensity to use service in the event of illness. Characteristics that are taken into account include age, sex, occupation, habits, and, directly or indirectly, race (33, pp. 463–474). Females are generally recognized to be more likely to use services. Certain occupations are conducive to illness or injury, while persons in other occupations are thought to be predisposed to excessive utilization or, in some cases, to fraudulent claims by virtue of their association with "low moral standards." Insurers recognize the crucial role of health status by obtaining data on height and weight, on familial illness, and on the applicant's past and present·health. In some instances a medical certificate may be required, or the applicant may be asked to submit to a medical examination.

But, since excessive rigor in underwriting discourages sales, it is more usual to introduce restrictions in the benefits themselves. Very frequently there are waiting periods following the acquisition of insurance, during which benefits are omitted or restricted. Equally frequent is the exclusion of preexisting conditions, which are diseases present at the time insurance is purchased. The presence of an early pregnancy or the purchase of maternity benefits in anticipation of a planned pregnancy is particularly subject to restrictions. Finally, as we have described earlier, the insurer may seek protection by reserving the options to cancel the policy or to refuse to renew it, either for an individual or for a category of individuals. Needless to say, to the extent that the provisions of the policy limit this option, the insurer will, accordingly, increase the rigor of the underwriting process. At the extreme, this process will involve the amassing of considerable information concerning the private affairs of individuals. In addition to statements made by the applicant and by the agent who wishes to sell him insurance, the insurer may conduct, or have conducted, an "inspection" which may involve checks on police and credit records, as well as more direct "inquiries in the neighborhood of the applicants' home or at his place of employment" (33, p. 560). Similar information may be available from other insurance companies under mutual agreements. Information may also be obtained from agencies that specialize in collecting and selling information to insurance companies, credit agencies, and the like. In addition to being a serious threat to privacy, such procedures add considerably to the cost of acquiring individual insurance, so that the returns in benefits are, as we have seen, very low compared to the premium charged.

Selling insurance to one person at a time is costly, besides being conducive to self-selection by the insured in a manner adverse to the insurer. As a result, a great deal of health insurance is sold under group policies. The insurer may take his first small step towards seeking safety in numbers through the practice of declaring "enrollment periods"—specified limited periods of time during which individuals may enroll while the insurer relaxes some of his precautions against the consequences of self-selection. The second, and much more important, step is the resort to "group insurance." This stipulates, in essence, that there be a group that is definable by virtue of some social affinity among its members other than that of purchasing insurance. To the extent that membership in the socially-defined group is itself dependent on the possession and maintenance of a reasonable level of health, so much the better for the insurer. The most usual group, and one that is particularly favorable to the insurer, is the employee group. However, there has been a tendency to extend the bases for grouping to include entities such as a labor union (with the union as policy holder), a creditor-debtor group (in which the policy is held by a bank, a finance company, a credit union, or even a retailer), and a variety of professional, fraternal, and other associations (254). In fact, the availability of group insurance of various kinds has become a favorite device for recruiting people and holding them in social aggregates—a practice that reintroduces the menace of self-selection, which grouping was supposed to avoid. The insurer must, therefore, be watchful that the group is a genuine, socially-defined entity and does not become predominantly a front for the collective purchase of insurance by individuals who either cannot be insured or can only obtain insurance as individuals under much less favorable terms. The careless or fraudulent recognition of groups for insurance purposes also poses a threat to some of the insured members, and is considered unfair competition to the individual sale of insurance. In consequence, most states regulate the definition of a group and any other conditions that must be satisfied before insurance may be purchased and sold on a group basis (240, 255). While such regulation offers reasonable safeguards, it can also be unnecessarily restrictive, so that access to group insurance is not open to many who might legitimately benefit from it (256).

As we have emphasized, a major safeguard in law as well as insurance practice is the stipulation that the group have a primary basis for membership other than the purchase of insurance. But this does not preclude the selection of members in a manner adverse to the insurer, especially in the smaller groups. Accordingly, a number of additional safeguards are usually in force (254). For example, there ought to be a flow of persons into and out of the group so that its characteristics remain reasonably constant. In the absence of this flow, the group is subject to the effects of aging and the other changes that we have considered under the rubric of seasoning. In order to minimize adverse selection within the group, a specified minimum proportion of employees (and of dependents, if these are covered) may be required to enroll. A further safeguard is for the employer to pay the entire premium or at least a significant part of it. This makes enrollment in the group "automatic," or as removed from the calculating, as possible, and discourages the selective withdrawal of those who find they do not use the benefits enough to justify the premiums. A reciprocal relationship may be established between the proportion of the premium paid by the employer and the proportion of employees who must enroll if the group is to qualify as a whole; the smaller the former is, the higher the latter will be (255, p. 86). Almost always, there is the additional requirement that all new employees (or new members of a nonemployee group) must enroll within a short period after joining the group. If they do not enroll within this period, enrollment is possible only during open enrollment periods, occurring once or twice a year. In addition to these controls on enrollment, benefits are specified and uniform for the entire group, or for categories within the group, so that adverse selection is as controlled in the choice of benefits as it is in the prior decision to enroll.

In all of this, the size of the group is a major and pervasive influence. State laws specify the minimum size of a group, although the permissible lower limit has become smaller over the years (255). Furthermore, as the size of the group grows smaller, the controls on adverse selection become increasingly stringent; in the vicinity of 5 or 10 members the controls become similar to those used in individual insurance. As we have said, the smaller the group the higher the proportion of members who must enroll before the group can qualify as a whole. In the smaller groups, the legitimacy of the group itself becomes an important question; it may be necessary to conduct inquiries on a sample of members to make sure, for example, that they are bona fide employees, and that a relative or friend of the owner has not been ostensibly added to the payroll only or mainly to make it possible for him to buy insurance. In the smallest groups it may be necessary to require that every member be enrolled and to add features such as medical questionnaires, exclusion of preexisting conditions, and waiting periods before insurance becomes effective (257, pp. 368–370). There is a striking contrast between the treatment of small groups and large groups. Furthermore, according to Pettengill, a group of 500 or more employees can be experience-rated by itself, so that it may be possible to determine the value of a given cost control procedure, which can be waived if the group wishes to pay an additional premium (253, p. 455).

A final set of controls on selective enrollment pertain to members who have severed their relationship with the group, usually because of retirement or loss of employment, and with or without attendant disability or ill health. Under these circumstances, original coverage may continue to be effective for only a specified period of time, after which the former group member may have the option to convert to individual insurance, with or without evidence of insurability, and subject to reduced benefits, an increase in premium, or both (253, pp. 459–461).

The third line of defense against unpredictable costs, as well as undesirably high costs, is to limit the tendency of those who have insurance to claim the benefits. For this tendency the insurers have another disapproving term: "moral hazard," a concept that has been discussed in an earlier chapter. In common usage, the distinction between moral hazard and adverse selection is not always clear, since moral hazard, while universal in some degree, is seen to be especially strong in persons with certain habits or in certain walks of life (33, pp. 463 ff). If so, then to insure persons who are particularly prone to moral hazard would represent adverse selection. There is at least an element of social value in moral hazard, as in adverse selection, since the social purpose of health insurance is, in part, to facilitate access to care. But from the point of view of the underwriter, anything that enhances the probability or the magnitude of the loss, or renders it less predictable, must be seen as a hazard rather than as a possibly desirable consequence. Perhaps we could prevail upon the underwriter to be less moralistic and more descriptive by calling it utilization hazard, or something to that effect.

The concept of moral hazard, is based on the notion that, while everyone having insurance is more likely to use services, the tendency is much stronger for certain people, under certain conditions, and under certain features of insurance benefits. The controls on moral hazard are both general and selective. The general controls are designed to curb excessive utilization by everyone who is insured; examples are deductibles and coinsurance. Selective controls focus on particular situations or groups of people. Among the selective controls are restrictions, and adjustments to the enrollment of those who are considered to be particularly prone to claim benefits, by virtue of habits, occupation or past insurance record. Pre-existing conditions may be excluded, along with diseases or injuries deliberately caused by the insured; waiting periods may be imposed before benefits become effective, partly to discourage those who want to buy insurance because they have an imminent need for care and those who are considered likely to defraud the plan. Under group insurance, it is generally recognized that workers who are laid off, or who are on strike, are much more likely to use service; so the insurer must either limit benefits during such periods, or add to the premium if benefits are to be maintained (253, p. 460).

The possession of multiple or duplicatory insurance policies is feared by insurers as a particularly potent inducement to moral hazard, since it raises the specter of the beneficiary's actually making a profit from insurance. The validity of this fear has been considered in a previous chapter; the remedy is a "coordination-of-benefits" agreement among insurers, which specifies an orderly procedure for assuming liability when more than one policy is in force, and which assures that benefits received by the client do not exceed the allowable expenses incurred. According to Dickerson, "the order of attachment of coverage involves primary coverage taking precedence over dependent; dependent coverage based on a male worker taking precedence on a female worker; and otherwise, attachment in the order of the time coverage commenced" (33, p. 213). Pettengill describes an "allowable expense" as "any necessary, reasonable and customary item of expense, at least a portion of which is covered under one of the specified plans insuring the person for whom claim is made" (253, p. 463). Under these terms, according to Pettengill, "much of the over-insurance hazard is completely removed . . . and the balance is under control" (253, p. 464).

The coordination of benefits plan is a specific example of the general principle that the benefit must rarely, if ever, be equal to the expenses incurred by the client. Insurance is considered unsound unless the client shares in the expense (33, p. 549). The provision of benefits is, therefore, always less than complete. Deductibles and coinsurance are a particular and highly visible expression of this general principle, and they enjoy almost universal support as safeguards against moral hazard.

The controls on adverse selection and moral hazard are indirect, in the sense that they operate on or through the client. But the unit primarily responsible for consumption, subject to a variety of external influences, is the client-physician dyad. The concept of moral hazard seems to discreetly ignore the contributions of the incompetent, careless, overly-accommodating, or venal physician. No doubt this is partly because the insurance companies have had negligible leverage on the practice of medicine and have not sought more. Blue Cross and Blue Shield may have greater influence, but not by much. Large public programs have the potential, through legislation for even more influence than the Blues. There has been a slowly developing methodology, and a gradually awakening social resolve, to exercise a greater degree of public control over the practice of medicine, so that quality and appropriate utilization may be assured. To pursue these developments would be to reopen a large, new area which we have already explored in another publication (103). What is more germane here is to note that should these direct public controls be successfully implemented, the need for the traditional insurance controls might no longer exist.

The insurer has a fourth set of defenses against unpredictability and high costs; those defenses can be seen as the final, definitive safeguards when all the preceding checks have failed to contain the threat. One of these is the placing of a dollar limit on the liability the insurer has for each person or for each family, during a specified benefit period. This is a common practice in major medical or catastrophic expense insurance. Needless to say, this limitation leaves the insured to his own devices at the time when he is most likely to need protection against further large expenditures. In purpose and effect, it is the precise opposite to the proposal that there be a limit on the liability of the *insured*, so that, after he has incurred reasonably large out-of-pocket expenses, any further expenses will be met by the insurance plan (109, 216). The clients' protection and the insurer's liability is even more sharply terminated by the cancellation of an individual policy, usually on a few day's notice, when it becomes apparent that a great deal of care is being used. The insurer may also refuse to renew, under various provisions that are somewhat less sudden, but equally final.

Another remedy against unpredicted high cost, which is open to provider-sponsored plans such as Blue Cross and Blue Shield, is a provision for "proration." Under this provision, participating physicians and hospitals agree to proportionate reductions in their charges should the resources of the plan fail to equal its obligations. This means that if something goes badly wrong, the physicians and hospitals will bear the loss, in effect. A final safeguard, open to all plans that insure large groups, is to be found in the experience rating practices that approximate a cost-plus arrangement: in this case, the insurer passes on to the insured group both the losses and the savings that result from any discrepancy between actual losses and predicted losses.

All of these provisions are calculated to safeguard the insurer, first against unpredictable loss, and then against a large amount of loss, even if predictable. As Dickerson points out in his discussion of underwriting: "The agent should endeavor to develop a market where he will find good risks, free of moral hazard, and in good physical condition, and of substantial financial strength" (33, p. 561). This is in keeping with the social function of private insurance, which is to offer protection against moderately large expenditures to those who are generally well and self-supporting. But it is a far cry from the social need to gather in the sick, the halt, and the poor of the world so that they may receive the care that they so desperately need. In pointing out the chasm that separates these two orientations it is not my intent to fault private insurance for not doing what it was not meant to do. My intent is, first, to brush away any illusions about the primary objectives of the insurance industry and, second, to point out how much more remains for the public sector to do. But whether a program is public or private the need for predictability and cost control remain essential objectives of the organization. What may differ is the means used to attain these objectives and the remedies available should the agency under-estimate the magnitude of its obligations.

Provider-Oriented Objectives

In our discussion of organization-oriented objectives, we noted that everyone is ostensibly committed to serving the client and everyone pays at least lip service to his interests. If this is true of the financing organization, it is even more true of the providers, whom society has entrusted with a fiduciary interest in the welfare of its members. We shall try to reach beyond the actual and alleged altruism and the interests they share with their patients, to tap those motivations that are more selfish and more specifically "provider-oriented." In doing so, we shall have in mind physicians and other professional providers, in particular. However, much that is said about physicians is also likely to be applicable to institutional providers, especially, but not exclusively, those organized for profit. Much of what is said will be tentative; the data that bear on our subject are so sparse and so widely dispersed that a definitive review would enlarge this project beyond its rather modest scope. We shall confine ourselves, therefore, to what might be regarded as reasonable speculation and extrapolation, based on partial knowledge.

The providers' first objective, in regard to insurance, would seem to be to have their services included among the benefits of any plans. The providers know that prepayment generates demand for more and better service, that payment to the provider is more certain, and that there are likely to be better prospects for raising prices. However, the pressure for inclusion would vary depending on a number of conditions. Providers who are very busy taking care of patients who can pay for their own care may not have an intense desire for inclusion, even though additional purchasing power would offer the prospect of higher prices, resulting in either greater revenue or more leisure. Inclusion is more ardently sought if the demand is low relative to the potential capacity to produce services, and particularly if poor patients who cannot be refused service account for a great deal of care. Since these attributes of supply and demand may vary by specialty and location, it is not surprising to find differences in the extent to which providers favor the extension of benefits. Thus, general practitioners in rural areas are more likely to support programs for low-income people than are specialists in urban practice.

For those in certain marginal occupations, such as chiropractors, inclusion in a public or quasi-public program signifies a degree of recognition and legitimation which has far reaching consequences. No wonder, then, that for marginal providers, inclusion becomes an object of intense political activity. The contrary phenomenon, concerted political pressure against inclusion, occurs when a proposed public program is seen as a threat to the autonomy and economic interest of an established profession, such as medicine, or to a category of institutions, such as hospitals. But their objection is not to inclusion itself so much as to the terms of inclusion. These terms are so important that the remaining provider-oriented objectives that we will consider will pertain exclusively to them.

Perhaps the most important objective providers have in setting the terms of inclusion is that there be no interference in the social organization and the established modes of practice of their profession. They want the option to be included without any compulsion to participate. A corollary objective is that the profession retain, and even expand, its control over the process of care and its economic and professional rewards. Ideally, the providers want to exploit the new demand for their services as they see fit. Accordingly, one would expect that physicians would insist on the most generous possible benefits so that they could prescribe or provide whatever services are needed by their patients and are professionally and economically rewarding to themselves. Strangely enough, this is not always the case. Physicians are not always averse to some limits on benefits, including deductibles and co-payments, even though these may constrain their own freedom to prescribe what they want. This may be, in part, because the release of the patient from all direct financial obligations is apt to make him more assertive, so that the ascendancy that the physician so jealously guards in his relationship with his patient would be in danger of being undermined. The power to exact payment appears necessary to the authoritarian mode.

A more important reason for the physicians' acquiescence in benefit limits could be that out-of-pocket payments are not likely to be limited to by provisions of a plan, and they offer an opportunity for revenue above what the plan itself has undertaken to pay. Some cynics have suggested that out-of-pocket payments are also easier to conceal from the pryings of the tax examiner. Physicians could have other reasons; like the rest of us, they are imbued with the ethic of personal responsibility, and are offended by the notion that the plan allows a "free ride" to some people, especially if the plan is tax supported. Their repugnance is intensified, no doubt, if the beneficiaries are seen as inherently less worthy by reason of poverty or other attributes that denote a lack of personal achievement or worth. Furthermore, since such people are less desirable as patients, impediments to their access to care can be viewed with equanimity, except where they are the only patients available.

Issues of remuneration, however disguised, are fundamental to the provider; control over the price of his services is paramount. Where complete control is not possible, the provider seeks as much influence over the setting of prices as the plan can be persuaded or pressured to allow. One feature that is sought is the option to make charges beyond the standard benefit allowed by the plan. This may be justified as an adjustment to the client's ability to pay or as a necessary requirement of an equitable system of rewards. Physicians are likely to contend that the lower fees that they have accepted for the less affluent beneficiaries of the plan are discounted prices, and that their regular, and more equitable, fees are those they charge the more affluent. If so, charging a higher fee to those who can pay permits the physician to accommodate the less affluent members of the plan. Needless to say, the option to levy extra charges according to the patient's ability to pay also allows the physician to improve his revenue by exacting a payment nearer the limit of what each patient is prepared to pay

(258). As we have pointed out, it also allows the physician to discourage those whom he does not wish to serve and to control those whom he does accept.

When individual physicians set the prices for their own services there is a presumption of equitability, in that higher prices are charged for more valued services. Beyond that, physicians seem willing to accept the market's judgment of what their services are worth, since this permits them to raise prices as long as they can find enough patients willing to pay. To the extent that the plan interferes with the ability of the physician to set his own fees, and test them in the market, issues of equitable remuneration assume great prominence for physicians. They demand a system that recognizes, among other distinctions, the qualifications of the physician, his experience, his effort, and his other inputs into care; the inconvenience he suffers due to peculiarities of time, place, or other factors in the delivery of service; the practitioner's investment in his practice and the geographic differences affecting general price levels and the balance of supply and demand. Physicians also want a payment system that allows the patient to have a free choice of physician and that provides prompt payment directly to the provider with a minimum of red tape. The possibility that charges might be disallowed after services have been given is particularly painful to professionals and institutions alike; sharing in the liabilities of the plan, through prorated reductions in revenue, is another feature assiduously to be avoided.

Abel-Smith has pointed out that, in addition to rational calculations, tradition seems to be a major determinant in the preference of physicians for one system over another: "Doctors often become attached to the system by which they are paid." In France they become attached to fee-for-service, in England to capitation, and in Israel to salary; "On the whole, doctors seem to like best the system to which they have become accustomed" (259). Nevertheless, some methods of payment are recognized to be more favorable to the physician than other methods, so that, as physicians have become more organized and politically effective, they have been able to obtain progressively better terms for their participation. "Each settlement with a government has been on terms more favorable than the last—from salary, to capitation, to fee-for-service, to reimbursement, to formal systems of price discrimination with published income classes" (259, p. 33). If this is true, the reader will recognize that the method of paying physicians under Medicare is the most favorable to the physician, short of reimbursing anything on demand. Under Medicare's system of "customary" and "prevailing" charges, individual physicians essentially determine their own rates of remuneration, as long as they are in reasonable step with the rest of their colleagues. The further option to accept or reject "assignment" on a case by case basis removes any limits on what the physician may collect from the patient, even though the plan will only pay the "reasonable" charge (260). It is no wonder that, in spite of serious initial reservations, a large proportion of physicians have become favorably disposed towards Medicare (261).

Collectivity-Oriented Objectives

Collectivity-oriented objectives are those that are meant to preserve the social system and its values. They serve the public interest rather than the narrower aims of the organization, the provider, or, even, subgroups of clients.

The most cursory review of the objectives of clients, providers and financing agencies reveals not only mutual interests, but also disagreements, the latter ranging from differences in emphasis to bitter conflict. It follows that society, through its legitimate institutions, must play the mediating role, balancing interest against interest to arrive at some compromise that seems acceptable, or at least tolerable, to all.

Fashioning this compromise is one aim of the collectivity. Some say it is the only one; others would contend that there is more to the notion of the public interest than mutual accommodation among partially or wholly divergent interests. They would hold that, at the collective level, the perspective is so different that a new set of social purposes and priorities emerge as guides to action. In this sense, we have said that public policy relevant to benefits in medical care programs has two objectives: to provide the public with financial protection against medical care expenditures that threaten economic security and to improve the production and distribution of health services and their benefits. We have conducted our analysis, so far, in the light of these two partly overlapping, but also partly diverging, objectives. In this concluding section we will recapitulate and round out our major themes, so that we can assess where we have been and in what directions we are likely to move.

Protection Against Unpredictable Expenses

The quest for protection has already been discussed in considerable detail from the vantage point of the client. We have suggested that clients face the prospect of either not receiving care and bearing the consequences, or of receiving care but at the cost of reducing their customary standard of living, depleting their financial reserves, incurring debts, or subjecting themselves to the indignity of receiving public assistance. What is sought in a health care plan is protection against being caught on the horns of this dilemma. From the social perspective, the major issues are whether a certain minimum degree of protection must be specified in order for a health plan to be acceptable, what this minimum should be, what, if anything, should be done to assure it, and for whom it should be assured. These issues are at least implicit in the formulation of public programs, as can be seen in the current debate on national health insurance and on the welter of proposals it has generated. But, in the private sector, the laissez-faire tradition remains supreme, so that the buyer must look out for himself with little legal protection. As Myerson has pointed out: "state law has been almost silent on the question of whether the benefits offered by individual health insurance policies are adequate to meet the needs of the policyholder. . . . The absence of such standards, coupled with widespread ignorance of the true cost of hospitalization and doctor's bills, has permitted some insurers to issue policies that can by no stretch of the imagination be considered as meeting the policyholder's coverage needs" (240, pp. 34, 35). In response to this situation, some states have adopted legislation that specifies minimum benefits and places limits on the cancellation of coverage. In addition, the Blue Cross and Blue Shield plans have regulated their own behavior by establishing minimum standards for themselves. According to Reed and Carr: "The American Hospital Association's approval program for hospital service plans requires that 'a plan shall cover on behalf of all member patients an average of not less than 75 percent of the total amount billed for usual and customary services rendered on an inpatient basis in multiple bed accommodations in contracting hospitals.' At a meeting of representatives of all plans in October 1968, the National Association of Blue Shield Plans amended its approval standards to require that 'each active member plan shall make available a paid-in-full program based upon the usual, customary and reasonable charges of physicians' " (244, pp. 20, 21).

In the formulation of public policy, more explicit consideration of the degree of protection has no doubt been hampered by the absence of a clearly formulated conceptual framework for the assessment of benefits. Such a framework would yield a reasonably precise and acceptable measure of the protective efficacy of alternative proposals. Without it, although we have descriptive information about the benefits proposed and very rough estimates of their cost, we have very little information about the degree of protection they provide. In some instances, this leads to the consideration of proposals that might reduce rather than augment the protection that is currently afforded to certain segments of the population (262).

The usual measure of protection that is used in public debate is the fraction of expenditures that is covered by a plan, whether private health insurance or some other form of third party payments. In assessing this measure, one must be careful to distinguish whether the denominator of the fraction is only medical care expenditures for services covered by the plan, or total medical care expenditures, including those for services that are not covered. Many insurance policies pay only a small share of the expenditures that are incurred for the services included as benefits. Even when the policy pays a very high percentage of the expenditures for covered services, it may pay a small proportion of the expenditures for *all* services, if few services are included as benefits.

Hospital benefits are the most usual feature of private health insurance. In 1972, 78 percent of consumer expenditures for hospital care were met by such insurance, compared to only 45 percent of consumer expenditures for physician's services, and an even smaller 42 percent of consumer expenditures for all health services (243, p. 38). Needless to say, public programs supplement and complement the protection offered by private health insurance, especially for the aged and the poor. As a result, only 35 percent of personal health expenditures in 1972 were paid directly by the consumer, while 37 percent were paid by federal and state government programs, 26 percent by private health insurance, and 2 percent by philanthropy and industry (263, p. 13).

These data raise several questions. One is whether a larger proportion of the protection that is now available should be provided under public rather than private auspices, and whether this protection should be provided in the form of insurance rather than some other basis for entitlement. This is a question of far-reaching importance but it does not concern us here; our focus is on the benefits themselves, irrespective of the auspices of the plan or the basis for eligibility. Our immediate concern is with a second question, whether it is a socially satisfactory situation to have 63 percent of personal health expenditures paid through insurance or public programs, and 37 percent paid out-of-pocket. The answer is that we do not know, partly because there is no consensus on what would be socially desirable partitioning of total expenditures between prepayment and direct payment. According to McNerney, "Excluding nonprescription drugs, cosmetic elements, and various nonessentials from the concept of the medical-care dollar, probably we will and should approach 80 percent [coverage] before the 1970's are very old" (256, pp. 57–58). But other authorities have advocated 67 percent, 90 percent or, even 100 percent; so, depending on what magic figure we adopt, we have either almost attained our objective or are a long way from it (264, p. 8). But even if we had already arrived at some social consensus concerning our goal, it is doubtful that we could state it simply as an average percentage of expenses covered. Any average value conceals a range of individual experiences, and it is necessary to see these in more detail in the form of a frequency distribution. More fundamentally, the degree of protection needs to be related, in some measure, to the ability to pay. What is an appropriate measure of the ability to pay is itself a matter for social determination. We must ask ourselves what percent of income, or of some other specified measure of wealth, should be allocated to medical care in the form of premiums, taxes, or direct payments. Average values are not enough; if we are truly committed to maintaining the economic and social integrity of all families at all times, there must be, for each class of income or ability to pay, a limit beyond which no further payments are exacted no matter how large medical expenses may become (216).

Production and Distribution of Health

We have postulated that a major objective, or class of objectives, pursued by the collectivity is the production and distribution of what we have called "health potential," which is the health status of individuals over a life time. The primary objective could be either generating the largest total increment of health potential, irrespective of its social distribution, or increasing health potential equally in all social classes, or achieving equal health potential in all social classes (2, p. 108). For each of these objectives there is a corresponding disposition of access to care, and appropriate health benefits are the key to achieving the desired level and social distribution of access. Thus, health benefits are a means to access, and access is a necessary, though not sufficient, means to health. But the restructuring of access in the pursuit of health opens up a set of concerns about equity, the efficiency of production, the efficiency of allocation, the integrity of the medical care process, and the quality of care. All of these are vital considerations to those who would restructure the medical care system itself in the design of health benefits. But, even those who have the more modest objective of providing financial protection cannot avoid these considerations. Whether we recognize it or not, the provision of benefits affects the use of service and the price, and these have profound consequences for the system as a whole.

We see, then, that at the level of the collectivity there must be concern for the entire range of issues that we have enumerated, whether the primary motivation is financial protection or the more fundamental reorganization of the medical care system. The difference, if there is any, is that from the narrower viewpoint of financial protection the effects of benefits on aspects of the medical care system—such as price, access, equity, quality, and efficiency—are seen as constraints on the achievement of protection, whereas, in the broader perspective of reorganizing the system, they are considered as objectives in their own right (265).

Equity

The concern for equity, as an objective, arises because those who are furthest behind in health status and, therefore, most in need of additional health services, are the least able to pay for these services. Hence, if health services are to be provided according to socially defined need, purchasing power must be transferred; and a collective decision must be made about the magnitude of these transfers as well as the means for achieving them. With respect to the means, we have seen that a competitive system of voluntary health insurance tolerates only limited transfers, achieved through community rating. Transfers of the required magnitude are possible only under some system of taxation, however it is disguised.

Efficiency of Production and Allocation

Achieving a high level of efficiency in the production and allocation of health services is obviously an objective of compelling force. It is also one that opens up enormous complexities of technical design and political management; inefficiencies flow from many sources, and their containment may require politically unpalatable remedies. At the most fundamental level, it could be said that prepayment itself, for all its advantages, introduces some degree of inefficiency by adding the cost of managing the prepayment system to the cost of producing care. These administrative costs are themselves related to the way clients are enrolled (for example, whether individually or in groups), the method of financing (through taxes or premiums), the nature of the benefits (for example, whether inpatient or outpatient), and the manner in which providers are reimbursed (for example, by fee-for-service or capitation). The containment of administrative costs is not simply a matter of managerial know-how, but also involves specifications of system design, the implementation of which depends on the social and political realities of the situation. The method of financing influences efficiency, partly because of its ease or difficulty of administration, and partly because of the "dead weight loss" that occurs from the distorting effect of taxation in a market economy. For the latter reason, Feldstein has suggested that an important objective of a national health scheme would be to avoid a large increase in the tax burden (216). This, of course, may also be the politically expedient thing to do. But the decision to use tax funds, and which particular taxes to tap, involves many additional considerations; not least among them is the effect on equity (201, pp. 151–158).

Closer to the level of production, we have seen that, unless the benefit package is properly designed, physicians, with the concurrence of their patients, could be encouraged to use more expensive substitutes for less expensive but equally effective services. One objective of benefit design should be, therefore, to encourage the use of less costly but still effective services. In part, this is a function of the range of services that are included as benefits; and in part, it depends on how the delivery of care is organized and paid for. Certain modes of organization and payment (for example, group practice or a health maintenance organization) may be more conducive to the efficient production and application of services (58, 59); if so, a choice must be made at the collective level: whether to offer inducements, through preferential treatment, that would encourage the development of the more efficient modes. Here again, technical merit is only one element in a decision that has pervasive political implications.

Inefficiencies in allocation are said to result when a lowering of the price of service at the point of consumption leads to the use of additional services that the consumer would not buy if he were paying the full price out-of-pocket (218, 246). These services are not considered to be worth the price; however, through the intermediacy of the prepayment program, consumers, individually or collectively, do pay the full price for all the services they use. In this way a consumer spends, as it were, with his left hand what he would not have spent with his right, and obtains less total satisfaction than he would if he had an equal sum of money to spend according to his own preferences. The reduction in the sum total of satisfaction under this formulation, is considered to be a "welfare loss" to individuals and to society.

As Pauly recognizes, and takes great pains to expound in a formal economic analysis, the welfare cost, or loss, is reduced to the extent that the additional services that are received under prepayment are valued at full price by society, even if they are not so valued by the consumer (3, 246). He concedes that many, though not necessarily all, of the additional services received by the poor meet a socially-defined need. He argues, however, that this is less likely to be true of the increment of services consumed by the rich because of prepayment. The object in benefit design, then, is to allow the poor to increase their consumption of services without allowing the rich to do the same.

But the consumption of socially-valued services is not the only welfare gain from prepayment, nor is the consumption of services that are not socially-valued the only loss. Feldstein argues that any assessment of the effects of insurance must include the gain through risk aversion and the loss through price inflation, plus the cost of administering the insurance program itself. When this assessment is made under certain assumptions, the net effect of the current level of insurance is a loss in welfare. In other words, the gain in protection against unpredictable expenses is probably more than offset by the higher cost of services and by the use of additional services that the consumer values less (218). But this assessment does not take into account the possibility that society may value this increment of services more highly than the consumer does, especially when the services go to those who would otherwise be underserved.

The upshot of these analyses is the recommendation of "variable subsidy" insurance in a form that would exact higher premiums and copayments from the rich and place a greater emphasis on protection against large expenditures rather than small (109, 216). It is hoped that such a scheme would dampen inflation by giving the consumer a stake in keeping prices low, would favor the use of service by the poor relative to the rich, would discourage everyone from using services for trivial reasons, and would offer protection against expenses that are very large relative to income. All this would be accomplished without excessively large increases in taxation, since a great share of the cost of health care, that part made up of expenditures that are small relative to income, would be borne directly by the consumer. Furthermore, the schedule of variable subsidies and of limits on the consumers' liability could be so graduated as to implement whatever equity objectives society wishes to pursue. Thus a variety of social objectives are achieved, through what seems to be a creative melding of planning and the market. Not least among these objectives is the smallest possible degree of interference with the established system of medical care. But, before we make any more comments on this seductive proposal, there are some further objective that we need to consider.

Maintaining the Integrity of the Medical Care Process

Among these objectives, maintaining the integrity of the medical care process would seem to occupy a key position. This concept was presented early in our introductory chapter; there we argued that medical care services must be regarded not as marbles in a bag but as a tissue of functionally interrelated parts. Some services are prerequisite to other services; the effectiveness of some services depends, in part on the concurrent or sequential use of other services; and some services can substitute for others, with various consequences for quality and cost. At best, medical care services can be separated into clusters or domains that are somewhat independent of each other; but within each domain the functional links are so vital that their disruption can be expected to have serious consequences. The chief consequences are a reduction in the efficiency of production and the effectiveness of care; a secondary, though still important, consequence is to alienate the physician who wishes to practice good medicine without artificial constraints on his judgment as to what are appropriate services. If this concern with the integrity of the medical care process is valid, it leads to the conclusion that the benefits in an optimal program must cover a comprehensive scope of service, at least within each domain of care, if these domains can indeed be distinguished.

Comprehensive Care and Benefits

There is wide agreement in the medical care field that the proper objective of medical care organization is to make available to all people all the medical care services they need. Comprehensive care is the ultimate objective. But comprehensive care, like love, is a remarkably difficult thing to define; nor is it certain, as has been said of pornography, that one would recognize comprehensive care if one saw it. Besides, it is not clear how comprehensive benefits are conceptually related to comprehensive care. It might be useful, therefore, to try to clarify both the definition and the relationship.

Although comprehensive care, like all potent symbols, has meant different things to different people, there are recurrent themes that, collectively, may be said to stand for the whole. In assembling these themes, we shall lean heavily on a masterly exposition by Franz Goldmann (266) and on a more recent formulation by the National Commission on Community Health Services (267). In these sources and elsewhere, one finds that an important element of comprehensive care is the availability of, and access to, a broad range of services. The range or scope of services is itself definable in terms of: (1) the number of services available, including less traditional auxiliary or supportive services; (2) the location of services, including the home, the office and a variety of outpatient and inpatient institutions; and (3) function, including prevention, early diagnosis, treatment, and rehabilitation, whether physical, vocational, or social. A second major theme of comprehensive care is the interrelationship among the components of care in terms of balance, continuity and coordination. Continuity and coordination imply attachment to a central source of care, which may be a personal physician, an institution, or both (268). It also implies a planned and orderly transfer of responsibility and information, so that the client remains in the charge of a competent source of care throughout his life, at all times and in all places. A corollary is that medical care services should be fitted within a larger framework of related personal services, such as social welfare and education. A third major theme of comprehensive care is that there should be a general orientation or philosophy of care, with emphasis on the constructive, preventive, anticipatory approach, and a concern for the whole person in his total social and economic milieu. And finally, Goldmann adds the elements of quantitative and qualitative adequacy to his exposition of comprehensive care (266).

Comprehensive care would seem to be the distillation of all that conventional wisdom has declared to be good and desirable in the financing and organization of health services (2). If so, comprehensive benefits must stand for that range and configuration of benefits that at least permits, and perhaps encourages, the delivery of comprehensive care. Thus, the range and scope of benefits to be provided is contingent on a prior agreement about the definition of health, the responsibilities and functions of the health care system, and the desirable attributes of that system. Consequently, as we have redefined our view of health and of the social responsibility for it, there has been a constant pressure to expand the purview of the health care system and to include a larger range and variety of services within it.

More concretely, comprehensive benefits can be specified as a list of services that explicitly or implicitly represent the attributes we have discussed. The National Council on Aging has put it as follows:

Medical care encompasses a broad spectrum of services. Such comprehensive care entails diagnosis, care of acute and chronic illness, ambulatory medical or dental care in private offices and clinics in hospitals, other institutions, and at home; psychiatric diagnosis, consultation, or treatment; home nursing services; coordinated home care programs; rehabilitation; and prescribed drugs and prostheses. Not least are personal health maintenance services—some given in physicians' offices and clinics and some through health department programs and the educational activities of voluntary agencies. For some patients additional services such as homemaker or other home help services, convalescent care, nursing home, foster home, or boarding home care, or transportation are indispensable to carrying out successfully the recommendations of the physician. They should thus be considered when estimating the cost of care. [269, p. 1749]

Reed and Carr report that at a special meeting of all Blue Shield plans held in October, 1968, a report was adopted recommending "that this Special Meeting establish the following as a comprehensive scope of benefits, to be available for purchase from or servicing by each Blue Shield plan not later than April 1, 1969:

1. Surgery—including routine pre- and post-operative care and assistant at surgery
2. Anesthesia services
3. Radiation therapy—in and out of the hospital
4. Diagnostic x-ray in-hospital
5. Laboratory and pathology in-hospital
6. In-hospital medical care, including concurrent care
7. Pulmonary tuberculosis, mental disorders, drug addiction and alcoholism
8. Obstetrical care
9. Emergency treatment for accidental injury
10. Consultation
11. Out of hospital diagnostic x-ray and laboratory and pathological service

12. Physical therapy
13. Home and office
14. Newborn care
15. Physical examinations
16. Out-patient psychiatric care
17. Inhalation therapy
18. Ambulance
19. Prosthetic appliances and orthopedic braces
20. Rental or purchase of durable equipment
21. Private duty nursing
22. Drugs
23. Dental
24. Vision care [270, footnote, pp. 108–109]

Table 43 gives an even longer list of the mandatory and optional services available under Medicaid in one state or another. Unfortunately, a long list of services is not a sufficient indication of comprehensiveness; stringent limits on the amount of each benefit can cripple the effectiveness of the whole, making window dressing of much of the list. Furthermore, impressive as these lists may be, they do not do full justice to the remarkable extensibility of the concept of comprehensive care. Witness the range of services that Richmond and Weinberger consider to be essential elements of comprehensive care for children and youth; in addition to the more traditional services, these include family planning; genetic counselling; amniocentesis; abortions; nutritional services; screening for developmental defects, including learning defects; mental health services; health education; prenatal care, family planning, and arrangements for maintaining schooling for pregnant adolescents; accident and poison control services; and a variety of "enrichment programs" including "home visits and 'tutoring' " and "head start" (271).

On the other hand, all these ambitious aspirations are in stark contrast to a more impoverished reality. Witness the rather modest standards that the Fifty-third International Labor Conference has set for sickness benefits under social security programs, even in the more affluent nations (272): in order to meet the standards of their new convention, medical care offered by developed countries must include general practitioner care in office and home; specialist care in the hospital and outside the hospital, as available; prescribed pharmaceutical supplies in and out of the hospital; medical aids such as eyeglasses; services for convalescents; and dental care and medical rehabilitation to the extent determined by the national legislatures of the member countries. To its credit, the convention does not seem to have called this range of services "comprehensive." Other programs have been less meticulous. Since comprehensive benefits has no standard meaning, all who wish it can claim that the services they provide are what is meant by comprehensive. Faced by this difficulty, Anne Sommers has suggested that, at least provisionally, the designation comprehensive benefits should stand for the range and quantity of benefits provided by certain of the more generous programs in actual operation. For this purpose, she singles out Medicare and the "high option" plans in the Federal Employees Health Benefits Program. Although she recognizes the limitations in both programs, Sommers contends that, at least for now, these benefits are a realistic representation of what comprehensive benefits might signify as an ideal (264).

Reasons for Providing Less Than Comprehensive Benefits

If comprehensive benefits are a necessary, though not sufficient, condition for the practice of good and effective medicine, one asks what justification there is for not providing them. Reed and Carr offer some of the reasons (270, pp. 109–111). The first is that the public is apparently unwilling to bear the high cost. While this may be true, there is also evidence that the public is willing to pay for more complete protection than is now usual. Under the Federal Employees Health Benefits Program, about 86 percent of the employees have chosen the more generous high option plans, and 75 percent have elected to include family members, both of these choices being made at greater cost to themselves (264, p. 9). Over 95 percent of Medicare beneficiaries have elected to participate in Part B of that program, and a large proportion have purchased supplementary insurance from private carriers; this is further evidence of the desire for greater protection (273). In their survey of the Detroit Metropolitan Area, Bashshur and Metzner found that the "importance of insurance coverage was judged high by many people. . . . A majority wanted insurance covering hospitalization, surgical services, medical services in the hospital, home, and office, drugs, dental services, home nursing, checkups, inoculations, and provision of group practice" (222, p. 86). While this list falls short of being comprehensive, it does include more benefits than the majority of people now enjoy, and suggests a greater readiness to accept expansions in insurance than one might suspect. Nevertheless, the high cost of comprehensive benefits is a major barrier that cannot be overcome without direct or indirect public subsidy, at least to certain segments of the population. Reed and Carr have suggested other, perhaps more easily remediable, barriers to the expansion of benefits: a lack of the technical, actuarial know-how necessary for the inclusion of new and untested benefits; custom, tradition and inertia; and legislation that hampers Blue Cross and Blue Shield plans in developing new benefits, or that forbids the "establishment and operation of consumer sponsored group practice plans."

Major additional barriers to comprehensive benefits are the traditional notion of an "insurable hazard" and the methods used to achieve "actuarial soundness"; these barriers are implicit, perhaps, in Reed's and Carr's explanations. They lead to the exclusion of certain benefits, and the inclusion of others, under conditions that impinge significantly on the degree of protection expected by the client. Allied to them is the high cost of covering small recurrent expenses under the traditional modes of medical practice.

There is such a close relationship between the organization of care and the appropriate and efficient use of services, that an inability to alter the organization of care, or a refusal to contemplate or support such a change, limits innovation in benefit design and creates a major obstacle to comprehensive care at an affordable price. This obstacle rests, of course, not only on the realities of political power but also on political ideology and on social values in general. Social values seem to have a more pervasive influence on health insurance than we are generally willing to admit. We have already discussed the value connotations of the concept of moral hazard. Not infrequently, one encounters the argument that it is good for people to help pay for the health services they receive, not only because this lessens their tendency to "abuse" the plan, but also because it contributes to a virtuous self-reliance; it also makes the patient more appreciative of the ministrations of his physician.

We suspect that moralistic valuations have hampered the inclusion of certain services among the benefits that are usually available; among these are coverage of self-inflicted injuries, alcoholism, and certain kinds of mental illness. These value judgments are even more likely to inhibit coverage of maternity services for unmarried women and of family planning and abortion services for all women. It is extraordinarily difficult to confirm these suspicions, and we are indebted to Charlotte Muller for painstakingly assembling some relevant information (274). Using her findings, we see that,with very few exceptions, Blue Cross and Blue Shield do cover abortions, either explicitly or implicitly, under the more general category of pregnancy and its complications. However, maternity coverage in all its aspects is almost always confined to "family contracts," which effectively excludes both the newlywed and the unwed. These maternity exclusions are also found in the plans that cover federal employees, with the exception of two large prepaid group practice plans. The most permissive of the plans surveyed appears to be CHAMPUS (the Civilian Health and Medical Program of the Uniformed Services), which, within the limits of state law, has offered abortion services not only to wives but also to unmarried daughters up to at least age 21, and up to age 23 if the daughters were students, all without a waiting period. Quite unexpectedly, the more generous group plans of the larger insurance companies were found to be intermediate between the Blues and CHAMPUS in their readiness to cover what might be regarded as a socially deviant hazard. Under these plans, maternity services and, by extension, abortion, are generally available not only to wives of workers, but also to female workers irrespective of marital status. However, the insurance companies, or their clients, usually appear to draw a line against such coverage for child dependents.

These findings of apparent moralistic valuations provide fuel for somewhat fanciful speculation. One wonders whether the quasi-public and government-sponsored plans are under a greater obligation to observe the mores of a society that they might appear to represent. By contrast, the commercial plans might be morally more neutral, being ready to provide whatever the customer is prepared to pay for. Along these lines, is it likely that the providers, who sponsor the Blues, are more moralistic and less permissive than the merchants? And what of the very permissive position taken by the armed services plan? A cynic might say that this is merely a recognition of the greater sexual hazards of the military vocation. A kinder interpretation, and one most probably nearer the mark, is that CHAMPUS benefits are a truer representation of enlightened professional opinion, which can express itself thanks to a kind of federal extraterritoriality enjoyed by military enclaves within the states.

The latter interpretation, and some of our earlier speculations, find support in a sequence of events described and analyzed by Curran (275). On July 1, 1970, an administrative order of the armed forces hospitals allowed the hospitals to perform abortions upon request of the patient, based on the clinical determination of the attending physician. According to Curran, the order was interpreted in at least some hospitals to allow "abortions on request" (275, p. 1042). This permissive policy was short lived. In April 1972, President Nixon, as Commander in Chief of the Armed Forces, revoked the prior directive, and ordered military hospitals to abide by the laws of the states in which they were located. In this way, the President reaffirmed both national morality and the deference of the federal government to state law.

A similar tendency for government to guard public morality and, in so doing, to come in conflict with professional reformism, may also be at work in decisions to provide or deny family planning and abortion services under Medicaid to the mothers of dependent children. This tendency is very difficult to document, beyond noting a general inadequacy in such services (276, 277). The policy may not be as self-defeating as it seems, since a more aggressive policy of birth control might inspire cries of "genocide." If this is part of the rationale, we can see it as evidence of the influence that more general political considerations have on the design of benefits under governmental programs. More pervasive, but equally elusive, is the principle of "lesser eligibility," which continues to linger since its apotheosis in the Elizabethan Poor Law. Part moral value, part political expediency, and part economic necessity, it holds that services for those who receive public assistance should not exceed those enjoyed by the poorest among the self-supporting.

It is possible that all of these interpretations are merely academic fancy, and that public welfare agencies simply don't know any better and don't give a darn—not until the prospective consumer has the power to call them to task. In any event, one can easily see glimpses of all these threads of thought in the sequence of actions and counteractions that have marked The Strange Case of Elective Abortions under Medicaid in New York State (278). When New York passed its liberal abortion legislation, abortions became available to Medicaid beneficiaries as to all residents of the state. But, within less than a year, the commissioner of social services ruled that the Medicaid benefit would be restricted to medically indicated abortions only, for the ostensible purpose of saving about $3 million a year. In the prolonged litigation that followed, the state supreme court initially struck down the commissioner's order; this ruling was initially upheld by the appellate division, then reversed by the state's highest court, the Court of Appeals and, finally, reaffirmed by a federal district court. The arguments in favor of the commissioner's order to restrict abortion services were, among others, that pregnancy was not a medical condition, and even if it were there was no obligation to provide Medicaid beneficiaries with every service available to the general population. The contrary arguments included the assertion that although pregnancy was not an abnormal condition, care for it was a medical service within the purview of the program, and that it was invidious discrimination to deny this service to some people because they were poor, and to deny it without due process and in violation of the constitutional guarantee of equal protection under the law. Furthermore, it was argued that there was no compelling public interest to justify the commissioner's order, since savings from withholding service would be more than offset by the need to care for the pregnant mother and the child, if pregnancy were not terminated. For all we know, the debate continues.

It is reasonable to conclude that certain benefits do bear the stigma of public opprobrium and are likely to be excluded as a result. Maternity benefits, besides being frowned upon for the unmarried, are also excluded or restricted for the married because pregnancy is considered to be an event at least partly under the volitional control of those who experience it. The same rationale excludes care for self-inflicted illness and injury, in general. Plastic surgery and other cosmetic procedures are excluded because they are "elective," which means that they can be planned for and that they are not necessary or indispensable, although for many people they may be critically important. The exclusion of plastic surgery opens up a fascinating area of exploration, concerning the importance of physical appearance to social and economic success, and the sometimes difficult distinction between the esthetically desirable and the functionally useful. But any benefit that involves the ambiguities of plastic surgery is likely to be excluded just for that reason. Mental illness is often excluded, or included only under severe restrictions, because both the definition of the disease and the specification of the treatment and type of therapist are matters of considerable difficulty. Nursing home care raises analogous difficulties of specifying what levels or intensities of care are covered, and where medical care ends and custodial care begins. Coverage of dental care is handicapped mainly by the very large backlog of unmet need that may be present when coverage begins; also, costs are hard to specify because comparable functional results can be obtained with treatments that have very different esthetic consequences and involve correspondingly different costs.

Drugs may be excluded because they appear to be supply-determined, so that physicians have a seemingly unlimited capacity to prescribe, and patients a corresponding capacity either to consume them or to accumulate them in their medicine cabinets. Certain drugs, such as antibiotics, stimulants and tranquilizers, are especially subject to abuse. Moreover, it is not easy at the fringes to distinguish the therapeutic use of certain pharmaceuticals from their use as a food supplement or as a fad; certain preparations that include vitamins and minerals are a good example. Laboratory tests are also considered subject to abuse by the physician, particularly if separate payment is made for tests performed by the physician himself or an employee in the physician's office. Care during the first few days of life is not particularly open to abuse, but it is excluded simply because it is always needed and, if the newborn is ill, injured, or deformed, care is likely to be expensive.

These selected examples do not constitute a complete list of problematic benefits, but they do indicate that certain features inherent in the services themselves, if they conflict with agency-oriented or collectivity-oriented objectives, can lead to a decision to exclude the services from coverage. As a result, benefits become less than comprehensive.

Consequences of Providing Less Than Comprehensive Benefits

We are already familiar with the consequences of less than comprehensive benefits. One consequence is that the cost of obtaining coverage is lowered, but protection is also reduced. Even though this lowered protection is reflected in the premium, the client may feel that it would be inequitable to have a system in which all make the same contributions, but the enjoyment of benefits depends on what illness happens to strike or what services happen to be needed (279, p. 62). When the range or quantity of benefits is severely restricted, physicians may refuse to offer their services unless they are assured that the patient is able to pay for any care additional to that included in the plan (280). If the physician is denied a relatively free choice in selecting the most appropriate mix of services, costs to the plan could be reduced, but they could also be increased if more expensive substitutes are used. The quality and effectiveness of care are reduced by the non-availability of certain services and by the use of less effective or more dangerous substitutes. It has been argued that in the long run, this results in greater cost to the plan, as well as losses to society.

Quality of Care

Assuring and promoting the quality of care is an objective to which providers, clients, and the collectivity are all ostensibly committed. The provision of benefits, by facilitating access to care, increases exposure both to what is good and to what is bad in our system of medical care. We have argued that proper benefit design should pose no barriers to the choice of the most appropriate modalities of care. Beyond that, good design might attempt to encourage those elements of care that are considered to be more desirable and discourage those that are less desirable, by selectively providing more or less generous benefits for each service covered. Nevertheless, the availability of benefits is also an invitation to the wasteful and inappropriate use of services. In some instances, inappropriate care can cause actual harm by exposing the patient to the considerable risks of hospitalization, improperly prescribed or controlled drug therapy, and unnecessary surgery. The machinery of medical care has a sinister potential for those who fall into it in the wrong place at the wrong time.

A Look to the Future

Every social mechanism appears to have a dual potential for good and evil. Prepayment for medical care is no exception. On the one hand, it provides assurance of necessary care as a safeguard to health, economic well-being, and peace of mind. On the other hand, it opens the way to wasteful and harmful care, to price inflation, and to concealed redistributions in socially undesirable directions. The problem is to devise a plan that allows us to reap the most advantages while we incur the fewest drawbacks. There are those who feel that this can be done through proper design of the prepayment mechanism itself. The proposed design usually takes the form of variable subsidy insurance, with limits on consumer liability so that both the subsidy and the limit on liability are adjusted to income, with an allowance for family size and composition. This design preserves the essential features of the medical care market, which is considered fully competent to adjust service to need.

As might be expected, there are those who strongly oppose the view that the medical care system, as it is now, is fundamentally sound, and that all a national health plan needs to do is to regulate consumer behavior through the selective application of financial incentives and barriers to care. To these advocates of more fundamental change, the test of income, as a necessary first step in determining what each family must contribute for the benefits it will receive, is ideologically repugnant and administratively unwieldy. Furthermore, these critics contend, as long as the client must make an initial out-of-pocket payment for care before the plan makes its benefits available, there is an impediment to early diagnosis and treatment. If the client must subsequently pay part of the cost of care he may be further inhibited from accepting the physician's recommendations. Finally, the medical care system itself is thought to require major reorganization before it can deliver quality care at reasonable cost. Consequently, these critics of the status quo would like to use the design of the prepayment mechanism as a means to bring about more fundamental change in the medical care system as a whole. This is in marked contrast to the position of those who believe that a national plan must not go beyond helping people to bear the burden of the unpredictable costs of care, and that the greatest emphasis must be on costs that are unusually high.

At their extremes, these two positions present the contrast between reform and revolution, but there is much ground in between. The political realities being what they are, we are likely to proceed in piecemeal fashion along both lines. On the one hand, we shall restructure the payment system so it conforms more closely to the objectives we have outlined. On the other hand, incentives will be provided to encourage the development and spread of new modes of delivering care. Hopefully, we shall see to it that the two lines of development are mutually sustaining; and that, as we proceed, we examine the consequences of our actions. If so, the future will be full of challenge, and of promise.

APPENDICES
REFERENCES
INDEX

APPENDIX A

Derivation of Values for Varieties of Price

1. *Proportion of population covered*

   According to reference 19, table 41, page 76, 66% of individuals had surgical-medical coverage in 1963.

2. *Use of Service*

   Feldstein, reference 169, page 123, says: "The ratio of U_I to U_N, derived from the Andersen and Anderson data on physician visits was taken to be 1.32."

3. *Expenditures*

   According to reference 20, table 73, page 139, mean expenditure of uninsured as percent of insured is 51 percent.

4. *Proportion of Expenditures not Covered by Insurance*

   According to reference 20, table 50, page 92: "percent aggregate expenditures for personal health services covered by aggregate health insurance benefits" is 25 percent, for services of physicians. Consequently:

$$\text{Proportion of Out-of-Pocket Expenditures} = \frac{\left(\begin{array}{c}\text{Out-of-Pocket}\\\text{Expenditures of Insured}\end{array}\right) + \left(\begin{array}{c}\text{Out-of-Pocket}\\\text{Expenditures of Uninsured}\end{array}\right)}{\left(\begin{array}{c}\text{Proportion}\\\text{Insured}\end{array}\right)\left(\begin{array}{c}\text{Expenditures}\\\text{for}\\\text{Insured}\end{array}\right) + \left(\begin{array}{c}\text{Proportion}\\\text{Uninsured}\end{array}\right)\left(\begin{array}{c}\text{Expenditures}\\\text{for}\\\text{Uninsured}\end{array}\right)}$$

$$0.75 = \frac{x + (0.34)(0.51)}{(0.66)(1.00) + (0.34)(0.51)}$$

$$0.75 = \frac{x + 0.1734}{0.66 + 0.1734} = \frac{x + 0.1734}{0.8334}$$

$$x = (0.75)(0.8334) - 0.1734 = 0.45$$

$$\text{Proportion of Expenditures Not Covered by Insurance, for Those Insured} = \frac{0.45}{0.66} = 0.68$$

5. *Actual Price*

The actual price paid by the insured is assumed to be equal to the "customary price" as reported by the Consumer Price Index. The actual price paid by the uninsured is derived as follows:

$$\frac{\left(\begin{array}{c}\text{Use of Service}\\\text{per Uninsured}\end{array}\right)\left(\begin{array}{c}\text{Price}\\\text{per Service}\end{array}\right)}{\left(\begin{array}{c}\text{Use of Service}\\\text{per Insured}\end{array}\right)\left(\begin{array}{c}\text{Price}\\\text{per Service}\end{array}\right)} = \frac{\begin{array}{c}\text{Expenditures}\\\text{per Uninsured}\end{array}}{\begin{array}{c}\text{Expenditures}\\\text{per Insured}\end{array}}$$

$$= \frac{(0.76)\,(x)}{1} = \frac{0.51}{1}$$

$$x = \frac{0.51}{0.76} = 0.67$$

The actual price paid by insured and uninsured combined is derived as follows:

$$\text{Average Actual Price} = \frac{\text{Total Expenditures}}{\text{Total Services}}$$

$$= \frac{\left(\begin{array}{c}\text{Proportion}\\\text{Insured}\end{array}\right)\left(\begin{array}{c}\text{Expenditures}\\\text{per Insured}\end{array}\right) + \left(\begin{array}{c}\text{Proportion}\\\text{Uninsured}\end{array}\right)\left(\begin{array}{c}\text{Expenditures}\\\text{per Uninsured}\end{array}\right)}{\left(\begin{array}{c}\text{Proportion}\\\text{Insured}\end{array}\right)\left(\begin{array}{c}\text{Services}\\\text{per Insured}\end{array}\right) + \left(\begin{array}{c}\text{Proportion}\\\text{Uninsured}\end{array}\right)\left(\begin{array}{c}\text{Services}\\\text{per Uninsured}\end{array}\right)}$$

$$= \frac{(0.66)\,(1.00) + (0.34)\,(0.51)}{(0.66)\,(1.00) + (0.34)\,(0.76)} = \frac{0.8334}{0.9184}$$

$$= 0.91$$

6. *Net Price*

The net price for the insured equals the proportion of expenditures covered by insurance. The net price for the uninsured is the same as the actual price for that category.

The net price for the uninsured plus the insured is derived as follows:

$$\text{Average Net Price} = \frac{\text{Total Out-of-Pocket Expenditures}}{\text{Total Services}}$$

$$= \frac{\left(\begin{array}{c}\text{Proportion}\\\text{Insured}\end{array}\right)\left(\begin{array}{c}\text{Out-of-Pocket}\\\text{Expenditures}\\\text{per Insured}\end{array}\right) + \left(\begin{array}{c}\text{Proportion}\\\text{Uninsured}\end{array}\right)\left(\begin{array}{c}\text{Out-of-Pocket}\\\text{Expenditures}\\\text{per Uninsured}\end{array}\right)}{\left(\begin{array}{c}\text{Proportion}\\\text{Insured}\end{array}\right)\left(\begin{array}{c}\text{Services}\\\text{per Insured}\end{array}\right) + \left(\begin{array}{c}\text{Proportion}\\\text{Uninsured}\end{array}\right)\left(\begin{array}{c}\text{Services}\\\text{per Uninsured}\end{array}\right)}$$

$$= \frac{(0.66)\,(0.68) + (0.34)\,(0.51)}{(0.66)\,(1.00) + (0.34)\,(0.76)} = \frac{0.6222}{0.9184} = 0.68$$

APPENDIX B

Health Plan Grading System *

Summary of Items

	Points Assigned
I. Organizational and administrative arrangements established to carry out the plan. (Decision-making in the collective bargaining process, responsibility and role of the joint trust, responsibility and role of the third-party or intermediary organization, and role and functions of any administrative office or agency.)	150 (I)
II. Extent of coverage. (Extent to which family members are covered by the health insurance contract.)	175 (II)
III. Scope of benefits. (What the contract pays for or provides, e.g., hospital room and board, laboratory and x-ray services, physician office visits.)	300 (III)
IV. Administrative provisions to assure quality of medical care provided under the plan. (The qualifications of physicians, the quality of hospitals and clinical laboratories providing services to those whom the plan benefits.)	250 (IV)
V. The amount of money which members of the plan spend for health services, in addition to the health insurance premium. (This considers the amount of money (sometimes called out-of-pocket costs) spent for health services, in addition to the health insurance premium—estimated now on the basis of previous studies, and to be estimated in the future on the basis of a data gathering system.)	125 (V)
Total Points	1,000

* *Source:* Reference 232, pages 19–24.

Detailed Description of Items

Points Assigned

I. Organizational and Administrative Arrangements Established to Carry Out the Plan.   150 (I)

  1. Continuity in the decision-making process, with free flow of information and effective coordination of action among collective bargaining negotiators, joint trustees, plan administrators, and the third party organization.

    —Problems are quickly referred to the appropriate decision-making level.

    —Problems which arise between periods of collective bargaining negotiations are not deferred until the next period of contract negotiations.   30 (1)

  2. Evidence of a focus on the total health needs of individuals and families.

    —There is no proliferation of separate plans with fragmented, uncoordinated specialized health care services.

    —The impact of "uncovered services" on the utilization of covered services is systematically analyzed.

    —The administration of various health plans covering the same population is coordinated.   25 (2)

  3. At all decision-making levels, up-to-date and reliable data are available.

    —Information concerning the age, sex, and employment status of the covered population.

    —Members' utilization of health care services of all kinds (not limited to those covered by the plan).

    —Members' expenditures for health care services of all kinds (not limited to those covered by the plan).

    —All costs of administration including those of third parties.   20 (3)

  4. At the operating levels, sufficient communication occurs with the covered population to determine their experience with and response to the plan.

—There is a grievance system and an educational program.

—The grievance system has appropriate fact-finding procedures and provides recourse to impartial arbitration.

—The educational program focuses on health care needs of the covered population.

—The policy makers continually reevaluate the effectiveness of the existing plan based on information retrieved by means of the educational program.

5. Policy standards or guidelines for administration of the plan have been formulated and are being followed.

—The system of claims review and surveillance is used to monitor both the cost and the quality of care.

—Reserves are maintained at a level reasonably related to incurred liabilities and to anticipated expenditures.

—Eligibility is systematically determined, including the eligibility of those who are not regularly employed.

—Data are reported to all persons involved in decision-making, including the covered population.

—Provision for employer delinquencies prevent liability of covered members. 25 (5)

6. Generally accepted principles of effective health care planning and programming are practiced.

—Choice of alternative plans, including group practice plans and those permitting free choice of physicians, is made available to the covered members whenever feasible.

—Qualified health care professionals who have no financial interest in any particular plans or programs are consulted regarding all key decisions.

—Consumer representatives are included on the top policy-making bodies of all third party or intermediary organizations involved in the plan.

Detailed Description of Items

Points Assigned

—Personnel involved in the plans are encouraged to participate in the solution of broader community health problems.

—Positive encouragement is given to the development of new or experimental health care programs, concepts, or "delivery systems," which might improve the health care of the covered population.   25 (6)

II. The Extent of Coverage Contained in the Contract.   175 (II)

    1. Employee and all dependents are covered.   175

    2. Employee and spouse only are covered.   60

    3. Employee only is covered.   30

III. Scope of Benefits Contained in the Contract—See chart on pages 398–399

IV. Administrative Provisions to Assure Quality of Medical Care   250 (IV)

    1. Either:

Physician services, in and out of hospital, are provided only by physicians with staff privileges in at least one accredited hospital.

Or:

Where services are provided by a group practice the following standards are met:

    a) There are at least 5 full time physicians with three specialists, including internal medicine and general surgery.

    b) There is at least one physician per 1,200 persons serviced by the group.

    c) The majority of physician services are provided by full time physicians   50 (1)

    2. Hospital services (except emergency services) are provided only in hospitals accredited by Joint Commission on Accreditation of Hospitals.   50 (2)

    3. Hospital services (except emergency services) are provided only in hospitals which conform to state and regional plans with respect to bed size and scope of services.   45 (3)

    4. Laboratory services are provided only in laboratories which participate in a perfor-

mance testing program approved by the
State Department of Public Health. 30 (4)

5. No services provided by chiropractors or
other nonscientific medical practitioners
are paid for by the plan. 25 (5)

6. A systematic medical audit of quality of
care (in addition to any audit of costs and
charges) is provided to the trustees and administrators of the health insurance plan.
The data, based on systematic statistical reporting and peer review, are reported on
the quality of service as a whole, not on individual physicians or other providers. 50 (6)

V. The Amount of Money Which Members of the
Plan Spend for Health Services, in Addition to the Health Insurance Premium. 125 (V)

1. Use of the plan results in no additional expenditures for health services per family
per year (beyond the cost of the health insurance premiums). 125 (1)

2. Use of the plan results in less than $50 ex-
penditures for health services per family
per year (beyond the cost of the health insurance premiums). 95 (2)

3. Use of the plan results in less than $100
but more than $50 in expenditures for
health services per family per year (beyond
the cost of the health insurance premiums). 90 (3)

4. Use of the plan results in less than $150
but more than $100 expenditures for health
services per family per year (beyond the
cost of the health insurance premiums). 75 (4)

5. Use of the plan results in less than $200,
but more than $150 total expenditures for
health services per family per year (beyond
the cost of the health insurance premiums). 60 (5)

6. Use of the plan results in less than $300,
but more than $200 total expenditures for
health services per family per year (beyond
the cost of the health insurance premiums). 40 (6)

7. Use of the plan results in less than $400,
but more than $300 total expenditures for
health services per family per year (beyond
the costs of the health insurance premiums). 20 (7)

Benefits	III. Scope of Benefits						Evaluation Points
Hospital Room and Board	Paid in full — 40	3 + bed ward rate paid up to 100 days — 35	3 + bed ward rate paid up to 70 days — 30	80% of costs paid up to limit $10,000 — 25	80% of costs paid up to limit $5,000 — 15	Paid up to limit $1,000 — 10	
Hospital Services	Paid in full — 30	Paid in full for period of hospitalization up to 70 days — 25	Paid in full with minor exceptions — 25	80% of costs paid up to $10,000 — 20	80% of costs paid up to $5,000 — 15	Paid up to $1,000 — 10	
Surgical	Paid in full — 35	80% of costs paid up to $10,000 — 25	80% of costs paid up to $5,000 — 20	Paid up to $1,000 — 20	Paid up to $750 — 15	Paid per schedule ** no limit 30 limited 15	
Anesthetist	Paid in full — 15	80% of costs paid up to $10,000 — 10	80% of costs paid up to $5,000 — 10	Paid up to $1,000 — 10	Paid up to $750 — 10	Paid per schedule ** no limit 10 limited 5	
Hospital, Diagnostic, X-Ray and Laboratory	Paid in full — 20	Paid in full up to 70 days in-hosp — 15	80% of costs paid up to $5,000 — 10	Paid up to $1,000 — 15	Paid up to $750 — 10	Paid per schedule ** no limit 15 limited 10	
Outpatient, Diagnostic, X-Ray and Laboratory	Paid in full — 20	80% of costs paid up to $10,000 — 15	80% of costs paid up to $5,000 — 10	Paid up to $1,000 — 15	Paid up to $750 — 10	Paid per schedule ** no limit 15 limited 5	
Doctor's Hospital Calls	Paid in full — 25	80% of costs paid up to $10,000 — 15	80% of costs paid up to $5,000 — 10	Paid up to $1,000 — 15	Paid up to $750 — 10	Paid per schedule ** no limit 20 limited 10	

Service						
Doctor's Office Calls	Paid in full — 20	80% of costs paid up to $10,000 — 10	80% of costs paid up to $5,000 — 10	Paid up to $1,000 — 15	Paid up to $750 — 10	Paid per schedule ** no limit 15 / limited 10
Doctor's Home Calls	Paid in full — 15	80% of costs paid up to $10,000 — 5	80% of costs paid up to $5,000 — 5	Paid up to $1,000 — 5	Paid up to $750 — 5	Paid per schedule ** no limit 10 / limited 5
Maternity	Paid in full — 15	80% of costs paid up to $10,000 — 5	80% of costs paid up to $5,000 — 5	Paid up to $1,000 — 5	Paid up to $750 — 5	Paid per schedule ** no limit 10 / limited 5
Ambulance	Paid in full — 5	Up to $50 per disability — 5				
Prescribed Medicines (Office or Home)	Paid in full — 10	Paid in full with minor exceptions — 5	80% of costs with $10,000 lifetime limit — 5	80% of costs with $5,000 lifetime limit — 5	Paid up to $750 — 5	Paid per schedule ** no limit 5 / limited 5
Dental Services	Paid in full — 15	Paid in full with minor exceptions — 10	Paid in full on approval — 10	80% of costs paid up to $5,000 — 10	Paid up to $750 — 5	Paid per schedule ** no limit 5 / limited 5
Psychiatric Services	Paid in full — 15	Paid in full with minor exceptions — 10	80% of costs with $10,000 lifetime limit — 5	80% of costs with $5,000 lifetime limit — 5	Paid up to $750 — 5	Paid per schedule ** no limit 10 / limited 5
Preventive Services *	Paid in full — 20	Some paid in full, others not at all — 10	All paid for but not in full — 10			

* (e.g., periodic health examination, well child supervision, immunization)

** As set forth in the insurance contract.

REFERENCES

1. Donabedian, Avedis, *Aspects of Medical Care Administration: Specifying Requirements for Health Care.* Cambridge: Harvard University Press, 1973, 649 pp.

2. Donabedian, Avedis, "Models for Organizing the Delivery of Personal Health Services and Criteria for Evaluating Them." *Milbank Memorial Fund Quarterly* 50: 103–154, October 1972, Part 2.

3. Pauly, Mark V., *Medical Care at Public Expense: A Study in Applied Welfare Economics.* New York: Praeger Publishers, 1971, 160 pp.

4. Kadushin, C., "Social Class and the Experience of Ill Health." *Sociological Inquiry* 24: 67–80, Winter 1964.

5. Antonovsky, A., "Social Class and Illness: A Reconsideration." *Sociological Inquiry* 37: 311–322, Spring 1967.

6. Antonovsky, A., "Social Class, Life Expectancy and Overall Mortality." *Milbank Memorial Fund Quarterly* 45: 31–67, April 1967, Part 1.

7. Lefcowitz, Myron J., "Poverty and Health: A Re-examination." *Inquiry* 10: 3–13, March 1973.

8. National Center for Health Statistics, *Selected Family Characteristics and Health Measures Reported in the Health Interview Survey.* P.H.S. Publication No. 1,000–Series 3, No. 7. Washington, D.C.: U.S. Government Printing Office, January 1967, 26 pp.

9. National Center for Health Statistics, *Chronic Conditions and Limitations of Activity and Mobility: United States, July 1965–June 1967.* P.H.S. Publication No. 1,000–Series 10, No. 61. Washington, D.C.: U.S. Government Printing Office, January 1971, 72 pp.

10. National Center for Health Statistics, *Disability Days, United States, 1971.* Vital and Health Statistics—Series 10, No. 90. Washington, D.C.: U.S. Government Printing Office, June 1974, 64 pp.

11. Feldstein, Paul J., and Carr, W. John, "The Effect of Income on Medical Care Spending." In *Proceedings of the Social Statistics Section, American Statistical Association*, pp. 93–105. Washington, D.C.: American Statistical Association, December 1964.

12. Feldstein, Paul J., "Research on the Demand for Health Services." *Milbank Memorial Fund Quarterly* 44: 128–162, July 1966, Part 2.

13. Friedman, Milton, *A Theory of the Consumption Function.* Princeton, New Jersey: Princeton University Press, 1957. Revised edition, 1967. (Cited in references 11 and 16.)

14. Klarman, Herbert E., "Economic Aspects of Projecting Requirements for Health Manpower." *Journal of Human Resources* 4: 360–376, Summer 1969.

15. Feldstein, Paul J., and Severson, Ruth, "The Demand for Medical Care." In American Medical Association, *Report of the Commission on the Cost of Medical Care; Volume 1, General Report,* pp. 57–76. Chicago: By the Association, 1964.

16. Silver, Morris, "An Economic Analysis of Variations in Medical Expenses and Work-Loss Rates." In Herbert E. Klarman, editor, *Empirical Studies in Health Economics,* pp. 121–140. Baltimore: The Johns Hopkins Press, 1970.

17. Robinson, W. S., "Ecological Correlations and the Behavior of Individuals," *American Sociological Review* 15: 351–357, June 1950.

18. Andersen, Ronald, and Benham, Lee, "Factors Affecting the Relationship between Family Income and Medical Care Consumption." In Herbert E. Klarman, editor, *Empirical Studies in Health Economics,* pp. 73–100. Baltimore: The Johns Hopkins Press, 1970.

19. Anderson, Odin W., and Feldman, Jacob J., *Family Medical Costs and Voluntary Health Insurance: A Nationwide Survey.* New York: The Blakiston Division, McGraw-Hill Book Company, Inc., 1956, 251 pp.

20. Andersen, Ronald, and Anderson, Odin W., *A Decade of Health Services: Social Survey Trends in Use and Expenditures.* Chicago: The University of Chicago Press, 1967, 244 pp.

21. Andersen, Ronald; Greeley, Rachel McL.; Kravits, Joanna; and Anderson, Odin W., *Health Service Use: National Trends and Variations—1953–1971.* DHEW Publications No. (HSM) 73-3,004. Washington, D.C.: U.S. Government Printing Office, October 1972, 57 pp.

22. Bice, Thomas W.; Eichhorn, Robert L.; and Fox, Peter D., "Socioeconomic Status and Use of Physician Services: A Reconsideration." *Medical Care* 10: 261–271, May–June 1972.

23. National Center for Health Statistics, *Physician Visits: Volume and Interval Since Last Visit, United States—1969.* Vital and Health Statistics–Series 10, No. 75. Washington, D.C.: U.S. Government Printing Office, July 1972, 58 pp.

24. Donabedian, Avedis, "The Nature and Magnitude of Unmet Need in Medical Care." In Richard F. Stoll, editor, *Institute on Planning and Administration of Nursing Services in Medical Care Programs: Selected Papers,* pp. 1–21. Ann Arbor: School of Public Health, The University of Michigan, 1968.

25. Wirick, Grover C., Jr., "A Multiple Equation Model of Demand for Health Care." *Health Services Research* 1: 301–346, Winter 1966.

26. Kalimo, Esko, *Determinants of Medical Care Utilization.* Helsinki: Publications of the National Pensions Institute, Finland, Series E: 11, 1969, 47 pp.

27. Kalimo, Esko; Kohn, Robert; and Branco, Benedić, "Interrela-

tionships in the Use of Selected Health Services: A Cross-National Study." *Medical Care* 10: 95–108, March–April 1972.

28. O'Donnell, Edward J., "The Neighborhood Service Center." *Welfare in Review* 6: 11–21, January–February 1968.

29. Geiger, H. Jack, "Health Center in Mississippi." *Hospital Practice* 4: 68–70, 75–77, and 81, February 1969.

30. This extension of the concept of a personal health service was brought to my attention by Professor Dorothy Donabedian, School of Nursing, The University of Michigan, Ann Arbor.

31. de Grazia, Alfred. *Politics and Government,* volume 1: *Political Behavior,* revised edition. New York: Collier Books, 1962, 388 pp. (Paperback.)

32. Monsma, George N., Jr., "Marginal Revenue and the Demand for Physicians' Services." In Herbert E. Klarman, editor, *Empirical Studies in Health Economics,* pp. 145–160. Baltimore: The Johns Hopkins Press, 1970.

33. Dickerson, O. D., *Health Insurance,* third edition. Homewood, Ill.: Richard D. Irwin Inc., 1968, 773 pp.

34. Phelps, Charles E., and Newhouse, Joseph P., "Effect of Coinsurance: A Multivariate Analysis." *Social Security Bulletin* 35: 20–29, June 1972.

35. National Center for Health Statistics, *Health Insurance Coverage, United States, July 1962–June 1963.* P.H.S. Publication No. 1,000–Series 10, No. 11. Washington, D.C.: U.S. Government Printing Office, August 1964, 37 pp.

36. Odoroff, M. E., and Abbe, L. M., "Use of General Hospitals, Variation with Methods of Payment." *Public Health Reports* 74: 316–324, April 1959.

37. National Center for Health Statistics, *Hospital and Surgical Insurance Coverage, United States—1968.* Vital and Health Statistics–Series 10, Number 66. Washington, D.C.: U.S. Government Printing Office, January 1972, 49 pp.

38. Rosenthal, Gerald, "Price Elasticity of Demand for Short-Term General Hospital Services." In Herbert E. Klarman, Editor, *Empirical Studies in Health Economics,* pp. 101–117 (comment by V. R. Fuchs, pp. 118–120). Baltimore: The Johns Hopkins Press, 1970.

39. Ro, Kong-Kyun, "Patient Characteristics and Hospital Use." *Medical Care* 7: 295–312, July–August 1969.

40. "Hospital Utilization and Covered Charges for Federal Employees Under Service Benefits." *Blue Cross Reports* Vol. 2, No. 1, January–February 1964.

41. Technical Data Services Staff, Division of Research and Development, Blue Cross Association, *The Use of Hospitals by Blue Cross Members in 1972.* Research Series 12. Chicago: Blue Cross Association, March 1974, 9 pp.

42. Luck, Elizabeth, "The Problem of Duplicate Coverage and Overinsurance." *Inquiry* 1: 21–34, August 1963.

43. Reed, Louis S., *The Extent of Health Insurance Coverage in the United States.* Office of Research and Statistics, Social Security Administration, Research Report No. 10. Washington, D.C.: U.S. Government Printing Office, 1965, 67 pp.

44. Wallace, Richard L., "Multiple Coverage by Health Insurance." *Medical Care Review* 25: 41–57, January 1969.

45. Ferber, Bernard, "The Relationship of Multiple Health Insurance Coverage and Hospital Utilization." *Inquiry* 3: 14–27, December 1966.

46. Andersen, R., and Riedel, Donald C., *People and Their Hospital Insurance: Comparisons of the Uninsured, Those with One Policy and Those with Multiple Coverage.* Research Series No. 23. Chicago: Center for Health Administration Studies, University of Chicago, 1967, 37 pp. (Also see *Blue Cross Reports*, Vol. 5, No. 1, January–March 1967, 8 pp.)

47. Mueller, Marjorie S., "Private Health Insurance in 1971: Health Care Services, Enrollment, and Finances." *Social Security Bulletin* 36: 3–22, February 1973.

48. Crowthers, Michael, "The Trouble with Overinsurance." *Medical Economics* 42: 191; March 8, 1965.

49. Anderson, Odin W., and Sheatsley, Paul B., *Comprehensive Medical Insurance: A Study of Costs, Use and Attitudes Under Two Plans.* Research Series No. 9. New York: Health Information Foundation, 1959, 105 pp.

50. Columbia University, School of Public Health and Administrative Medicine, *Family Medical Care Under Three Types of Health Insurance.* New York: Foundation on Employee Health, Medical Care and Welfare, Inc., 1962, 202 pp.

51. Committee for the Special Research Project in the Health Insurance Plan of Greater New York, *Health and Medical Care in New York City.* Cambridge: Harvard University Press, 1957, 275 pp.

52. Roemer, Milton I.; Hetherington, Robert W.; Hopkins, Carl E.; Gerst, Arthur E.; Parsons, Eleanor; and Long, Donald M., *Health Insurance Effects.* Research Series No. 16. Ann Arbor: Bureau of Public Health Economics, School of Public Health, The University of Michigan, 1972, 70 pp.

53. Greenlick, Merwin R., *A Comparison of General Drug Utilization in a Metropolitan Community with Utilization Under a Drug Prepayment Plan.* Doctoral Dissertation, The University of Michigan, Ann Arbor, 1967, 194 pp.

54. Waller, Julian A.; Garner, Richard; and Lawrence, Robert, "Utilization of Ambulance Services in a Rural Community." *American Journal of Public Health* 56: 513–520, March 1966.

55. Weisbrod, Burton A., and Fiesler, Robert J., "Hospitalization Insurance and Hospital Utilization." *American Economic Review* 51: 126–132, March 1961.

56. Klarman, Herbert E., "Effect of Prepaid Group Practice on Hospital Use." *Public Health Reports* 78: 955–965, November 1963.

57. Donabedian, Avedis, *A Review of Some Experiences with Prepaid Group Practice*. Research Series No. 11. Ann Arbor: Bureau of Public Health Economics, School of Public Health, The University of Michigan, 1965, 74 pp.

58. Donabedian, Avedis, "An Evaluation of Prepaid Group Practice." *Inquiry* 6: 4–27, September 1969.

59. Roemer, Milton I., and Shonick, William, "HMO Performance: The Recent Evidence." *Health and Society (Milbank Memorial Quarterly)*, Summer 1973, pp. 271–317.

60. Densen, Paul M.; Jones, Ellen W.; Balamuth, Eve; and Shapiro, Sam, "Prepaid Medical Care and Hospital Utilization in a Dual Choice Situation." *American Journal of Public Health* 50: 1,710–1,726; November 1960.

61. Densen, Paul M.; Shapiro, Sam; Jones, Ellen W.; and Baldinger, Irving, "Prepaid Medical Care and Hospital Utilization." *Hospitals* 36: 63–68 and 138; November 16, 1962.

62. Densen, P. M.; Balamuth, E.; and Shapiro, S., *Prepaid Medical Care and Hospital Utilization*. Hospital Monograph Series, No. 3. Chicago: American Hospital Association, 1958, 55 pp.

63. Dozier, D.; Krupp, M.; Melinkoff, S.; Schwarberg, C.; and Watts, M., *Report of the Medical and Hospital Advisory Council to the Board of Administration of the California State Employees' Retirement System*. Sacramento, 1964, 110 pp.

64. Dozier, D., and others, *Final Report on the Survey of Consumer Experience Under the State of California Employees' Hospital and Medical Care Act*. Sacramento, June 1968, 105 pp.

65. Hastings, J. E. F.; Mott, F. D.; Barclay, A.; and Hewitt, D., "Prepaid Group Practice in Sault Ste. Marie, Ontario: Part I: Analysis of Utilization Records." *Medical Care* 11: 91–103, March–April 1973.

66. Mott, F. D.; Hastings, J. E. F.; and Barclay, A. T., "Prepaid Group Practice in Sault Ste. Marie, Ontario: Part II: Evidence from the Household Survey." *Medical Care* 11: 173–188, May–June 1973.

67. Penchansky, Roy, and Rosenthal, Gerald, "Productivity, Price and Income Behaviour in the Physicians' Services Market—A Tentative Hypothesis." *Medical Care* 3: 240–244, October–December 1965.

68. National Advisory Commission on Health Manpower. "The Kaiser Foundation Medical Care Plan." In *Report of the National Advisory Commission on Health Manpower, Volume II*, appendix IV, pp. 197–228. Washington, D.C.: U.S. Government Printing Office, November 1967.

69. Newhouse, Joseph P., *The Economics of Group Practice*. Santa Monica, Calif.: The Rand Corporation, February 1971, 26 pp.

70. Richardson, A. Leslie, "The Methods of Distribution of Income." *Medical Group Management* 8: 15–17, September 1961.

71. This point was brought to my attention by Professor Roy Penchansky, School of Public Health, The University of Michigan, Ann Arbor.

72. Freidson, E., *Patients' Views of Medical Practice.* New York: Russell Sage Foundation, 1961, 268 pp.

73. Densen, P. M., and Shapiro, S., "Hospital Use Under Varying Forms of Medical Organization." In *Conference on Research in Hospital Use,* P.H.S. publication No. 930-E-2, pp. 14–16. Washington, D.C.: U.S. Public Health Service, Division of Hospital and Medical Facilities, 1963.

74. Perkoff, Gerald T.; Kahn, Lawrence; and Mackie, Anita, "Medical Care Utilization in an Experimental Prepaid Group Practice Model in a University Medical Center." *Medical Care* 12: 471–485, June 1974.

75. United Steelworkers of America; Insurance, Pension and Unemployment Department, *Special Study on the Medical Care Program for Steelworkers and Their Families.* Pittsburgh, Pa.: The Department, 1960, 108 pp.

76. Alexander, C. A., "The Effects of Change in Method of Paying Physicians: The Baltimore Experience." *American Journal of Public Health* 57: 1,278–1,289; August 1967.

77. Shapiro, S.; Weiner, L.; and Densen, P., "Comparison of Prematurity and Perinatal Mortality in a General Population and in the Population of a Prepaid Group Practice, Medical Care Plan." *American Journal of Public Health* 48: 170–187, February 1958.

78. Columbo, Theodore J.; Saward, E. W.; and Greenlick, Merwyn R., "The Integration of an OEO Health Program Into a Prepaid Comprehensive Group Practice Plan." *American Journal of Public Health* 59: 641–650, April 1969.

79. Greenlick, Merwyn R.; Freeborn, Donald K.; Colombo, Theodore J.; Prussin, Jeffrey A.; and Saward, Ernest W., "Comparing the Use of Medical Care Services by a Medically Indigent and a General Membership Population in a Comprehensive Prepaid Group Practice Program." *Medical Care* 10: 187–200, May–June 1972.

80. Weiss, James; Freeborn, Donald K.; and Lamb, Sara, "Use of Mental Health Services by Poverty and Nonpoverty Members of a Prepaid Group Practice Plan." *Health Services Reports* 88: 653–662, August–September 1973.

81. Richardson, William C., "Measuring the Urban Poor's Use of Physicians' Services in Response to Illness Episodes." *Medical Care* 8: 132–142, March–April 1970.

82. Fitzpatrick, Thomas B.; Riedel, Donald C.; and Payne, Beverly C., "Appropriateness of Admission and Length of Stay." In McNerney, Walter J., and study staff, *Hospital and Medical Economics: A Study of Population, Services, Costs, Methods of Payment and Controls,* volume 1, pp. 471–494. Chicago: Hospital Research and Educational Trust, 1962, 716 pp.

83. Nassau County Medical Society, Voluntary Health Insurance Committee, *Pilot Study of Hospital Use in Nassau County.* Garden City, N.Y.: The Society, November 1963, 76 pp.

84. Sparling, J. F., "Measuring Medical Care Quality: A Comparative

Study." *Hospitals* 36: 62–68, March 16, 1962; and 56–57, 60–61, April 1, 1962.

85. Stewart, William H., and Enterline, Philip E., "Effects of the National Health Service on Physician Utilization and Health in England and Wales." *New England Journal of Medicine* 265: 1,187–1,194; December 14, 1961.

86. Purola, T.; Kalimo, E.; Nyman, K.; and Sievers, K., "National Health Insurance in Finland: Its Impact and Evaluation." *International Journal of Health Services* 3: 69–80, Winter 1973.

87. Nyman, Kauko, and Kalimo, Esko, "National Sickness Insurance and the Use of Physicians' Services in Finland." *Social Science and Medicine* 7: 541–553, July 1973.

88. Donabedian, Avedis, and Thorby, Jean A., "The Systemic Impact of Medicare." *Medical Care Review* 26: 567–585, June 1969.

89. Lowenstein, R., "Early Effects of Medicare on the Health Care of the Aged." *Social Security Bulletin* 34: 3–20 and 42, April 1971.

90. Payne, Beverly C., "Medicare in Michigan." *Michigan Medicine* 69: 15–21, January 1970.

91. Pettengill, Julian H., "Trends in Hospital Use by the Aged," *Social Security Bulletin* 35: 3–15, July 1972.

92. Enterline, Philip E.; Salter, Vera; McDonald, Alison D.; and McDonald, J. Corbett, "The Distribution of Medical Services Before and After 'Free' Medical Care—The Quebec Experience." *New England Journal of Medicine* 289: 1,174–1,178; November 29, 1973.

93. Enterline, Philip E.; McDonald, J. Corbett; McDonald, Alison D.; Davignon, Lise; and Salter, Vera, "Effects of 'Free' Medical Care on Medical Practice—The Quebec Experience." *New England Journal of Medicine* 288: 1,152–1,155; May 31, 1973.

94. The possibility of the attrition of health care events in a panel population was brought to my attention by Professor Benjamin Darsky, School of Public Health, The University of Michigan, Ann Arbor.

95. Avnet, Helen H., *Physician Service Patterns and Illness Rates.* New York: Group Health Insurance, Inc., 1967, 452 pp.

96. Alpert, Joel J.; Heagarty, Margaret C.; Robertson, Leon; Kosa, John; and Haggerty, Robert J., "Effective Use of Comprehensive Pediatric Care: Utilization of Health Resources." *American Journal of Diseases of Children* 116: 529–533, November 1968.

97. Bellin, Seymore S.; Geiger, H. J.; and Gibson, Count D., "Impact of Ambulatory-Health-Care Services on the Demand for Hospital Beds. A Study of the Tufts Neighborhood Health Center at Columbia Point in Boston." *New England Journal of Medicine* 280: 808–812; April 10, 1969.

98. Strauss, Mark A., and Sparer, Gerald, "Basic Utilization Experience of OEO Comprehensive Health Services Projects." *Inquiry* 8: 36–49, December 1971.

99. Sparer, Gerald and Anderson, Arne, "Utilization and Cost Experi-

ence of Low-Income Families in Prepaid Group-Practice Plans." *New England Journal of Medicine* 289: 67–72; July 12, 1973.

100. Social Security Administration, Office of Research and Statistics, *Medicare: Health Insurance for the Aged, 1971, Section 2: Enrollment.* Washington, D.C.: U.S. Government Printing Office, 1973, 27 pp. plus 59 pages of tables.

101. Feldstein, Paul J., "A Proposal for Capitation Reimbursement to Medical Groups for Total Medical Care." In *Reimbursement Incentives for Hospital and Medical Care: Objectives and Alternatives,* pp. 61–72. Social Security Administration, Research Report No. 26. Washington D.C.: U.S. Government Printing Office, 1968.

102. Ellwood, Paul M. Jr.; Anderson, Nancy N.; Billings, James E.; Carlson, Rick J.; Hoagberg, Earl J.; and McClure, Walter, "Health Maintenance Strategy." *Medical Care* 9: 291–298, May–June 1971.

103. Donabedian, Avedis, *A Guide to Medical Care Administration, Volume II: Medical Care Appraisal.* New York: American Public Health Association, Inc., 1969, 176 pp.

104. U.S. Congress, Senate and House of Representatives, 92nd Congress, *Social Security Amendments of 1972.* P.L. 92-603. Washington, D.C.: U.S. Government Printing Office, 1972, 165 pp.

105. Egdahl, R., "Foundations for Medical Care." *New England Journal of Medicine* 288: 491–498; March 8, 1973.

106. Brian, E. W., "Government Control of Hospital Utilization: A California Experience." *New England Journal of Medicine* 286: 1,340–1,344; June 22, 1972.

107. Flashner, Bruce A.; Reed, Shirley; Coburn, Robert W.; and Fine, Philip R., "Professional Standards Review Organizations: Analysis of Their Development and Implementation Based on a Preliminary Review of the Hospital Admission and Surveillance Program in Illinois." *Journal of the American Medical Association* 223: 1,473–1,484; March 26, 1973.

108. Feldstein, Martin, "A New Approach to National Health Insurance." *The Public Interest,* Spring 1971, pp. 93–105.

109. Pauly, M. V., "A Variable Subsidy Insurance Proposal." In *National Health Insurance: An Analysis,* pp. 33–48. Washington, D.C.: American Enterprise Institute, Special Analysis No. 8, August 1971.

110. Lerner, Monroe; and Fitzgerald, Sandra W., "A Comparative Study of Three Major Forms of Health Care Coverage: A Review." *Inquiry* 2: 37–60, June 1965.

111. Wolfe, Gretchen Y., "Current Medicare Survey Report, Medical Insurance Sample, January–December 1969." *Health Insurance Statistics,* Social Security Administration, Office of Research and Statistics, CMS-14; July 12, 1971; 27 pp.

112. Sellers, A. H., "The Influence of Waiting Periods on the Costs of Hospital Care Insurance." *Canadian Medical Association Journal* 77: 1,132–1,133; December 15, 1957.

113. Ackart, R. J., "Prepaid Medical Care: Deductibles and Co-Insurance." *Virginia Medical Monthly* 88: 276–277, May 1961.

114. Straight, Byron W., "Reducing the Incidence of Office and Home Visits in a Medical Service Plan by Use of Coinsurance Charges." In *Conference of Actuaries in Public Practice. The Proceedings, 1961–1962,* Volume 11, pp. 73–79. Chicago.

115. Hall, Charles P., "Deductibles in Health Insurance: An Evaluation." *The Journal of Risk and Insurance* 33: 253–263, June 1966.

116. Williams, Robert, "A Comparison of Hospital Utilization and Costs by Type of Coverage." *Inquiry* 3: 28–42, September 1966.

117. Jesmer, Shirley, and Scharfenberg, Robert J., "Problems in Measuring The Effect of Deductibles Upon Hospital Utilization." *Blue Cross Reports,* volume 6, October 1968, 7 pp.

118. Heaney, Charles T., and Riedel, Donald C., "From Indemnity to Full Coverage: Changes in Hospital Utilization." *Blue Cross Reports* Research Series 5. Chicago: Blue Cross Association, October 1970, 13 pp.

119. *The Effect of Deductibles, Coinsurance and Copayment on Utilization of Health Care Services—Opinions and Impressions from Blue Cross and Blue Shield Plans.* Chicago: Blue Cross Association and National Association of Blue Shield Plans, September 28, 1971, 13 pp. (Mimeo.)

120. Hardwick, C. Patrick; Shuman, Larry; and Barnoon, Shlomo, "Effect of Participatory Insurance on Hospital Utilization." *Health Services Research* 7: 43–57, Spring 1972.

121. Scitovsky, Anne A., and Snyder, Nelda M., "Effect of Coinsurance on Use of Physician Services." *Social Security Bulletin* 35: 3–19, June 1972.

122. Luft, Harold A., *Effects of Coinsurance on the Use of Physician Services: Comment.* Boston: Harvard Center for Community Health and Medical Care, Program on Health Care Policy, Health Care Policy Discussion Paper Number 9, June 1973, 6 pp. (Mimeo.)

123. Peel, Evelyn, and Scharff, Jack, "Impact of Cost-Sharing on Use of Ambulatory Services Under Medicare, 1969." *Social Security Bulletin* 36: 3–24, October 1973.

124. Koropecky, Orest, and Huang, Lien-fu, "The Effects of the Medicare Method of Reimbursement on Physicians' Fees and on Beneficiaries' Utilization: Volume II, Part II, Effects on Beneficiaries' Utilization." In Health Insurance Benefits Advisory Council, *A Report on the Results of the Study of Methods of Reimbursement for Physicians' Services Under Medicare,* appendix A, pp. 1–71. S.S. Publication No. 92-73 (10-73). Washington, D.C.: Social Security Administration, July 1973.

125. Bailey, Richard M., "Economics of Scale in Medical Practice." In Klarman, H. E., Editor, *Empirical Studies in Health Economics,* pp. 255–273. Baltimore: The Johns Hopkins Press, 1970.

126. Scheff, Thomas J., "Preferred Errors in Diagnosis." *Medical Care* 2: 166–172, July–September 1964.

127. Steep, Mary Ann, and Tilley, Thomas J., "Outpatient Diagnostic Benefits and the Effects on Inpatient Experience: A Three Part Study." *Inquiry* 2: 3–12, June 1965.

128. Kelly, Denwood N., "Experience with an Outpatient Diagnostic Program." *Hospitals* 34: 50–51; August 1, 1960.

129. Kelly, Denwood N., "Experience with a Program of Coverage for Diagnostic Procedures Provided in Physicians' Offices and Hospital Outpatient Departments—Maryland Blue Cross and Blue Shield Plans (1957–1964)." *Inquiry* 2: 28–44, November 1965.

130. Fogel, Neil L., "Outpatient Presurgical Care Conserves Inpatient Days." *Hospitals* 43: 51–54; January 1, 1969.

131. Roemer, Milton I., "The Influence of Prepaid Physician's Service on Hospital Utilization." *Hospitals* 32: 48–52; October 16, 1958.

132. Shipman, George A.; Lampman, Robert J.; and Miyamoto, S. Frank, *Medical Service Corporations in the State of Washington*. Cambridge: Harvard University Press, 1962, 215 pp.

133. Avnet, Helen Hershfield, "Hospital Use Under Comprehensive vs. Limited Physician Insurance Coverage." In *Physician Service Patterns and Illness Rates*, pp. 372–376. Group Health Insurance, Inc., 1967.

134. Hill, Daniel B.; and Veney, James E., "Kansas Blue Cross/Blue Shield Outpatient Benefits Experiment." *Medical Care* 8: 143–158, March April 1970.

135. Lewis, Charles E. and Keairnes, Harold W., "Controlling Costs of Medical Care by Expanding Insurance Coverage: Study of a Paradox." *New England Journal of Medicine* 282: 1,405–1,412; June 18, 1970.

136. Moles, Oliver; Hess, Robert F.; and Fascione, Daniel, "Who Knows Where to Get Public Assistance?" *Welfare in Review* 6: 8–13, October 1968.

137. Moles, Oliver, "Predicting Use of Public Assistance: An Empirical Study." *Welfare in Review* 7: 13–19, November–December 1969.

138. Alexander, Raymond S.; and Podair, Simon, "Educating New York City Residents to Benefits of Medicaid." *Public Health Reports* 84: 767–772, September 1969.

139. Bashshur, Rashid L.; and Metzner, Charles, A., "Vulnerability to Risk and Awareness of Dual Choice of Health Insurance Plan." *Health Services Research* 5. 106–113, Summer 1970.

140. Newhouse, Joseph P., "A Design for a Health Insurance Experiment." *Inquiry* 11: 5–27, March 1974.

141. Kisch, Arnold I.; and Torrens, Paul R., "Health Status Assessment in the Health Insurance Study." *Inquiry* 11: 40–52, March 1974.

142. Orr, Larry L., "The Health Insurance Study: Experimentation and Health Financing Policy." *Inquiry* 11: 28–39, March 1974.

143. Hester, James; and Leveson, Irving, "The Health Insurance Study: A Critical Appraisal." *Inquiry* 11: 53–60, March 1974.

144. Shain, Max, and Roemer, Milton I., "Hospital Costs Relate to the Supply of Beds." *Modern Hospital* 92: 71–73 and 168, April 1959.

145. Roemer, Milton I., "Bed Supply and Hospital Utilization: A Natural Experiment." *Hospitals* 35: 36–42; November 1, 1961.

146. Feldstein, Martin S., "Effects of Differences in Hospital Bed Scarcity on Type of Use." *British Medical Journal* 2: 561–564; August 29, 1964.

147. Feldstein, Martin S., "The Supply and Use of Inpatient Care." In *Economic Analysis for Health Service Efficiency*, pp. 187–228. Amsterdam: North-Holland Publishing Company, 1967.

148. Feldstein, Martin S., "An Aggregate Planning Model of the Health Care Sector." *Medical Care* 5: 369–381, November–December 1967.

149. Feldstein, Martin S., "Hospital Cost Inflation: A Study of Nonprofit Price Dynamics." *American Economic Review* 61: 853–872, December 1971.

150. Fuchs, Victor R., and Kramer, Marcia J., *Determinants of Expenditures for Physicians' Services in the United States 1948–68*. DHEW Publication No. (HSM) 73-3,017; National Bureau of Economic Research, Occasional Paper 117. Washington, D.C.: U.S. Government Printing Office, 1973, 63 pp.

151. Lenzer, Anthony, and Donabedian, Avedis, "Needed . . . Research in Home Care." *Nursing Outlook* 15: 42–45, October 1967.

152. Bakst, Henry J., and Marra, Edward F., "Experience with Home Care for Cardiac Patients." *American Journal of Public Health* 45: 444–450, April 1955.

153. Hanchett, Effie, and Torrens, P. R., "A Public Health Home Nursing Program for Outpatients with Heart Disease." *Public Health Reports* 82: 683–688, August 1967.

154. Stone, Joseph R.; Patterson, Elizabeth; and Felson, Leon, "The Effectiveness of Home Care for General Hospital Patients." *Journal of the American Medical Association* 205: 145–148; July 15, 1968.

155. Katz, Sidney; Vignos, Paul J.; Moskowitz, Roland W.; Thompson, Helen M.; and Svec, Kathryn H., "Comprehensive Outpatient Care in Rheumatoid Arthritis: A Controlled Study." *Journal of the American Medical Association* 206: 1,249–1,254; November 4, 1968.

156. Katz, Sidney; Ford, Amasa B.; Downs, Thomas D.; Adams, Mary; and Rusby, Dorothy I., *Effects of Continued Care: A Study of Chronic Illness in the Home*. DHEW Publication No. (HSM) 73-3,010. Washington, D.C.: U.S. Government Printing Office, 1973, 168 pp.

157. Greenlick, Merwyn R.; Burke, Donald W.; and Hurtado, Arnold V., "The Development of a Home Health Program Within a Comprehensive Prepaid Group Practice Plan." *Inquiry* 3: 31–39, October 1967.

158. Hurtado, Arnold V.; Greenlick, Merwyn R.; and Saward, Ernest W., "The Organization and Utilization of Home-Care and Extended-Care Facility Services in a Prepaid Comprehensive Group Practice Plan." *Medical Care* 7: 30–40, January–February 1969.

159. Hurtado, Arnold V.; Greenlick, Merwyn R.; and Saward, Ernest

W., *Home Care and Extended Care in a Comprehensive Prepayment Plan.* Chicago: Hospital Research and Educational Trust, 1972, 127 pp.

160. Roemer, Milton I., "Hospital Utilization and the Supply of Physicians." *Journal of the American Medical Association* 178: 989–993; December 19, 1961.

161. Haldeman, Jack C., and Abdellah, Faye G., "Concepts of Progressive Patient Care." *Hospitals* 33: 38–42, 142 and 144; May 16, 1959; and 41–46, June 1, 1959.

162. Griffith, John R.; Weeks, Lewis E.; and Sullivan, James H., *The McPherson Experiment: Expanded Community Hospital Services.* Ann Arbor: The University of Michigan, Bureau of Hospital Administration, 1967, 337 pp. (The study and its findings are summarized in Weeks, L. E., *The Complete Gamut of Progressive Patient Care in a Community Hospital,* pp. 28–47. Battle Creek, Mich.: The W. K. Kellogg Foundation.)

163. Griffith, John R.; Weeks, Lewis E.; and DeVries, Robert A., *A Reappraisal of the McPherson Experiment in Progressive Patient Care.* Ann Arbor: The University of Michigan, Bureau of Hospital Administration, 1970, 69 pp. (For a brief account, see DeVries, Robert A., "Progressive Patient Care." *Hospitals* 44: 43–48; June 16, 1970.)

164. Goldberg, I. D.; Krantz, G.; and Locke, B. Z., "Effect of a Short-Term Outpatient Psychiatric Therapy Benefit on the Utilization of Medical Services in a Prepaid Group Practice Medical Program." *Medical Care* 8: 419–428, September–October 1970.

165. Follette, William, and Cummings, Nicholas A. "Psychiatric Services and Medical Utilization in a Prepaid Health Plan Setting." *Medical Care* 5: 25–35, January–February 1967.

166. Cummings, Nicholas A., and Follette, William T., "Psychiatric Services and Medical Utilization in a Prepaid Health Plan Setting: Part II." *Medical Care* 6: 31–41, January–February 1968.

167. Donabedian, Avedis, "The Quality of Medical Care." In Corey, Lawrence; Saltman, Steven E.; and Epstein, Michael F., editors, *Medicine in a Changing Society,* pp. 83–101. Saint Louis: The C. V. Mosby Company, 1972.

168. Goss, Mary E. W., "Organizational Goals and the Quality of Medical Care: Evidence from Comparative Research on Hospitals." *Journal of Health and Social Behavior* 11: 255–268, December 1970.

169. Feldstein, Martin S., "The Rising Price of Physicians' Services." *The Review of Economics and Statistics* 52: 121–133, May 1970.

170. Feldstein, Martin S., *The Rising Cost of Hospital Care.* Washington, D.C.: Information Resources Press, 1971, 88 pp.

171. Rice, Dorothy P., and Horowitz, Loucele A., "Trends in Medical Care Prices." *Social Security Bulletin* 30: 13–28, July 1967.

172. Klarman, Herbert E., *The Economics of Health.* New York: Columbia University Press, 1965, 200 pp.

173. Scitovsky, Anne A., "An Index of the Cost of Medical Care—A Proposed New Approach." In *The Economics of Health and Medical*

Care, pp. 128–142. Proceedings of The Conference on the Economics of Health and Medical Care, May 10–12, 1962. Ann Arbor: The University of Michigan, Bureau of Public Health Economics and Department of Economics, 1964.

174. Scitovsky, Anne A., "Changes in The Costs of Treatment of Selected Illnesses, 1951–1965." *American Economic Review* 57: 1,182–1,195; December 1967.

175. Health Insurance Benefits Advisory Council, *Annual Report on Medicare, July 1, 1966–December 31, 1967.* Washington, D.C.: Social Security Administration, July 1969, p. 36.

176. Klarman, Herbert E.; Rice, Dorothy P.; Cooper, Barbara S.; and Stettler, H. Louis III., *Sources of Increase in Selected Medical Care Expenditures, 1929–1969.* Washington, D.C.: U.S. Department of Health, Education and Welfare, Social Security Administration, Office of Research and Statistics, Staff Paper No. 4, April, 1970, 69 pp.

177. Thomas, Lewis, *Aspects of Biomedical Science Policy.* Washington, D.C.: Institute of Medicine, National Academy of Sciences, 1972, 16 pp.

178. Fein, Rashi, *The Doctor 'Shortage: An Economic Diagnosis.* Washington, D.C.: The Brookings Institution, 1967, 199 pp.

179. Gouldner, Alvin W., "Cosmopolitans and Locals: Toward an Analysis of Latent Social Roles." Parts I and II. *Administrative Science Quarterly* 2: 281–306 and 444–480, December 1957 and March 1958.

180. Horowitz, Loucele A., "Medical Care Price Changes 1967–1971." Research and Statistics Note No. 6. Washington, D.C.: Social Security Administration. Office of Research and Statistics, March 24, 1972, 12 pp.

181. Horowitz, Loucele A., "Medical Care Price Changes Under The Economic Stabilization Program." Research and Statistics Note No. 8. Washington, D.C.: Social Security Administration, Office of Research and Statistics, May 15, 1973, 17 pp.

182. Rice, Dorothy P.; and Cooper, Barbara S., "National Health Expenditures, 1950–67." *Social Security Bulletin* 32: 3–20, January 1969.

183. Department of Health, Education, and Welfare, Social Security Administration, Office of Research and Statistics, *Medical Care Costs and Prices: Background Book.* DHEW (SSA) 72-11,908. Washington, D.C., January 1972, 148 pp.

184. Huang, Lien-fu, and Koropecky, Orest, "The Effects of the Medicare Method of Reimbursement on Physicians' Fees and on Beneficiaries' Utilization: Volume II, Part I, Effects on Physicians' Fees." In Health Insurance Benefits Advisory Council, *A Report on the Results of the Study of Methods of Reimbursement for Physicians' Services Under Medicare,* appendix A, pp. 1–67. S.S. Publication No. 92-73 (10-73). Washington, D.C.: Social Security Administration, July 1973.

185. Goodman, Leo A., "Ecological Regressions and the Behavior of

Individuals." *American Sociological Review* 18: 663–664, December 1953.

186. Goodman, Leo A., "Some Alternatives to Ecological Correlation." *American Journal of Sociology* 64: 610–625, May 1959.

187. Horowitz, Loucele A., "Medical Care Price Changes in Medicare's First Five Years." *Social Security Bulletin* 35: 16–29, March 1972.

188. Feldstein, Paul J., and Waldman, Saul, "The Financial Position of Hospitals in the First Two Years of Medicare." *Inquiry* 6: 19–27, March 1969.

189. Davis, Karen, *Net Income of Hospitals 1961–1969.* Washington, D.C.: Social Security Administration, Office of Research and Statistics, Staff Paper No. 6., December 1970, 78 pp.

190. Pettengill, Julian, "Financial Position of Private Community Hospitals, 1961–1971." *Social Security Bulletin* 36: 3–19, November 1973.

191. Spitzer, Walter O., "The Small General Hospital: Problems and Solutions." *Milbank Memorial Fund Quarterly* 48: 413–447, October 1970.

192. Horowitz, Loucele A., "Magnitude and Frequency of Physicians' Fee Increases for Selected Procedures, December 1965–December 1969." Research and Statistics Note No. 11. Washington, D.C.: Social Security Administration, Office of Research and Statistics, July 16, 1970, 7 pp. plus tables.

193. Staff to the Committee on Finance, United States Senate, *Medicare and Medicaid: Problems, Issues, and Alternatives.* Committee Print, 91st Congress, 1st Session. Washington, D.C.: U.S. Government Printing Office, February 9, 1970, 323 pp.

194. deVise, Paul, "Physician Migration from Inland to Coastal States: Antipodal Examples of Illinois and California." *Journal of Medical Education* 48: 141–151, February 1973.

195. Pine, Penelope L., "Current Medicare Survey Report. Supplementary Medical Insurance: 1967–71 Trends and Fourth Quarter 1971." *Health Insurance Statistics.* Washington, D.C.: Social Security Administration, Office of Research and Statistics. CMS-26, August 15, 1973, 7 pp.

196. Rimlinger, C. V. and Steele, H. B., "An Economic Interpretation of the Spatial Distribution of Physicians in the U.S." *The Southern Economic Journal* 30: 1–12, July 1963.

197. Health Insurance Advisory Council, *A Report on the Results of the Study of Methods of Reimbursement for Physicians' Services Under Medicare.* S.S. Publication No. 92-73 (10-73). Washington, D.C.: Social Security Administration, July 1973. Not paginated consecutively.

198. Cooper, Barbara; Worthington, Nancy; Pettengill, Julian; Dyckman, Zachary; Fitzmaurice, Michael; Horowitz, Loucele; Piro, Paula; and Mueller, Marjorie, *Medical Care Expenditures, Prices, and Costs: Background Book.* Social Security Administration, Office of Research and Sta-

tistics, DHEW Publication No. (SSA) 74-11,909. Washington, D.C.: U.S. Government Printing Office, September 1973, 90 pp.

199. American Hospital Association, *Service Benefits or Cash Indemnity in Hospital Prepayment*. Chicago: American Hospital Association, 1960, 9 pp.

200. Eckstein, Otto, "Taxation: Principles and Issues of Fairness." In *Public Finance*, pp. 51–69. Englewood Cliffs, New Jersey: Prentice-Hall, Inc., 1964.

201. Burns, Eveline M., *Social Security and Public Policy*. New York: McGraw-Hill Book Company Inc., 1956, 291 pp.

202. Titmuss, Richard M., "The Role of Redistribution in Social Policy." *Social Security Bulletin* 28: 14–20, June 1965.

203. Stuart, Bruce C., and Bair, Lee A., *Health Care and Income: The Distributional Impacts of Medicaid and Medicare Nationally and in the State of Michigan*. Lansing, Michigan: Michigan Department of Social Services. Research Paper No. 5, second edition, September 1971, 329 pp.

204. Stuart, Bruce C., *The Impact of Medicaid on Interstate Income Differentials*. Lansing, Michigan: Michigan Department of Social Services, January 1971, 29 pp.

205. Stuart, Bruce, "Equity and Medicaid." *Journal of Human Resources 7: 162–178*, Spring 1972.

206. Feldstein, Martin S., and Allison, Elizabeth, *Tax Subsidies of Private Health Insurance: Distribution, Revenue Loss and Effects*. Boston, Mass.: Harvard Center for Community Health and Medical Care, Program on Health Care Policy, Health Care Policy Paper Number 2, October 1972, 21 pp. plus appendix.

207. In Department of the Treasury, Internal Revenue Service, *Your Federal Income Tax, 1974 Edition, For Individuals*, pp. 85–89. Washington, D.C.: U.S. Government Printing Office, 1973.

208. MacIntyre, Duncan M., "Pricing Health Insurance." In *The Economics of Health and Medical Care*, pp. 148–169. Proceedings of the Conference on the Economics of Health and Medical Care, May 10–12, 1962. Ann Arbor, Michigan, Bureau of Public Health Economics and Department of Economics, The University of Michigan, 1964.

209. MacIntyre, Duncan M., *Voluntary Health Insurance and Rate Making*. Ithaca, N.Y.: Cornell University Press, 1962, 301 pp.

210. Institute of Medicine, National Academy of Sciences, *Selected Issues in Mandated Health Insurance*. Minutes of Seminar, November 20, 1972. Washington, D.C.: National Academy of Sciences, 1973, 14 pp. and Appendices.

211. Brewster, Agnes W., *Health Insurance and Related Proposals for Financing Personal Health Services: A Digest of Major Legislation and Proposals for Federal Action, 1935–1957*. Washington, D.C.: Social Security Administration, 1958, 54 pp.

212. Department of Health, Education, and Welfare, *Analysis of*

Health Insurance Proposals Introduced in the 92nd Congress. Printed for the Use of the Committee on Ways and Means, 92nd Congress, First session. Washington, D.C.: U.S. Government Printing Office, August 1971, 129 pp. plus attachments.

213. Waldman, Saul, *National Health Insurance Proposals: Provisions of Bills Introduced in the 93rd Congress as of July 1974.* DHEW Publication No. (SSA) 75-11,920. Washington, D.C.: U.S. Government Printing Office, 1974, 227 pp.

214. Shain, Max, "The Change to Experience Rating in the Michigan Blue Cross Plan." *American Journal of Public Health* 56: 1,695-1,698; October 1966.

215. U.S. Congress, Senate and House of Representatives, 93rd Congress. *Health Maintenance Organization Act of 1973.* P.L. 93–222. Washington, D.C.: U.S. Government Printing Office, 1973, 23 pp.

216. Feldstein, Martin S., "A New Approach to National Health Insurance." *The Public Interest* 23: 93–105, Spring 1971.

217. Feldstein, Martin S.; Friedman, Bernard; and Luft, Harold, *Distributional Aspects of National Health Insurance Benefits and Finance.* Boston, Mass.: Harvard Center for Community Health and Medical Care, Program on Health Care Policy, Health Care Policy Paper Number 3, October 1972, 37 pp.

218. Feldstein, Martin S., "The Welfare Loss of Excess Health Insurance." *Journal of Political Economy* 81: 252–280, March–April 1973.

219. Pratt, J. W., "Risk Aversion in the Small and in the Large." *Econometrica* 32: 122–136, January–April 1964.

220. Arrow, Kenneth J., *Aspects of the Theory of Risk Bearing.* Yrjo Jahnsson Lectures. Helsinki: Yrjo Jahnsson Foundation, 1965. Reissued in 1971 as *Essays in the Theory of Risk-Bearing.* Chicago: Markham Publishing Co., 1971, 278 pp.

221. Bashshur, Rashid L., and Metzner, Charles A., "Patterns of Social Differentiation Between Community Health Association and Blue Cross-Blue Shield." *Inquiry* 4: 23-44, June 1967.

222. Bashshur, Rashid L., and Metzner, Charles A., "Demand for Health Insurance Coverage In a Metropolitan Population." *Public Health Reports* 83: 81–86, January 1968.

223. Bashshur, Rashid L., and Metzner, Charles A., "Vulnerability to Risk and Awareness of Dual Choice of Health Insurance Plan." *Health Services Research* 5: 106–113, Summer 1970.

224. Richie, Nicholas D., *Vulnerability to Risk and Level of Information Concerning Features of Health Care Plans: A Study of Consumer Information.* Doctoral Dissertation. Ann Arbor: The University of Michigan, 1972, 228 pp.

225. Metzner, Charles A.; Bashshur, Rashid L.; and Shannon, Gary W., "Differential Public Acceptance of Group Medical Practice." *Medical Care* 10: 279–287, July–August 1972.

226. Moustafa, A. Taher; Hopkins, Carl E.; and Klein, Bonnie, "Determinants of Choice and Change of Health Insurance Plan." *Medical Care* 9: 32–41, January–February 1971.

227. Hochbaum, Godfrey M., *Public Participation in Medical Screening Programs: A Sociopsychological Study.* P.H.S. Publication No. 572. Washington, D.C.: U.S. Government Printing Office, 1958, 23 pp.

228. Rosenstock, Irwin M., "Why People Use Health Services." *Milbank Memorial Fund Quarterly* 44: 94–127, July 1966, Part 2.

229. Denenberg, Herbert S., *A Shopper's Guide to Health Insurance.* Harrisburg, Pa.: Pennsylvania Insurance Department, December 1973, 16 pp.

230. Commonwealth of Massachusetts, Office of Comprehensive Planning, Executive Office of Human Services, *Consumer's Guide to Health Insurance.* Boston, Mass.: Office of Comprehensive Health Planning, 1974, 17 pp.

231. Shapiro, Mildred B., *Grading of Health Insurance Plans.* Albany, N.Y.: New York State Department of Health, February 1972, 4 pp.

232. Breslow, Lester; Rich, Shirley; Procter, Donald; Vial, Don; and Poyer, Bruce, *HPGS, Health Plan Grading System: A System for Evaluating Health Insurance Plans.* Los Angeles: School of Public Health, University of California, 1969, 24 pp.

233. Loebs, Stephen, F., *Variations Among States in Selected Optional Decisions in the Medicaid Program.* Doctoral dissertation. Ann Arbor: The University of Michigan, 1974, 327 pp.

234. Berg, Robert L., editor, *Health Status Indexes.* Chicago: Hospital Research and Educational Trust, 1973, 262 pp.

235. Lee, R. I., and Jones, L. W., *The Fundamentals of Good Medical Care.* Publication of the Committee on the Costs of Medical Care, No. 22. Chicago: The University of Chicago Press, 1933, 302 pp.

236. Falk, I. S.; Schonfeld, H. K.; Harris, B. R.; Landau, S. J.; and Milles, S. S., "The Development of Standards for the Audit and Planning of Medical Care, I. Concepts, Research Design and the Content of Primary Care." *American Journal of Public Health* 57: 1,118–1,136; July 1967.

237. Schonfeld, H. K., "Standards for the Audit and Planning of Medical Care: A Method for Preparing Audit Standards for Mixtures of Patients." *Medical Care* 8: 287–297, July–August 1970.

238. White, Gladys O., *Simplified Methods of Determining Needs.* U.S. Department of Health, Education, and Welfare, Welfare Administration, Bureau of Family Services. Washington, D.C.: U.S. Government Printing Office, 1964, reprinted 1965, 8 pp.

239. The Community Council of Greater New York, Budget Standards Service, Research Department, *How to Measure Ability to Pay for Social and Health Services,* revised edition. New York: The Council. 1967, 39 pp.

240. Mayerson, Allen L., "State Laws and Health Insurance." In U.S.

Department of Health, Education and Welfare, Social Security Administration, Office of Research and Statistics, *Private Health Insurance and Medical Care: Conference Papers,* pp. 19–41. Washington, D.C.: U.S. Government Printing Office, 1968.

241. Blue Cross Association, "Group and Nongroup Hospital Utilization and Charges." *Blue Cross Reports* vol. 1, no. 1, July 1963, 11 pp.

242. Olendzki, Margaret; Goodrich, Charles H.; and Reader, George G., "The Significance of Welfare Status in the Care of Indigent Patients." *American Journal of Public Health* 53: 1,676–1,684; October 1963.

243. Mueller, Marjorie Smith, "Private Health Insurance in 1972: Health Services, Enrollments and Finances." *Social Security Bulletin* 37: 20–40, March 1974.

244. Reed, Louis S.; and Carr, Willine, "Private Health Insurance in the United States, 1967." *Social Security Bulletin* 32: 3–22, February 1969.

245. Darsky, Benjamin J.; Sinai, Nathan; and Axelrod, Solomon J., "Problems in Voluntary Insurance: Some Answers from the Windsor Experience." *American Journal of Public Health* 48: 971–978, August 1958.

246. Pauly, Mark V., "A Measure of the Welfare Cost of Health Insurance." *Health Services Research* 4: 281–291, Winter 1969.

247. Smith, David B.; and Metzner, Charles A., "Differential Perceptions of Health Care Quality in a Prepaid Group Practice." *Medical Care* 8: 264–275, July–August 1970.

248. Ehrlich, J.; Morehead, M. A.; and Trussell, R. E., *The Quantity Quality and Costs of Medical and Hospital Care Secured by a Sample of Teamster Families in the New York Area.* New York: Columbia University, School of Public Health and Administrative Medicine, 1964, 98 pp.

249. Pollack, Jerome, "The Voice of the Consumer: Cost, Quality and Organization of Medical Service." In Knowles, J. H., editor, *Hospitals, Doctors and the Public Interest,* pp. 167–186. Cambridge: Harvard University Press, 1965.

250. Goldberg, Theodore, "A Consumer Looks at Medical Care." *Medical Care* 5: 9–18, January–February 1967.

251. We have paraphrased McIntyre, who ascribes the "half-dragged, half-lured" formulation to C. A. Kulp. See Reference 209, page 24.

252. Eilers, Robert D., and Crowe, Robert M., editors, *Group Insurance Handbook.* Homewood, Ill.: Richard D. Irwin, Inc., 1965, 972 pp.

253. Pettengill, Daniel W., "Cost Control Through Contractual Provisions." In Eilers, Robert D. and Crowe, Robert M., editors, *Group Insurance Handbook,* pp. 455–473. Homewood, Ill.: Richard D. Irwin, Inc., 1965.

254. Gregg, Davis W., "Fundamental Characteristics of the Group Technique." In Eilers, Robert D. and Crowe, Robert M., editors, *Group Insurance Handbook,* pp. 31–44. Homewood, Ill.: Richard D. Irwin, Inc., 1965.

255. Browning, Arthur M., "Legal Environment of Group Insur-

ance." In Eilers, Robert D. and Crowe, Robert M., editors, *Group Insurance Handbook*, pp. 85–100. Homewood, Ill.: Richard D. Irwin, Inc., 1965.

256. McNerney, Walter J., "Improving the Effectiveness of Health Insurance and Prepayment." In U.S. Department of Health, Education and Welfare, Social Security Administration, Office of Research and Statistics, *Private Health Insurance and Medical Care: Conference Papers*, pp. 43–73. Washington, D.C.: U.S. Government Printing Office, 1968.

257. Cody, Donald D., "Underwriting Group Medical Expense Coverage." In Eilers, Robert D. and Crowe, Robert M., editors, *Group Insurance Handbook*, pp. 354–372. Homewood, Ill.: Richard D. Irwin, Inc., 1965.

258. Kessel, Reuben A., "Price Discrimination in Medicine." *Journal of Law and Economics* 1: 20–53, October 1958.

259. Abel-Smith, Brian, "Paying the Family Doctor." *Medical Care* 1: 27–35, January–March 1963.

260. Department of Health, Education, and Welfare, Social Security Administration, Health Insurance Program for the Aged, "Criteria for Determination of Reasonable Charges; Reimbursement for Services of Hospital Interns, Residents, and Supervising Physicians." *Federal Register* 32: 12,599–12,603; August 31, 1967.

261. Colombotos, John, "Physicians and Medicare: A Before and After Study of the Effects of Legislation on Attitudes." *American Sociological Review* 34: 318–334, June 1969.

262. Stuart, Bruce C., "National Health Insurance and the Poor." *American Journal of Public Health* 62: 1,252–1,259; September 1972.

263. Cooper, Barbara S., and Worthington, Nancy L., "Age Differences in Medical Care Spending, Fiscal Year 1972." *Social Security Bulletin* 36: 3–15, May 1973.

264. Somers, Anne R., "What Price Comprehensive Care?" *Archives of Environmental Health* 17: 6–20, July 1968.

265. Simon, H. A., "On the Concept of Organizational Goal." *Administrative Science Quarterly* 9: 1–22, June 1964.

266. Goldmann, Franz, "Comprehensive Medical Care: Basic Issues." *The Social Science Review* 29: 267–284, September 1955.

267. National Commission on Community Health Services, Task Force on Comprehensive Personal Health Services, *Comprehensive Health Care: A Challenge to American Communities*. Washington, D.C.: Public Affairs Press, 1967, 94 pp. (See especially the section on "Comprehensive Personal Health Services Defined," pages 16–21.)

268. The notion of a central source of care is developed in Solon, Jerry A.; Sheps, Cecil G.; and Lee, Sidney S., "Delineating Patterns of Medical Care." *American Journal of Public Health* 50: 1,105–1,113; August 1960.

269. National Council on Aging, "Principles and Criteria for Determining Medical Indigency: Report of the National Committee for the

Project of the National Council on the Aging." *American Journal of Public Health* 54: 1,745–1,765; October 1964.

270. Reed, Louis S., and Carr, Willine, *The Benefit Structure of Private Health Insurance,* 1968. U.S. Department of Health, Education, and Welfare, Social Security Administration, Office of Research and Statistics, Research Report No. 32. Washington, D.C.: U.S. Government Printing Office, 1970, 111 pp.

271. Richmond, Julius B., and Weinberger, Howard L., "Essential Elements for Comprehensive Health Care for Children and Youth." In North, Frederick A., editor, *The Role of Maternal and Child Health and Crippled Children's Programs In Evolving Systems of Health Care,* pp. 14–51. Conference Proceedings, March 23–25, 1970. An Arbor: The University of Michigan, 1970.

272. Yoffee, William M., "New International Standards for Medical Care and Sickness Benefits Under Social Security Programs." *Social Security Bulletin* 32: 21–28, October 1969.

273. Ruther, Martin, "Medicare: Number of Persons Insured, July 1, 1972." Health Insurance Statistics, H1-59, June 19, 1974. Washington, D.C.: U.S. Department of Health, Education and Welfare, Social Security Administration, Office of Research and Statistics. DHEW Publication No. (SSA) 74-11,702, 21 pp.

274. Muller, Charlotte, "Health Insurance for Abortion Costs: A Survey." *Inquiry* 7: 51–64, September 1970. This paper in slightly different form has appeared as Muller, Charlotte F., "Health Insurance for Abortion Costs: A Survey." *Family Planning Perspectives* 2: 12–20, 1974.

275. Curran, William J., "Public Health and the Law: Presidential Morality, Abortion, and Federal-State Law." *American Journal of Public Health* 61: 1,042–1,043; May 1971.

276. Rosoff, Jeannie I., "Family Planning, Medicaid and the Private Physician: Survey of a Failure." *Family Planning Perspectives* 1: 27–332, October 1969.

277. Wallace, Helen M.; Hyman, Goldstein; Gold, Edwin M.; and Oglesby, Allan C., "A Study of the Title 19 Coverage of Abortion." *American Journal of Public Health* 62: 1,116–1,122; August 1972.

278. Kane, Stanley D., "A Tangled Case: Medicaid for Elective Abortions." *Modern Medicine* 41: 94–96, January 8, 1973.

279. Advisory Planning Committee on Medical Care to the Government of Saskatchewan, *Interim Report.* Regina, Saskatchewan: Lawrence Amon, Printer to the Queen's Most Excellent Majesty, September 1961, 123 pp.

280. Notkin, Herbert, "Medical Care for the Needy." *New York State Journal of Medicine* 60: 1,593–1,599; May 1, 1961.

SUBJECT INDEX

Access: barriers to, by class, 143-144; benefits and, 25; to dental care, 24-25; equalization of, 109; to hospital care, 23-24; income and, 19-20, 23-25; measurement of, 14; Medicare and, 19, 95; to physician care, 19-20; Quebec Health Insurance, 99; race and, 14; social class and, 143-144

Actual price, 219-221

Admissions. *See* Hospitals—admissions

Adverse selection, 354-355

Age: and access to dental care services, 24-25; disability and, 11-12; and hospital services, used under Medicare, 93; and effect of insurance on use of physician surgical services, 75-76; need and, 14, 25; and use of physician services, 28-29; and physician visits, 20-23

"Aging" effect: coinsurance and, 145-146; seasoning and, 102-103

Allocation of resources, 107-108

Allocation of services, 44-45, 130-131

Ambulance services, 61-62

Ambulatory care benefits, 152-155

Ambulatory care services: use of, coinsurance and, 47-48, 142-143; under Finnish National Health Insurance Scheme, 86-87; insurance and, 61-62; Medicare and, 91-93, 138-139; prepaid group practice and, 69-71; psychiatric care benefits and, 193-197

Ambulatory psychiatric care services, 193-197

"Arithmetic" effect: coinsurance and, 146; in deductibles and copayment, 119-120; of substitution, 150

"Attrition" effect, 104-105

Average price, 216-218; average net price and average actual price, 219-220; effect on physician production of services, 226; for physician services under Medicare, 239-240

Barriers to care. *See* Access

Bed supply: use of services and, 228-229. *See also* Hospital—bed supply

"Behavioral" effects: of deductibles and copayment, 119-126, 146

Benefit design, 3, 27, 32, 330-331

Benefits:
—abuse of: "discovery" effect and, 199; effect on medical staff, 193-194
—access and, 25
—ambulatory care: effect on hospital costs, 153-154
—"benefit principle," 277-278, 303-304
—"benefit to burden" ratio, 288
—comprehensive, 199, 376-386
—comparability under dual choice, 66-67
—consumer knowledge of, 198
—coordination and moral hazard, 359-360
—costs: effect on hospital costs of ambulatory care benefits, 153-154; under Medicare/Medicaid, 284; prices and, 201-275; relative prices and increases in, 218-219
—coverage and, 271
—dollar limits, 360-361
—extended, 197-200, 206-207
—implementation of, 4
—limitations on, 364-365
—"multiplier" effect and, 42
—"price" effect and, 41-42
—prices and, 206-207
—program objectives of, 321-322
—provider decisions and, 42
—rating of health insurance through, 334-335, 337-341
—returns, individual versus group purchase, 347-348
—"revenue" effect and, 42
—scope of, 197-200
—substitution effect of, 152-155, 193-198

—types of, 270-275
Blue Cross and Blue Shield: community rating and, 308-309; as Medicare carriers, effect on prices, 257-258. *See also* author index
British National Health Insurance: effects, 66; use of physician services under, 86

Capacity to produce services, 199-200
Carrier selection under Medicare, 257
Carry-over provision: deductibles and effect under Medicare, 137-138
Cash indemnity, 270-271
Charges: reasonable, and physician income, 265-266
Clients: controls on, 110-111; decisions, 41-42; preference change, 43
Client-oriented objectives, 323-349; degree of protection, 323-324, 326; provider stability and continuity, 343-346; value for money spent, 346-349
Coinsurance: "aging" effect and, 145-146; prices and, 262-264; "turnover" effect and, 145-146; use of services and, 142-148. *See also* Participatory payments
Collectivity-oriented objectives: comprehensive care and benefits, 376-385; economic security, 368-371; efficiency of production and allocation, 373-375; equity, 372-373; integrity of the medical care process, 376-388; public interest, 368; quality of care, 386
Commercial insurance, 130-131. *See also* Insurance
Community rating, 306-309
Community size: home visits and, 250; physician pricing behavior and, 248-252
Complementarity of services: in dental care, 242; post-Medicare price increases and, 254. *See also* Health Services
Comprehensive benefits. *See* Benefits—comprehensive
Comprehensive care, 376-379
Consumers behavior, 206; knowledge of benefits, 198. *See also* Clients, Patients
Consumer Price Index, 202-204
"Continuation" effect, 142-143
Controls on use of services, 110-111
Coordination of benefits, 359-360. *See also* Benefits

Copayment, 112-147; differential effects of, 126; and income differentials in use of services, 72-73; hospital use and, 127-130; Medicare and, 112-113; use of services and, 123-126
"Cosmopolitan" practice organization, 209-210. *See also* Organization of practice
Costs: and deductibles and copayment, 114, 116, 146; and direct benefits under Medicare/Medicaid, 284; home care benefits and, 183; hospital, effect of ambulatory care benefits on, 153-155; hospital, effect of extended care benefits on, 191-193; out-of-pocket, and insurance, 76-77; under Quebec Health Insurance, 99 (*see also* Quebec Health Insurance); scale as determinant of, 38; substitution effect on, 33; technology and, 207-209; third party payments and, 259-260
Cost-plus premiums and inflation, 272-273. *See also* Insurance
Cost reimbursement and hospital price trends, 235
Customary fees, 255; Medicare and, 257-258; policies for, 267; prices and, 211-212. *See also* Physicians—fees
Customary Prices, 216-221. *See also* Prices; Hospitals—prices

Deductibles, 111-112, and care, 113, 146; carry-over provision in, 137-138; controls on use of services through, 112-147; hospital use and, 128-130; and income differentials in use of services, 72-73; Medicare and, 112-113; prices and, 262-264. *See also* Deductibles and Copayment; Participatory Payments
Deductibles and copayment, 112-147; administrative costs to the insurer of, 146, advantages, 114; allocation of services through, 130-131; "arithmetic" effect of, 119-120, 146; "behavioral" effects of, 146; consequences of, 117-118; costs of, 116; disadvantages, 115-116; distinctions between, 117-118; effects of, 113-114, 138-140; empirical observations, 116-147; function of self-selection, 118-119; graded response, 118; and Medicare, 133-140; and social objectives, 115-116; transfers of obligations and, 119-120.

264-266; variation in physician charges, 258-259

Government intervention: price trends and, 216; in voluntary health insurance, 279

Graded response and participatory payment, 118

Gross price. *See* Prices—gross

Gross transfers: among income classes, 291-293. *See also* Redistribution

Group practice, 67-71, 78-79. *See also* Organization of practice

"Halo" effect, 166

Health: definition, 35-36; measurement, 7-8

Health improvement or maintenance effect, 102-103

Health maintenance organization, 111

Health potential and redistribution, 280, 310-311

Health services, 32-38

Health status: and benefits, 43; and home care benefits, 178-179

High option insurance, 54. *See also* Insurance

Home care benefits: "discovery" effect and, 178-179; effects on costs of care, 183; community size and, 250; hospital use and, 176-184, 186; under Medicare, 250; progressive patient care and, 187-188

"Horizontal equity" in taxation, 278. *See also* Taxation

Hospitals:

—accommodations: effect of 'more' insurance on, 58-60

—admissions: effect of ambulatory care benefits on, 152-153; group practice and, 66; effect of insurance on, 49-52, effect of "more" insurance on, 58-60; experience under Medicare, 93-94

—bed supply: Medicare and, 95; occupancy and, 53-54; in relation to need and demand, 187

—costs: effect of ambulatory care benefits on, 153-155; effect of progressive patient care on, 191-193

—demand for, 210-212

—expenditures for: income elasticities of, 18

—for-profit: plant assets under Medicare, 236

—length of stay: interaction of admission and, 51-52; effect of insurance on,

49-52, 75; payment source and, 53-54; price and, 52

—nonprofit: plant assets under Medicare, 236

—occupancy, 53-54

—patient-days: income elasticities for, 18; Medicare and, 93

—prices: cost reimbursement and, 235; daily hospital service charges and physician fees compared, 240-241; trends in, 214; pre-and-post Medicare/Medicaid, 232-238

—transfers of technical functions, 230

Hospital services—use: according to admissions and length of stay, 51-52; effect of ambulatory care benefits on, 152-153; coinsurance and, 47-48, 142-143; copayment and, 127-130; deductibles and, 128-130; extended care facilities and, 184-193; extended home care benefits and, 176-184; insurance and, 53-54, 73-75, 227-229; length of stay, 49-54, 75, 106-107; and Medicare, 93-94; effect of organized care, 168-170; payment source and, 53-54; effect of physician outpatient benefits, 156-158; physician services and, 168-176; prepaid group practice and, 69-71; effect of price on, 227-229; related services and, 49; relative gross price and, 229; relative net price and, 228-229; seasoning effect and length of stay, 106-107; substitution, 151-197; trends in, 23-24

Hospital-sparing effect: of ambulatory care benefits, 194-195; of diagnostic benefits, 198; of home care, 186-187. *See also* Substitution

Illness: cost-effectiveness of care, chronicity and extended benefits, 199, distribution by social class, 9-11; income and, 11-14; and price of care, 210, problems of definition, 11; severity and effect of insurance on use of service, 81. *See also* Disability

Incentives: for geographic redistribution of services, 265-266; physician, nonfinancial, 187; for substitution of services, 150-151

Income: definition and measurement, 12-14, 17; differential in use of services, 71-81; expenditures and, 18 (*see also* Income Elasticities); and hospital use as affected by insurance, 73-75; illness

AUTHOR INDEX

(Numbers refer to pages)